STAY HEALTHY AT EVERY AGE

STAY HEALTHY AT EVERY AGE

What Your Doctor Wants You to Know

SHANTANU NUNDY, M.D.

THE JOHNS HOPKINS UNIVERSITY PRESS   *Baltimore*

Notes to the reader: This book is not meant to substitute for the medical advice or care provided by a physician, and testing and treatment should not be based solely on its contents. Instead, treatment must be developed in a dialogue between the individual and his or her physician. This book has been written to help with that dialogue. The services of a competent medical professional should be obtained whenever medical advice is needed.

© 2010 The Johns Hopkins University Press
All rights reserved. Published 2010
Printed in the United States of America on acid-free paper
9 8 7 6 5 4 3 2 1

The Johns Hopkins University Press
2715 North Charles Street
Baltimore, Maryland 21218-4363
www.press.jhu.edu

Library of Congress Cataloging-in-Publication Data

Nundy, Shantanu.
   Stay healthy at every age : what your doctor wants you to know / Shantanu Nundy.
      p. cm.
   Includes bibliographical references and index.
   ISBN-13: 978-0-8018-9393-3 (hardcover : alk. paper)
   ISBN-10: 0-8018-9393-3 (hardcover : alk. paper)
   ISBN-13: 978-0-8018-9394-0 (pbk. : alk. paper)
   ISBN-10: 0-8018-9394-1 (pbk. : alk. paper)
   1. Self-care, Health—Popular works. 2. Medicine, Preventive—Popular works. I. Title.
   RA776.95.N86 2009
   613—dc22   2009014458

Figures I.1, 1.1, 3.1, 4.1, 5.1, 6.1, 8.1, 9.1, 9.2, 11.1, 12.1, 16.1, 18.1, and 22.3
are by Jacqueline Schaffer.

Special discounts are available for bulk purchases of this book. For more information, please contact Special Sales at 410-516-6936 or specialsales@press.jhu.edu.

The Johns Hopkins University Press uses environmentally friendly book materials, including recycled text paper that is composed of at least 30 percent post-consumer waste, whenever possible. All of our book papers are acid-free, and our jackets and covers are printed on paper with recycled content.

To my parents,
whose constant love and support allow me to dream

CONTENTS

This book was born of conversations between a mother and her concerned son. As a medical student in Baltimore, I frequently had the opportunity to visit my parents at our home in Washington, D.C. My mother, then in her early fifties, and having struggled with type 2 diabetes for several years, was beginning a stage in her life where her health was a more prominent concern and less of a given.

I would come home to my mom's cooking, with my huge medical textbooks in tow and my mind chock full of new ideas to keep my mother healthy. When my classmates and I studied diseases of the gastrointestinal system, I taught her that all adults over age 50 should be screened for colon cancer. When we studied cardiovascular disease, I reminded her that the number one cause of death in people with diabetes is coronary heart disease and that she should talk to her doctor about taking aspirin every day to lower her risk. When we studied infectious diseases, I pointed out that annual flu shots are recommended for all adults over age 50 and for younger adults with chronic diseases like diabetes. Much to my surprise, even though my mother saw a doctor regularly and had health insurance, many of these recommendations were new to her.

My efforts at improving her preventive care redoubled after I left the classroom and joined the medical wards. There I took care of patients who were sick or dying of illnesses that could have been prevented by the very measures I counseled my mother about: a 64-year-old grandfather with late-stage colon cancer who had never been screened for it; a 43-year-old businessman with diabetes, admitted for a massive heart attack, who was not on aspirin therapy; and a 55-year-old newly retired secretary, hospitalized for the flu, who had missed her influenza shot that year. As I shuttled back and forth from the hospital, I would call my mother and list the preventive measures she needed to talk about with her doctor.

In return, she went from welcoming my suggestions to feeling overwhelmed by them. "Another test! How many more are you going to ask me to get?" she would lament. She appreciated my efforts but needed my recommendations to be presented in a way that allowed her to better understand and more easily follow them. Instead of receiving one suggestion at a time, she wanted a complete list of all the screening tests, medications, and counseling services she needed to discuss with her doctor—in short, a checklist of preventive health care. This checklist would contain all the preventive services she needed based on her risk factors. She wanted the list to be comprehensive yet include only the preventive measures that were proven to benefit her. (After all, she reminded me, she didn't like going to the doctor!) With such a list, she could check off the items as she and her doctor addressed them, to make sure they were staying on top of her health needs and enabling her to continue to get the most out of life.

Her request was not easy to fill. Despite a rigorous search, I could not find the checklist she wanted. Various medical organizations made recommendations about preventive services, but few of these were comprehensive, and many presented conflicting information. Newspapers and popular magazines occasionally ran stories about vaccines or mammograms, but the stories were scattered and short. The published books on health promotion either covered the gamut of preventive health and provided limited information about proven preventive services or were written for doctors and would not answer my mother's needs.

I decided to make the checklist myself. I talked to my mentors at medical school, reviewed the recommendations of major medical organizations, and read all the books on preventive medicine I could get my hands on. In the end, I came up with the checklist she wanted and additional reading materials to help her understand each of the preventive services on her list. Along the way, I realized that my mother was not alone in needing a checklist. Clearly, some of the patients I had cared for would have benefited from lists of their own. If I could help my mother get the preventive services she needed, surely there was a way to help others as well.

The result of this humbling and rewarding journey is this book. It was written by a newly minted medical doctor and internal medicine resident and is based on the recommendations of scientific panels and expert doctors; but it is, I can proudly say, still grounded in the attempts of a loving son trying his best to help his mother stay healthy.

This is for you, Mama.

Shantanu

ACKNOWLEDGMENTS

I would like to acknowledge some of the people who helped me write this book.

Each chapter has been reviewed by a faculty member at a major academic medical institution, many of whom are nationally if not internationally renowned experts in their fields. These individuals offered their time and expertise to me without reservation, and for this I am grateful. From Johns Hopkins, I would like to acknowledge Dr. Bimal Ashar (Aspirin to Prevent Cardiovascular Disease), Dr. Dominique Ashen (Healthy Eating), Dr. Michele Bellantoni (Osteoporosis), Dr. Roger Blumenthal (Cholesterol), Dr. Lawrence Cheskin (Obesity), Dr. Joseph Cofrancesco (HIV), Dr. Robert Dudas (Early Childhood), Dr. Emily Erbelding (Syphilis), Dr. Thomas Finucane (Introduction), Dr. Thomas Koenig (Depression), Dr. Elizabeth Ratchford (Abdominal Aortic Aneurysm), Dr. Reed Riley (Blood Pressure), Dr. Dorothy Rosenthal (Cervical Cancer and HPV), Dr. Daniel Salmon (Adult Vaccines), Dr. Jonathan Samet (Tobacco Use), Dr. Christopher Saudek (Diabetes), Dr. Rosalyn Stewart (Adult Vaccines), Dr. Sayeedha Uddin (Pregnancy), and Dr. Jonathan Zenilman (Gonorrhea). I would like to acknowledge, from the University of Chicago, Dr. William Harper (Alcohol Misuse), Dr. Funmi Olopade (Breast Cancer), Dr. Nancy Reau (Hepatitis B), Dr. David Rubin (Colon Cancer), and Dr. Matthew Sorrentino (illustrations for Blood Pressure and Aspirin chapters). Although they reviewed the chapter contents, any errors within them are entirely my own. I would also like to acknowledge my friends Dr. Richard Lerner and Dr. Amit Vora, who provided less formal guidance on many of the chapters in this book.

More generally, this book had the support of several people who advised, mentored, and sometimes counseled me through its development. I am lucky to count Dr. John Burton, Dr. Bimal Ashar, and Dr. Miriam Alexander as some of my mentors. I am also indebted to the Paul and Daisy Soros Fellowship for New Americans, which helped fund my graduate studies and gave me the confidence I needed to pursue this project.

I cannot express enough my appreciation for my editor, Jacqueline Wehmueller. In the late spring of 2007, she entertained a call from a bright-eyed medical student who had an idea for a book that would "save lives." Instead of laughing at me, as I fully expected, she graciously listened and then encouraged me to get started. Through the book's entire writing, rewriting, and further rewriting, I benefited from her honesty, her patience, and her talent. More broadly, I would like to thank the Johns Hopkins University Press for taking a chance on a young author and for supporting this book through all its stages.

I would also like to acknowledge my illustrator, Jacqueline Schaffer, and my copyeditor, Melanie Mallon. After reading an early draft of the book, Jackie became almost as excited as I am about publishing a book that would finally put evidence-based preventive medicine into the mainstream, and she brought that enthusiasm to her illustrations. Melanie brought much-needed energy late in this book's development as well as her expert eyes and ready pen.

This book would literally not exist without my mother, Anju Nundy. It was my love for her and my desire to keep her as healthy as possible that compelled me to write it. She was a constant source of support throughout the writing and was one of my most valued reviewers. I have my father, Rajiv Nundy, to thank for his guiding hand and his unfailing belief that I could really pull this off. And I thank my sister, Neeti Nundy, for being my most vocal advocate (as always) and for talking me through the many challenges I faced in writing this book.

Finally, I must acknowledge my best friend and life partner, Dr. Sonali Rudra. Through college, medical school, residency training, and life, she has been my constant friend and my muse of good deeds. All my readers have her to thank for keeping the focus of this book exactly where it should be—on helping everyday folks get the preventive health care they need to lead fuller, healthier lives.

STAY HEALTHY AT EVERY AGE

About This Book

WHY THIS BOOK MATTERS

When you were growing up, someone probably told you that "an ounce of prevention is worth a pound of cure." Many of us have learned from experience how much better it is to prevent a bad thing from happening than to try to fix the consequences once it has happened. Most people can agree that prevention is the way to go. This concept applies to our health as much as it applies to other areas of our lives: it is far better to prevent disease than to treat it. And if disease is already present, it is better to catch it early than to treat its complications. In health, an ounce of prevention is truly worth a pound of cure.

Yet the sad fact is that many people fail to take advantage of the available means of preventing disease. As a result, thousands of Americans die or become sick from preventable illnesses. According to the 2007 report by Partnership for Prevention,

▸ 45,000 additional lives would be saved each year if we increased to 90 percent the portion of adults who take aspirin daily to prevent heart disease. Today, fewer than half of American adults take aspirin preventively.

▸ 42,000 additional lives would be saved each year if we increased to 90 percent the portion of smokers who are advised by a health professional to quit and are offered medication or other assistance. Today, only 28 percent of smokers receive such services.

▸ 14,000 additional lives would be saved each year if we increased to 90 percent the portion of adults age 50 and older who are up to date with any recommended screening for colorectal cancer. Today, fewer than 50 percent of adults are up to date with screening.

▸ 12,000 additional lives would be saved each year if we increased to 90 percent the portion of adults age 50 and older immunized against influenza annually. Today, 37 percent of adults have had an annual flu vaccination.

▸ Nearly 4,000 additional lives would be saved each year if we increased to 90 percent the portion of women age 40 and older who have been screened for breast cancer in the past 2 years. Today, 67 percent of women have been screened in the past 2 years.[1]

More than 100,000 lives would be saved annually in the United States just by increasing the use of these five preventive measures. And these statistics do not include the countless people who would benefit from lower rates of disease, lower costs of health care, and higher quality of life. Just think what would happen if we included all the dozens of other recommended preventive services!

The causes for these failures are many—outdated medical practices, inconsistent preventive health guidelines, poor health insurance coverage, low public awareness, and, frankly, a broken system that is designed more for "sick care" than for "health care." Regardless of the cause, the patient stands to suffer most. It is the person with the preventable disease, not the doctors or the health care system, who suffers. And it is for this person that this book was written.

The purpose of this guide is simple: to arm you with the tools and know-how you need to take charge of your preventive health care so that you don't become one of these statistics. It focuses not on fad diets, unregulated supplements, or too-good-to-be-true advice but rather on those preventive services that are proven to save lives and prevent disease. The philosophy of this book is that with the right information, anyone can get the preventive services he or she needs to live a longer, healthier life.

SCOPE

From the latest blockbuster drugs to ancient remedies, MRI scans to yoga, and daily exercises to celebrity diets, preventive health is a huge subject. It encompasses an incredible number of approaches to leading a healthier life, each with its own value and place. But this book is focused. In the vast world of health promotion, it stakes out a small but important territory.

This book is about medical services that can help you *stay* healthy. These services include the screening tests, medications, and counseling that doctors provide to prevent disease or complications from disease. The focus is on promoting health, not on promoting medicine. This book is not about diagnosing diseases for the sake of diagnosing them or about recommending medicines that doctors think you should take. Books on preventive health already cover diets to lose weight, fat-burning exercises, and tips for quitting smoking, and although this book talks about healthy lifestyle choices, it does so in a different way. Instead of telling you what healthier choices to make—many of which you probably know—it tells you about medical services your doctor can provide, such as weight-loss counseling and assistance to quit smoking, to help you make those choices and stick with them. In addition, dozens of other topics, such as cardiovascular disease, infectious diseases, and cancer, are covered from a preventive health care perspective. This book looks at the entire lifespan, including childhood and pregnancy, and is intended to be a one-stop guide for you and your family.

The recommendations on the pages that follow are based on hard science and expert opinions. Only those preventive services that have passed the highest standards of evaluation are included here, which means that every recommendation in this book is proven to prevent disease and save lives. For every measure that is recommended, several others were not because they did not meet these strict criteria. Nothing discussed in this volume is experimental or controversial. Only those measures most likely to improve your health are included so that you get the most out of preventive health care without spending all your time at the doctor's office or all your money on unproven services and products that don't live up to their promises.

PHILOSOPHY

The philosophy of this book stems from the realization that preventive health care is like car maintenance. If we can take good care of our cars by following simple checklists, then we can better take care of ourselves by following similar checklists for disease prevention.

Sometimes I take my car to the mechanic because I feel that something is wrong—like a sick visit to my doctor. But often I take my car to the shop even though everything seems to be running smoothly, because it's often hard to tell whether the brake pads are wearing out until it is too late. Rather than risk injury or a breakdown, I take my car to the mechanic for regular maintenance checks.

The human body is similar, because many diseases (such as high blood pressure, diabetes, and cancer) don't cause any symptoms in the early stages. It may seem pointless going to the doctor when there is nothing wrong, but just as your car runs fine until the moment you completely run out of gas, certain things can go wrong with your body that you don't see until you bother looking—or until it's too late. That's why regular checkups with your doctor are as important as routine maintenance for your car.

I don't know much about cars (just ask my wife), but I still take good care of mine. The trick is having a checklist of maintenance services my car needs. The checklist tells me that every three months my car needs an oil change, every year it needs its wheels realigned, and every two years it needs a complete tune-up. That I don't know how to do these things doesn't matter. What matters is that I have my checklist, and that when it's time for a checkup, I remember to take my car to the mechanics who do know what to do.

Until now, most Americans have functioned without having a health maintenance plan. In addition, our health care system isn't designed for preventive health in the way the automobile industry is for car maintenance. So it's no wonder many people do a better job getting their car's oil changed than they do getting their blood pressure checked.

Just as a checklist for car maintenance includes regular services your car needs regardless of how it's running, the checklists in this book include health services every person needs regardless of symptoms. The chapters that follow the checklists explain the what, the why, and the how behind them, describing each preventive service in a reader-friendly way. By letting you know when you need to go to the doctor for which preventive services, this book will put you in charge of your health.

ORGANIZATION

Using this guide, you will be able to identify the preventive services that are recommended for you and understand what's involved with them so that you and your doctor can make sure you are getting the most out of preventive health opportunities. This book is divided into three parts:

- ▶ Part I provides an overview of preventive health and gives you tools to understand the recommendations that follow.

- ▶ Part II contains checklists organized by age. Some of the checklist items apply to everyone within the age range; others apply only to men or only to women; and still others apply to people with certain risk factors. At a glance, you can identify the preventive services that apply to you.

- ▶ Part III, by far the longest section, explains each preventive service and checklist item. In general, there is one chapter for each group of related services. By the end of each chapter, you will have a general understanding of the related disease, the rationale behind the checklist item, and what following the recommendation will mean for you.

HOW TO USE THIS BOOK

Start by reading part I, which explains where the recommendations come from, how to make the leap from "sick care" to "health care," and the basic terminology and concepts of preventive health. Then turn to part II and find the checklist designed for you. For example, if you are 52 years old, turn to the checklist titled "Ages 50 to 64." Identify which preventive services apply to you.

Next, read the chapters in part III that explain the preventive services that apply to you. If your checklist includes colon cancer screening, for example, read chapter 9. Pay attention to the section of the chapter that discusses the potential benefits and harms of the preventive measure. Develop a sense of whether this service is right for you and what questions you want your doctor to answer before you make your decision.

If you are interested in preventive services that are not recommended for you, such as those that will apply when you are older, read those chapters as well. For example, if you are a 35-year-old woman and want to learn more about breast cancer screening, even though screening is not recommended until age 50, read chapter 5.

Always keep in mind: the recommendations in this book are just that—recommendations. In the end, it is up to you and your doctor to decide which ones you follow and which preventive services are right for you and when.

THE SOURCE OF THE RECOMMENDATIONS

The United States Preventive Services Task Force (USPSTF) is the major source for the recommendations in this book. It would usually appear in each chapter's reference list, but to avoid repetition, I instead acknowledge this source here. (See www.ahrq.gov/clinic/USpstfix.htm for all USPSTF recommendations, which are periodically updated.) Only the recommendations on adult and pediatric immunizations come from another source, the Advisory Committee on Immunization Practices (ACIP) of the Centers for Disease Control and Prevention (CDC).

The USPSTF is a government-sponsored panel of independent experts in prevention and primary care. Their job is to conduct rigorous, impartial assessments of the scientific evidence for the effectiveness of clinical preventive services. Their recommendations are regarded as the gold standard in preventive health. The CDC is an agency of the U.S. Department of Health and Human Services that works to protect the public health and safety of the American people. ACIP comprises experts in the field of immunization who have been selected by the CDC to provide advice and guidance on the control of vaccine-preventable diseases.

WHAT THIS BOOK IS NOT

This book is not a substitute for a proper medical consultation. Rather, it is an informational guide to preventive services, including the potential benefits and harms. The recommendations in these pages represent expert consensus on the relative weights of these potential benefits and harms. How you weigh them is extremely important, however, and your feelings and preferences must play a role in the open discussion you will have with your doctor about any preventive care suggested for you here.

The recommendations are based on the highest standards of evaluation by the USPSTF. Only services that have been tested in large-scale clinical studies are considered. This means that the USPSTF has not evaluated some preventive services routinely performed by physicians—such as annual physical exams. The suggestions in this book should therefore be seen as the minimum preventive health care that should be offered to every American.

The advice reflects the risk factors of the average American, and in many circumstances, these recommendations may not apply to you. Some of these situations are described in the "How to Read the Checklists" section at the beginning of part II. That these circumstances exist underscores the need for medical consultation before undergoing any preventive service.

The original USPSTF and CDC recommendations are intended for use by physicians and other health care professionals, so I have adapted them for the average reader. Therefore, the suggestions in this book should not be considered direct reflections of the opinions of these organizations.

The information in this volume is up to date as of November 2009 and is subject to change. The USPSTF and CDC periodically revise and add to their guidelines as new scientific information becomes available and prevailing expert opinions shift. The most reliable and up-to-date recommendations can be obtained directly from these organizations and from physicians and other health care professionals.

The content of this book does not reflect the opinions of the author per se but presents the prevailing views of the larger medical community. In instances where the author holds opinions contrary to that community, the views of the latter are expressed because the intent of this book is to present generally accepted truths and not individuals' opinions. The vast majority of the content is widely accepted. However, there is some controversy and debate about certain sections (e.g., dietary advice, weight-loss management). Where points of contention exist, you and your doctor are left to reconcile them.

PART I

Introduction to Preventive Services

It's tough to get our heads around the idea of preventive health. We aren't accustomed to going to the doctor when we're well or receiving medical care to prevent an illness rather than to treat one. In prevention, everything is turned upside down, because instead of waiting for diseases to happen to us, we go after diseases before they even start. Getting into the preventive health mode requires a shift in the way we approach medical care. It also requires a new language and a set of tools for understanding common preventable diseases such as cancer and cardiovascular disease.

Preventive health also requires us to become active participants in our health care. Every medical service has the potential to help or to hurt. Although experts recommend only those preventive services for which they believe the benefits outweigh the harms, only you can decide which preventive care options are right for you. When we rely entirely on our doctors to track our preventive health, we often miss out on the services we need. Therefore, prevention must be deliberately scheduled into our lives. We owe it to ourselves to take responsibility for our well-being.

Preventive health care can be frustrating and confusing, but it doesn't have to be. When presented in the right way, it is one area of medicine that is accessible to everyone, regardless of medical knowledge. Getting you up to speed on preventive health is what this part of the book is all about.

DEFINING PREVENTIVE SERVICES

Preventive services are the medical services your doctor provides to help prevent disease or the complications from disease. They are also called *preventive health care, preventive health measures,* or *health maintenance.* There are three basic types of preventive services:

1. *Screening.* The purpose of screening is to detect disease before symptoms or complications develop. Many diseases begin years before the first symptoms are noticed. By the time symptoms develop, the disease may have already caused significant harm or progressed to an advanced stage, when treatments are less effective. Through screening, diseases can be detected early, when treatment can better slow or even halt their progression. Examples include high blood pressure screening, depression screening, and cancer screening.

2. *Preventive medicine.* The purpose of preventive medicine, also called *prophylactic medicine,* is to prevent disease before it develops. Preventive medicine is usually prescribed to high-risk individuals to lower their chances of developing disease or to prevent disease altogether. Examples include vaccines to prevent infectious diseases, aspirin to prevent heart attacks, and tamoxifen to prevent breast cancer.

3. *Counseling.* The purpose of counseling is to change habits that negatively affect health. Counseling may involve a combination of education, behavioral therapy, and medications (e.g., smoking cessation medications). Examples include counseling to quit smoking, to promote breastfeeding, or to aid in weight loss.

SHIFTING FROM "SICK CARE" TO "HEALTH CARE"

Usually you go to the doctor when you're sick. You have a symptom, go to the clinic, find out what's wrong, and get treated. It's the pattern we are most accustomed to and the pattern the health care system is designed to deal with best.

But preventive health care is different—you go to the doctor when you're healthy. You schedule a visit with your doctor months in advance, find out what diseases you're at risk for, and get the preventive services that will help you stay healthy. It's a whole different approach to medicine, and one that requires you to completely change how you think about medical care. Preventive health means shifting your thinking

from symptoms to risk factors,
from diagnosis to screening,
from treatment to prevention, and
from doctor's responsibility to shared responsibility.

From Symptoms to Risk Factors

"Sick care" focuses on symptoms. Symptoms are easy to understand because they are something you experience. You *feel* sick, so you go to the doctor. But "health care" is not about symptoms. If you have symptoms, then from a prevention point of view, you're already too late.

Health care is all about *risk factors,* those attributes that increase your chances, or risk, of having a disease or getting it in the future. Smoking is a risk factor for lung cancer because smoking increases your chances, or your risk, of developing lung cancer compared with nonsmokers. Being a woman is a risk factor for breast cancer because women have a greater chance of developing breast cancer than men do. So risk factors are things about you—your age, your gender, your habits, your genes, and your medical history—that put you at increased risk for certain diseases.

From Diagnosis to Screening

Symptoms are unreliable. Many diseases, such as sexually transmitted infections and cancers, have no symptoms in the early stages; other diseases, such as high blood pressure, do not have symptoms even in their late stages. That's why the first symptom of many diseases is a complication, such as a heart attack in people with high blood pressure. Sick care steps in when symptoms occur.

In health care, however, diseases are diagnosed before symptoms arise. Doctors use screening tests to detect diseases that are quietly causing harm to the body, and then they treat the illness before complications develop. To maximize their chances of finding diseases you have without subjecting you to unnecessary tests for those you most likely do not have, doctors decide which diseases to screen you for based on your risk factors.

From Treatment to Prevention

In sick care, the goal of treatment is to eliminate symptoms of disease. If symptoms improve, you know the treatment is working, and you continue it until the symptoms go away. If symptoms don't improve, you stop the treatment and try a new one.

In health care, the goal of prevention is to eliminate the risks of disease. If a disease is successfully prevented, you will never know it. The decision to continue prevention depends not on successful prevention but on the benefits of prevention continuing to exceed the harms. If you take aspirin to prevent heart attacks, you will never know if the aspirin saved you from having a heart attack. But because you continue to be at the same or increased risk of heart attacks, you continue taking the aspirin (unless you are having intolerable side effects). Instead of relying on physical evidence that the aspirin is working for you personally, you rely on medical research showing that for men at increased risk of heart disease, aspirin prevents up to one-third of heart attacks.

From Doctor's Responsibility to Shared Responsibility

In sick care, you rely on your doctor for medical care. When you are sick, your doctor decides what tests to run and what treatments to give.

In health care, you and your doctor share responsibility. Our health care system is poorly equipped to provide preventive services, but by partnering with your doctor, you can overcome these deficiencies and stay on top of your preventive health. You keep track of your preventive services and schedule appointments with your doctor when it's time for your mammogram or when you want to discuss aspirin therapy. Your doctor counsels you about the pros and cons of each option to help you make an informed decision and then provides the medical care and referrals you need to get the services you want.

BARRIERS TO PREVENTIVE HEALTH

Shifting to preventive health is not easy. We are all accustomed to thinking about health care through the sick care model. Below are some of the common barriers in our way. See if recognizing them can help get you over the hump.

Barrier: I don't like going to the doctor unless I have to.

Normally, you go to the doctor when you're sick, and even then, you usually wait an extra day or two before going in. But in preventive health, you will probably go to the doctor more often (or have longer visits), including when you are feeling healthy and have no symptoms. A major reason you probably don't like going to the doctor is that you feel there isn't much he or she can do to help you. Much of what doctors do is a mystery, and you might see little value in going to the clinic unless you have a compelling reason to go.

But with this book, you will have a reason to seek medical care even when you're not sick. The goal is for you to be able to say to your doctor, "Hey, Doc. I just turned 50 years old, and this book tells me that I need to get screened for colon cancer because screening will reduce my risk of dying from colon cancer by over 30 percent. I looked at the three options for screening it talks about, and I've decided to go with option 2. What do you think?" This is an entirely different doctor's appointment than the one many of us dread. With this book, you will know exactly what you will be getting out of each visit and will often be the one setting the terms.

Barrier: I don't like getting medical tests.

Nobody likes to get medical tests. But a major problem with the way things are done now is that we often have no idea what the test is for, let alone how it will improve our health. But in this book, a test is recommended only if major scientific studies show that it prevents disease and saves lives. While this does not make getting the test any less uncomfortable, knowing that the test may lead to an improvement in health and even longer life at least makes the discomfort worthwhile.

Barrier: I don't want to know if I'm sick.

Being screened for diseases like diabetes and cancer is scary. Because of this fear, people commonly say, "If I have cancer or some other terrible disease, I don't want to know about it." For diseases for which there are no good treatments, this approach makes some sense, because there is little value in being diagnosed with a disease unless diagnosis leads to treatments that improve health. However, the recommendations in this book are not subject to this reasoning. Every screening recommendation is based on evidence that screening for the disease actually improves health.

This book does not recommend routine prostate cancer screening, for example, because there is insufficient evidence that screening for prostate cancer improves health. Screening leads to more diagnoses of the disease, but studies have not shown that men who are screened for prostate cancer live longer than men who are not screened. Finding out that you have a disease is scary, but with the tests in this book, you will not be simply getting a diagnosis; you'll be getting the chance to slow or eliminate the disease and give yourself a healthier future.

Barrier: I don't like taking medicines.

Medicines are one component of preventive health care, albeit an important one. As with medical tests, part of our distaste for medicines is that we often take them with uncertain benefits. Cholesterol-modifying medicines are a good example. With this book you will understand the hazards of abnormal cholesterol and be given the tools to assess your own risk for coronary heart disease (CHD). That way, when you take a cholesterol-modifying medication (as part of a broader risk-reduction strategy), you will better appreciate the benefit in terms of CHD prevention. Knowing the value of the medicines you are taking will, I hope, make them easier to swallow.

TERMS AND CONCEPTS

Understanding the preventive health terminology and concepts that are used throughout this book will help you grasp the finer points of preventive care. This in turn will make it easier to decide with confidence which services are right for you.

Primary, Secondary, and Tertiary Preventive Measures

Primary preventive measures are interventions that prevent the onset of disease. Examples include immunizations to prevent infections, aspirin to prevent heart attacks, and weight-loss counseling to prevent obesity-related medical conditions. *Secondary preventive measures* are interventions that prevent symptoms and complications in people who have already developed disease but in whom the disease has not yet become clinically apparent. Examples of secondary prevention include cancer screening, blood pressure screening, and osteoporosis screening. The goal of primary prevention is to avert disease. The goal of secondary prevention is to identify and treat disease in its earliest stages, to prevent symptoms or complications from developing.

This book covers both primary and secondary prevention, but not tertiary prevention. The goal of *tertiary prevention* is to prevent the further progression of diseases that are already clinically apparent. Because tertiary prevention pertains to diseases that have already been diagnosed and are being treated, it falls outside the scope of this book.

Asymptomatic versus Symptomatic

Asymptomatic means not symptomatic, or without symptoms. Being asymptomatic means having no symptoms related to the medical condition being considered. It doesn't necessarily mean being completely healthy and having no symptoms of any disease. Thus a woman without symptoms of breast cancer would be considered asymptomatic for breast cancer, even if she had symptoms of a urinary tract infection at the time. This term matters because *the guidelines in this book apply only to asymptomatic individuals.* Although breast cancer screening is recommended every two years in women ages 50 to 74, a 56-year-old woman who develops breast cancer symptoms should be evaluated by a doctor even if her last mammogram was done six months ago. Once she becomes *symptomatic* for breast cancer—that is, she develops symptoms related to the disease—the screening recommendation no longer applies.

Screening Tests versus Diagnostic Tests

Screening tests are medical tests or standardized examinations given to asymptomatic individuals to identify the need for further medical evaluation. In contrast, *diagnostic tests* are given to symptomatic individuals to identify the cause of their symptoms. *The goal of screening tests is to identify people who need further medical evaluation.* It is not *necessarily* to make a definitive diagnosis. Various screening tests are available to help us prevent disease or catch it early, including blood tests to screen for diabetes, medical procedures to screen for colon cancer, and questionnaires to screen for depression. The distinction between the two types of tests sometimes blurs, but the concepts are still useful to keep in mind.

Sensitivity, Specificity, False Negatives, and False Positives

No medical test is perfect; with each test, there is a chance that the disease will be missed or that a healthy person will be diagnosed with a disease he or she does not have.

The *sensitivity* of a medical test is the chance that the test will be positive, or abnormal, among patients who have the disease. Sensitivity can be thought of as the detection rate. Mammograms have a sensitivity of 80 percent. That means 80 percent of breast cancers are detected through routine mammography, and that 20 percent of breast cancers are missed. A mammogram that fails to detect a breast cancer is *falsely negative*, or gives a negative, or normal, result even though the person has the disease. The higher the sensitivity of a test, the higher the detection rate, and the less likely it is to give a false-negative result.

The *specificity* of a medical test is the chance that the test will be negative, or normal, among patients who do not have the disease. Mammograms have a specificity of 95 percent. That means that 5 percent of mammograms are *falsely positive*, or give a positive, or abnormal, result even though the patient does *not* have the disease. False positives are like false alarms, because they suggest that the disease is present even though it is not. The higher the specificity of a test, the less likely it is to give a false-positive result.

Screening Interval

The *screening interval* is the length of time between consecutive screening tests. Some recommendations specify a screening interval (e.g., routine mammography every two years in women ages 50 to 74). Other recommendations leave it up to you and your doctor to decide how often you should be screened. In general, shorter screening intervals increase overall sensitivity because the chance of detecting disease increases with the number of screening tests performed. However, shorter screening intervals also decrease overall specificity and increase false positives.

SPECIAL SECTION ON CARDIOVASCULAR DISEASE

The leading cause of morbidity and mortality in the United States is cardiovascular disease. *Cardiovascular disease* is a term that refers to any disease involving the heart or blood vessels (the arteries and veins that carry blood between the heart and the body). It includes major diseases such as coronary heart disease and stroke, which are the number one and number three leading causes of death in the United States. More than 60 million Americans suffer from some form of cardiovascular disease, and nearly 2,600 die every day from it—or one person every thirty-three seconds. Because cardiovascular disease is such an important topic, and because the preventive services that pertain to it are spread across multiple chapters, this section is intended to provide a brief background on cardiovascular disease and to define some important terms and concepts.

When doctors talk about cardiovascular disease, they are usually referring to a disease called *atherosclerosis* (ath-er-o-skle-RO-sis). Atherosclerosis is the fatty buildup of plaque inside the arteries that causes them to become narrower, much as grease can clog kitchen pipes. The disease can occur in any blood vessel in the body. *Coronary heart disease,* or CHD, is a common term for atherosclerosis that occurs in the vessels that supply the heart.

Over time, the more plaque buildup there is, the narrower the vessels become. The most dangerous consequence of atherosclerosis is plaque rupture leading to complete blockage of a blood vessel. This blockage prevents the flow of essential nutrients and oxygen and causes the tissues relying on the blood vessel to die. When plaque rupture occurs in a vessel that provides

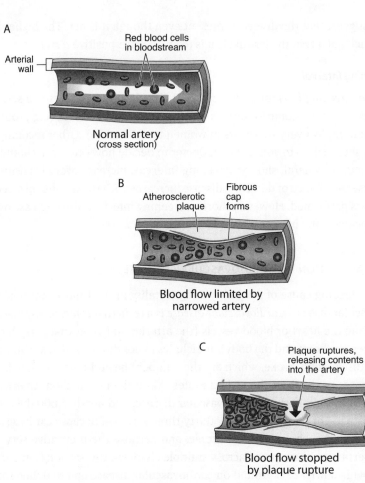

Figure I.1. Atherosclerosis is the fatty buildup of plaque inside the arteries. (A) In a healthy artery, blood flow is uninhibited, allowing for the effective delivery of nutrients and oxygen. (B) In an atherosclerotic artery, plaque may form within the arterial wall. Plaque can limit the delivery of nutrients and oxygen, which may cause health problems. For example, plaque in the arteries of the heart can cause angina, or chest pain. (C) The dreaded complication of atherosclerosis is plaque rupture. Plaque rupture causes an acute stoppage in blood flow. When this occurs in the heart, it leads to a heart attack.

blood to the heart, it causes a *heart attack*. When it occurs in a vessel that provides blood to the brain, it causes a *stroke*.

Heart attacks and strokes rarely occur in the absence of the major risk factors for cardiovascular disease—tobacco use, cholesterol disorders, high blood pressure, and diabetes. Additional risk factors include older age, obesity, unhealthy eating, sedentary lifestyle, and a family history of early cardiovascular disease. The best way to prevent cardiovascular disease is through healthy lifestyle choices. This means maintaining a healthy weight, exercising regularly, eating right, not smoking, and, for people with diabetes, keeping blood sugar under control. For those who cannot optimize their risk factors through lifestyle choices, medication is a good complement. A wide range of medications are available: cholesterol-modifying medications, blood pressure–lowering medications, medicines to help people quit smoking, and medicines for controlling diabetes. Lifestyle modifications and medications together can improve a person's risk factors and lower the chances of heart attack, stroke, and death from cardiovascular disease.

To control the risk factors, you first must understand what they are and determine whether you have any of them. Three chapters in this book present the United States Preventive Services Task Force (USPSTF) screening recommendations for the major risk factors that cause atherosclerosis and cardiovascular disease. Chapter 4 discusses screening for high blood pressure; chapter 8, cholesterol screening; and chapter 11, screening for diabetes. Knowledge of these risk factors can then be used to estimate one's overall risk of cardiovascular disease. Chapter 3 discusses methods for estimating 10-year risk of CHD along with the guidelines on aspirin use for the prevention of cardiovascular events.

SPECIAL SECTION ON CANCER

Few words in the English language evoke as much fear and anxiety as the word "cancer." It is arguably the most dreaded diagnosis in medicine, distressing enough that the thought of being diagnosed with cancer sometimes deters us from getting screened for it, even if screening is proven to prevent cancer and save lives. Part of the problem is that we mostly learn about cancer from the popular media or our family and friends, and so it is a terribly misunderstood disease.

The goal of this section is to dispel common myths about cancer and introduce concepts to explain the cancer-related recommendations in this book. It starts with five facts everyone should know about cancer, and then defines common cancer terms.

Fact 1: Cancer is not one disease but many diseases. Breast cancer, brain cancer, lung cancer—these are all different diseases with different risk factors, different treatments, and different expected outcomes. For example, the cancer that Lance Armstrong had, testicular cancer, is curable in most men and has a greater than 95 percent ten-year survival rate. In contrast, lung cancer is usually fatal and has a 5 percent ten-year survival rate.

Fact 2: The major causes of cancer-related deaths are preventable. So much attention is placed on new treatments for cancer that often we overlook the incredible advances in cancer prevention. It surprises many people to find out that serious morbidity and death from the three most common cancers in the United States—lung cancer, colon cancer, and breast cancer—are largely preventable.

Fact 3: Cancer is not a death sentence. A major reason that people do not want to be screened for cancer is that they think it is untreatable. But for many cancers, screening is often the first step to treating and even curing the disease.

Fact 4: Cancer is not an all-or-nothing disease. What cancer means in terms of treatment and outcomes is closely tied to its stage (see below). The goal of screening is to detect cancer at a stage when treatments are more effective and cure is more likely.

Fact 5: Cancer matters to everyone. It is the second leading cause of mortality in the United States, accounting for one in every four deaths. It's not just a disease of older adults. Cancer affects people of all ages, and the cancers that affect our health in older age often result from choices we make in early adulthood (e.g., smoking). It's also not a disease that only people with a family history should worry about. Not having a family history of cancer reduces but does not eliminate your risk of developing it.

Benign versus Malignant Tumors

A cancer, or malignant tumor, is a mass of abnormal cells that develops from normal tissue. Normally, cells grow and divide to form new cells as the body needs them. When cells grow old, they die, and new cells take their place. But sometimes this orderly process goes wrong. New cells form when the body does not need them, and old cells do not die as they should. These extra cells form a mass of tissue called a growth, or *tumor*. Tumors can be either benign or malignant. The difference between benign and malignant tumors is that *malignant tumors* can invade adjacent tissues and other parts of the body; *benign tumors* cannot. Benign tumors are not considered cancers; only malignant tumors are cancers. The terms cancer and malignant tumor are interchangeable.

Cancer versus Precancer

Cancer is a progressive disease. It develops from normal cells, but the transition is not instantaneous; it is gradual and occurs in phases. During the in-between period, when the cells are no longer normal but not yet cancer, they are called *precancerous,* or *precancers*. Unlike cancer cells, precancers cannot invade nearby tissues or spread to other parts of the body. As a result, they are much easier to remove and treat. Not all precancers will become cancers, but because they have a risk of becoming cancerous, doctors generally treat them.

Stage, Metastasis, and Prognosis

The extent of a cancer is called its *stage*. The larger the cancer and the greater its spread, the more advanced its stage. The most advanced stage of cancer is when it has spread to distant organs, called *metastatic cancer,* or *metastasis*. Staging matters because *prognosis*—the likely outcome or course of the disease—is closely tied to stage. The earlier the stage at diagnosis, the more favorable the prognosis. The goal of cancer screening is to detect cancer at a stage when its prognosis is better and there is hope of effective treatment and even cure.

THE RATIONALE BEHIND THESE RECOMMENDATIONS

The major source of recommendations in this book is the United States Preventive Services Task Force (USPSTF). Because the recommendations in this book may differ from what your doctor advises, it is important to understand why this book follows the USPSTF and what the implications are for you.

The USPSTF guidelines have three major advantages:

1. *Impartiality.* The USPSTF is a government-sponsored panel of independent experts. Other organizations that put forth guidelines on preventive health care, such as the American College of Cardiology and the American College of Surgeons, have professional interests and are therefore more likely to be biased.

2. *Comprehensiveness.* The USPSTF evaluates preventive services across diseases and demographic groups, including children and pregnant women. In contrast, other organizations are oriented toward a particular medical specialty or disease group (for example, the American Cancer Society primarily evaluates cancer-related preventive services). Following the USPSTF recommendations allows for the use of one consistent set of guidelines.

3. *Reputability.* The USPSTF recommendations are considered the gold standard in preventive services. The task force sets the highest bar for

recommending a preventive service and recommends only services that are clearly proven to prevent disease and reduce mortality.

Because of its high standards, the USPSTF tends to make recommendations that are more conservative than those of other organizations. In some cases, this means recommending a preventive service to fewer people (for example, screening only women with risk factors for sexually transmitted infections rather than screening all women) or less often (for example, mammography every two years rather than every year). In other cases, it means not recommending a preventive service that other organizations routinely support (for example, prostate cancer screening). This is because the task force bases its recommendations on hard data: if the evidence for a preventive measure is insufficient or not compelling enough, the measure is not recommended.

That this book gives you only the "most proven" preventive services has important implications for you. It means that by following this book, you can make sure you are not missing out on preventive health care that is most likely to benefit you. At the same time, it doesn't preclude you from getting additional preventive services. Just because a preventive measure is not supported by the USPSTF does not mean it has no value—it may simply mean that there is not yet enough data to recommend it widely. In the end, the guidelines in this book were chosen in a way that allows you to benefit from the advice and expertise of your doctor and new developments in the field while ensuring that you are getting the preventive health care that the data best support and that the experts recommend.

THE BENEFITS AND HARMS OF PREVENTIVE HEALTH

More than anything else, this book is about helping you become an informed consumer of preventive health care. To better participate in your health care, you need to know both the potential benefits and the potential harms of every recommendation that applies to you. While the specific benefits and harms of each preventive service are covered in part III, table I.1 provides a broad overview.

Since breast cancer can affect women in their thirties, even though it's rare, people sometimes wonder why screening for breast cancer is not recommended to start at age 30. Many assume the reason is cost. But as table I.1 shows, cost is a minor consideration out of many. Screening average-risk women ages 30 to 39 may pick up a few more cases of breast cancer, but, as

Table I.1: Potential benefits and harms of preventive services

Type of preventive service	Potential benefits	Potential harms
Screening	Earlier detection and treatment of diseases, leading to better health outcomes (e.g., colon cancer screening reduces death from colon cancer by 33%). Reduced anxiety with a negative, or normal, test result.	Direct harms of the screening test: for many tests (such as blood tests or questionnaires), these harms are minimal; for others (such as colonoscopy) they may be significant. Indirect harms from further testing: most screening tests require further testing before a definitive diagnosis can be made; these follow-up tests have potential for harm. Treatment of diseases that without detection would not have caused any harm. Unnecessary testing and anxiety after a false positive. A false sense of security and delayed diagnosis because of a false negative. Feeling stigmatized by a diagnosis. Cost.
Preventive medicine	Reduced risk or prevention of disease (e.g., tamoxifen prevents up to 50% of breast cancers in high-risk women).	Side effects from medications or vaccination. False sense of security. Cost.
Counseling	Reduced risk of injury or disease (e.g., people who smoke are more than twice as likely to quit if they receive assistance from their doctors).	Less time for other medical care. Cost.

discussed in greater detail in chapter 5, it would also lead to unnecessary biopsies and treatments for breast cancers that would never cause any harm.

Even counseling services have potential harms. To make the most out of the ten to fifteen minutes you spend with your doctor, it is best for your doctor to provide only the counseling services that will benefit you. If instead of counseling you on smoking cessation, for example, which has proven health benefits, he or she counsels you on seatbelt safety, which may be valuable but has not been shown to improve health outcomes, then the counseling session has detracted from proven medical services that could have been offered to you, and in doing so, has inadvertently caused harm by depriving you of those services.

Every preventive service has potential harms. That is why this book recommends only those measures that have been shown through well-conducted medical studies to improve health. With this approach, the potential benefits of preventive health can be realized while minimizing unnecessary harms.

PLANNING FOR PREVENTION

Most people's system for preventive health is to rely on their doctors and the health care system to provide them with the preventive services they need. But as health statistics show, for most of us, the current system is not working. To best use the information in this book, you need to develop a more robust system, in which prevention is planned for and built into your routine.

There is no one-size-fits-all approach to planning for prevention, but everyone should keep in mind two general ideas.

One is to engage your doctor in a discussion about how best to arrange for your preventive health care. Every doctor and medical practice has a different approach. Some doctors schedule separate "prevention visits." Others schedule time at the end of their regular appointments. And still others use a team of health care professionals to provide preventive care. With your doctor, you will need to find a mutually agreeable system that enables you to get the services you need while working within the norms of your doctor's practice.

Second, create a personal system for tracking your preventive health. This can be challenging, because you will receive multiple services, often from various health care providers. It is not uncommon for the same patient to receive smoking counseling from her primary care doctor, Pap smears from her gynecologist, and mammograms from her radiologist. However, the decentralized nature of these services makes it even more essential for you to have a system for scheduling and keeping appointments and following up on test results. Do not simply rely on your doctors—you need your own preventive health medical record. That way, if you move or change doctors, or your doctor simply loses track, you will still receive the services you need. It is a good idea to integrate preventive health into your current organizational system—whether on a PDA, on a desktop computer, or in an appointment diary. That way you have one system for all your organizational needs. For those who don't have an organizational system, now is as good a time as ever to start one!

Please, find a system that works and use it. By partnering with your doctor early and staying organized, you can plan for prevention and make sure you are getting the most out of preventive health care.

PART II

Healthy Checks Guidelines

HOW TO READ THE CHECKLISTS

The checklists presented in this section are called "Healthy Checks" because they describe preventive health recommendations. Healthy Checks are provided here for each age group and for pregnancy. Before turning to the checklists, review the following guidelines to help you decide which advice is relevant to you.

A recommendation generally applies to you if:

▸ *You have one or more of the applicable risk factors.* For some recommendations, the only pertinent risk factor is age (for example, adults over age 18 are advised to get screened for high blood pressure). For others, age and gender determine applicability (for example, women ages 50 to 74 are advised to have mammography screenings for breast cancer). Still others are based on multiple risk factors (for example, children over 6 months old whose primary source of water is fluoride deficient should receive oral fluoride supplements).

▸ *You do not have any symptoms consistent with the disease.* Screening is by definition for people who are asymptomatic; if you have symptoms, then the guidelines no longer apply. For example, screening for colon cancer is recommended for adults over age 50, but if you are under age 50 and have symptoms consistent with colon cancer, such as blood in the stools and unintentional weight loss, then you should be evaluated by a doctor and, if necessary, be tested for colon cancer.

▸ *You have not been diagnosed with the disease or a related condition.* Preventive services are intended for people without established disease. If you have a history of the disease or a related condition, *the guidelines no longer apply.* For example, the recommendations on breast cancer screening do not apply to women with a history of breast cancer. Likewise, the guidelines on aspirin do not apply to people with a history of coronary heart disease.

A recommendation *may not* apply to you if:

▸ *You are age 65 or older.* Most of the recommendations are based on studies of people younger than 65 years. Therefore, in general, the potential benefits and harms of many preventive services are unknown for people over age 65. This does not mean that people over age 65 should not receive any preventive services. Rather, it means that in this age group, decisions about preventive services should be made individually and with a physician.

▸ *You have a terminal or major medical illness.* The benefits of preventive measures accrue over a period of years such that people with terminal or major medical illness may not experience the full benefit. At the same time, they are at greater risk of harm from preventive health care. The resulting circumstances may tip the balance of risks and benefits against certain preventive measures.

▸ *You were born or reside outside the United States.* The recommendations in this book are from the United States Preventive Services Task Force (USPSTF) and the United States Centers for Disease Control and Prevention (CDC). The advice is intended for people living in the United States and may not apply to someone born or residing elsewhere. For example, in some areas of the world, additional vaccinations against common infectious diseases such as yellow fever and tuberculosis may be required. Similarly, in some countries, colon cancer is much less common than in the United States such that the benefits of routine screening may not outweigh the risks.

A Note on Vaccinations

On the following pages, you may notice that only a handful of vaccines are listed. The vaccine guidelines in this book apply to healthy people without any additional risk factors for infectious diseases. If you have certain medical conditions or risk factors, then you may need additional vaccinations. For example, all healthy people are recommended to receive the vaccine against pneumonia at age 65. Thus, this recommendation is listed in the "Healthy Checks: Age 65 or Older" checklist. However, people with certain chronic conditions, such as asthma or diabetes, are advised by the CDC to receive the pneumonia vaccine at an earlier age.

Everyone benefits from the complete CDC recommendations, so each page includes "Vaccines as recommended by the latest CDC guidelines" as a checklist item. This item should prompt you to review with your doctor the latest CDC guidelines to determine which vaccines are right for you. The 2009 CDC immunization schedule and the most up-to-date CDC vaccine information sheets are included in the appendix for your reference. See chapter 23 for more information on adult vaccines or chapter 12 for more details on childhood vaccines.

HEALTHY CHECKS: EARLY CHILDHOOD

- ☐ Eye drops in newborns to prevent gonococcal ophthalmia neonatorum (See chapter 12 for more information on all recommendations in this checklist.)

- ☐ Newborn screening for congenital hypothyroidism (CH)

- ☐ Newborn screening for phenylketonuria (PKU)

- ☐ Newborn screening for sickle cell disease

- ☐ Newborn screening for hearing loss

- ☐ Iron supplementation for children ages 6 to 12 months at increased risk for iron deficiency anemia
  - ‣ preterm birth (born before 37 weeks)
  - ‣ low birthweight (under 5.5 lb at birth)

- ☐ Oral fluoride supplementation for preschool children older than 6 months whose primary water source is deficient in fluoride

- ☐ Screening to detect amblyopia, strabismus, and defects in visual acuity in children younger than 5 years

- ☐ Vaccinations as recommended by the latest CDC guidelines (see appendix)

HEALTHY CHECKS: ADOLESCENCE TO AGE 19

All Adolescents

☐ Blood pressure screening for everyone age 18 and over (see chapter 4)

☐ Depression screening (see chapter 10)

☐ Vaccinations as recommended by the latest CDC guidelines (see chapter 23 and appendix)

Additional Measures for Women

☐ Cervical cancer screening: if sexually active begin three years after first sexual intercourse (see chapter 6)

☐ Chlamydia screening for sexually active women 24 years of age or younger (see chapter 7)

☐ Gonorrhea screening for sexually active women 24 years of age or younger (see chapter 13)

☐ HPV vaccine for women ages 13 to 26 (unless already vaccinated; see chapter 6)

☐ Preventive services for pregnant women (see "Healthy Checks: Pregnancy," p. 48)

Additional Measures for At-Risk People

☐ HIV screening if at risk for infection (see chapter 16):
  ‣ men and women who have unprotected sex with multiple partners
  ‣ men who have sex with men
  ‣ people being treated for a sexually transmitted infection (e.g., syphilis, gonorrhea, or chlamydia)
  ‣ injection drug users
  ‣ people who exchange sex for drugs or money
  ‣ sexual partners of anyone with one or more of the above risk factors

☐ Sexually transmitted infection (STI) counseling if sexually active (see chapter 20)

☐ Syphilis screening if at risk for infection (see chapter 21):
  ‣ men who have sex with men
  ‣ people who exchange sex for drugs or money
  ‣ people in adult correctional facilities

HEALTHY CHECKS: AGES 20 TO 29

Everyone Ages 20 to 29

☐ Blood pressure screening (see chapter 4)

☐ Depression screening (see chapter 10)

☐ Obesity screening and counseling (see chapter 17)

☐ Tetanus vaccine every ten years (see appendix and chapter 23)

☐ Vaccinations as recommended by the latest CDC guidelines (see appendix and chapter 23)

Additional Measures for Women

☐ BRCA genetic counseling and evaluation referral for women with certain family history patterns of breast and ovarian cancer (See chapter 5 for a list of applicable family history patterns.)

☐ Cervical cancer screening: at least every three years beginning three years after first sexual intercourse but no later than age 21 (see chapter 6)

☐ Chlamydia screening for sexually active women 25 years or younger, and older women at risk for infection (see chapter 7):
  ‣ new or multiple partners
  ‣ history of sexually transmitted infection
  ‣ inconsistent condom use
  ‣ exchange of sex for drugs or money

☐ Gonorrhea screening for sexually active women 25 years or younger, and older women at risk for infection (see chapter 13):
  ‣ new or multiple partners
  ‣ history of sexually transmitted infection
  ‣ inconsistent condom use
  ‣ exchange of sex for drugs or money

☐ HPV vaccine for women ages 13 to 26 (unless already vaccinated; see appendix and chapter 6)

☐ Preventive services for pregnant women (see "Healthy Checks: Pregnancy," p. 48)

Additional Measures for At-Risk People

☐ Alcohol misuse screening for people who consume alcohol (see chapter 2)

☐ Cholesterol screening if at risk for cardiovascular disease (see chapter 8):
- diabetes
- tobacco use
- high blood pressure
- obesity (body mass index [BMI] ≥30 kg/m²)
- family history of early heart disease (before age 50 in first-degree male relatives or before age 60 in first-degree female relatives)
- personal history of cardiovascular disease

☐ Diabetes screening if sustained blood pressure ≥135/80 mmHg (see chapter 11)

☐ Healthy eating counseling if at risk for cardiovascular and diet-related chronic disease (see chapter 14):
- cholesterol disorder
- high blood pressure
- diabetes
- obesity (BMI ≥30 kg/m²)
- overweight (BMI 25–29.9 kg/m²)
- abdominal obesity (weight circumference ≥40 inches in men or ≥35 inches in women)

☐ HIV screening if at risk for infection (see chapter 16):
- men and women who have unprotected sex with multiple partners
- men who have sex with men
- people being treated for a sexually transmitted infection (e.g., syphilis, gonorrhea, or chlamydia)
- injection drug users
- people who exchange sex for drugs or money
- sexual partners of anyone with one or more of the above risk factors

☐ Sexually transmitted infection (STI) counseling if at risk for STI (chapter 20):
- multiple current sexual partners
- current STI or history of infection in past year

☐ Syphilis screening if at risk for infection (see chapter 21):
- men who have sex with men
- people who exchange sex for drugs or money
- people in adult correctional facilities

☐ Tobacco use counseling for people who smoke or use tobacco products (see chapter 22)

HEALTHY CHECKS: AGES 30 TO 39

Everyone Ages 30 to 39

☐ Blood pressure screening (see chapter 4)

☐ Depression screening (see chapter 10)

☐ Obesity screening and counseling (see chapter 17)

☐ Tetanus vaccine every ten years (see appendix and chapter 23)

☐ Vaccinations as recommended by the latest CDC guidelines (see appendix and chapter 23)

Additional Measures for Women

☐ BRCA genetic counseling and evaluation referral for women with certain family history patterns of breast and ovarian cancer (See chapter 5 for a list of applicable family history patterns.)

☐ Breast cancer chemoprevention: considered in women at high risk of breast cancer and at low risk of adverse effects from therapy (see chapter 5)

☐ Cervical cancer screening at least every three years, except women who have had a total hysterectomy for benign disease (see chapter 6)

☐ Chlamydia screening in women at risk of infection (see chapter 7):
  ‣ new or multiple partners
  ‣ history of sexually transmitted infection
  ‣ inconsistent condom use
  ‣ exchange of sex for drugs or money

☐ Cholesterol screening in women at risk for cardiovascular disease (see chapter 8):
  ‣ diabetes
  ‣ tobacco use
  ‣ high blood pressure
  ‣ obesity (body mass index [BMI] ≥30 kg/m^2)
  ‣ family history of early heart disease (before age 50 in first-degree male relatives or before age 60 in first-degree female relatives)
  ‣ personal history of cardiovascular disease

☐ Gonorrhea screening in women at risk for infection (see chapter 13):

  ‣ new or multiple partners
  ‣ history of sexually transmitted infection
  ‣ inconsistent condom use
  ‣ exchange of sex for drugs or money

☐ Preventive services for pregnant women (see "Healthy Checks: Pregnancy," p. 48)

Additional Measures for Men

☐ Cholesterol screening in men over age 35 and in younger men at risk for cardiovascular disease (see chapter 8):

  ‣ diabetes
  ‣ tobacco use
  ‣ high blood pressure
  ‣ obesity (BMI ≥30 kg/m^2)
  ‣ family history of early heart disease (before age 50 in first-degree male relatives or before age 60 in first-degree female relatives)
  ‣ personal history of cardiovascular disease

Additional Measures for At-Risk People

☐ Alcohol misuse screening for people who consume alcohol (see chapter 2)

☐ Diabetes screening if sustained blood pressure ≥135/80 mmHg (see chapter 11)

☐ Healthy eating counseling if at risk for cardiovascular and diet-related chronic disease (see chapter 14):

  ‣ cholesterol disorder
  ‣ high blood pressure
  ‣ diabetes
  ‣ obesity (BMI ≥30 kg/m^2)
  ‣ overweight (BMI 25–29.9 kg/m^2)
  ‣ abdominal obesity (weight circumference ≥40 inches in men or ≥35 inches in women)

☐ HIV screening if at risk for infection (see chapter 16):

  ‣ men and women who have unprotected sex with multiple partners

(continues)

(Ages 30–39, Additional Measures for At-Risk People, continued)

- ‣ men who have sex with men
- ‣ people being treated for a sexually transmitted infection (e.g., syphilis, gonorrhea, or chlamydia)
- ‣ injection drug users
- ‣ people who exchange sex for drugs or money
- ‣ sexual partners of anyone with one or more of the above risk factors

☐ Sexually transmitted infection (STI) counseling if at risk for STI (chapter 20):

- ‣ multiple current sexual partners
- ‣ current STI or history of infection in the past year

☐ Syphilis screening if at risk for infection (see chapter 21):

- ‣ men who have sex with men
- ‣ people who exchange sex for drugs or money
- ‣ people in adult correctional facilities

☐ Tobacco use counseling for people who smoke or use tobacco products (see chapter 22)

HEALTHY CHECKS: AGES 40 TO 49

Everyone Ages 40 to 49

☐ Blood pressure screening (see chapter 4)

☐ Depression screening (see chapter 10)

☐ Obesity screening and counseling (see chapter 17)

☐ Tetanus vaccine every ten years (see appendix and chapter 23)

☐ Vaccinations as recommended by the latest CDC guidelines
(see appendix and chapter 23)

Additional Measures for Women

☐ BRCA genetic counseling and evaluation referral for women with
certain family history patterns of breast and ovarian cancer (See
chapter 5 for a list of applicable family history patterns.)

☐ Breast cancer chemoprevention: considered in women at high
risk of breast cancer and at low risk of adverse effects from
therapy (see chapter 5)

☐ Cervical cancer screening at least every three years, except for
women who have had a total hysterectomy for benign disease
(see chapter 6)

☐ Chlamydia screening in women at risk for infection
(see chapter 7):
  ‣ new or multiple partners
  ‣ history of sexually transmitted infection
  ‣ inconsistent condom use
  ‣ exchange of sex for drugs or money

☐ Cholesterol screening in women at risk for cardiovascular disease
(see chapter 8):
  ‣ diabetes
  ‣ tobacco use
  ‣ high blood pressure
  ‣ obesity (body mass index [BMI] $\geq$30 kg/m^2)
  ‣ family history of early heart disease (before age 50 in first-
    degree male relatives or before age 60 in first-degree female
    relatives)
  ‣ personal history of cardiovascular disease

(continues)

(Ages 40–49, Additional Measures for Women, continued)

☐ Gonorrhea screening in women at risk for infection
(see chapter 13):
  - new or multiple partners
  - history of sexually transmitted infection
  - inconsistent condom use
  - exchange of sex for drugs or money

☐ Preventive services for pregnant women (see "Healthy Checks:
Pregnancy," p. 48)

Additional Measures for Men

☐ Aspirin to prevent cardiovascular disease in men over age
45—discuss potential benefits and harms with a doctor
(see chapter 3)

☐ Cholesterol screening (see chapter 8)

Additional Measures for At-Risk People

☐ Alcohol misuse screening for people who consume alcohol
(see chapter 2)

☐ Diabetes screening if sustained blood pressure ≥135/80 mmHg
(see chapter 11)

☐ Healthy eating counseling if at risk for cardiovascular and diet-
related chronic disease (see chapter 14):
  - cholesterol disorder
  - high blood pressure
  - diabetes
  - obesity (BMI ≥30 kg/m^2)
  - overweight (BMI 25–29.9 kg/m^2)
  - abdominal obesity (weight circumference ≥40 inches in men
    or ≥35 inches in women)

☐ HIV screening if at risk for infection (see chapter 16):
  - men and women who have unprotected sex with multiple
    partners
  - men who have sex with men
  - people being treated for a sexually transmitted infection
    (e.g., syphilis, gonorrhea, or chlamydia)
  - injection drug users
  - people who exchange sex for drugs or money
  - sexual partners of anyone with one or more of the above risk
    factors

☐ Sexually transmitted infection (STI) counseling if at risk for STI
  ‣ multiple current sexual partners
  ‣ current STI or history of infection in past year

☐ Syphilis screening if at risk for infection (see chapter 21):
  ‣ men who have sex with men
  ‣ people who exchange sex for drugs or money
  ‣ people in adult correctional facilities

☐ Tobacco use counseling for people who smoke or use tobacco products (see chapter 22)

HEALTHY CHECKS: AGES 50 TO 64

Everyone Ages 50 to 64

☐ Blood pressure screening (see chapter 4)

☐ Colon cancer screening—one of the following three options (see chapter 9):
- ▸ high-sensitivity fecal occult blood testing (FOBT) every year
- ▸ flexible sigmoidoscopy every five years, with high-sensitivity FOBT every three years
- ▸ colonoscopy every ten years

☐ Depression screening (see chapter 10)

☐ Obesity screening and counseling (see chapter 17)

☐ Seasonal influenza vaccine every year (see appendix and chapter 23)

☐ Shingles vaccine once after age 60 if not received earlier (see appendix and chapter 23)

☐ Tetanus vaccine every ten years (see appendix and chapter 23)

☐ Vaccinations as recommended by the latest CDC guidelines (see appendix and chapter 23)

Additional Measures for Women

☐ Aspirin to prevent cardiovascular disease in women over age 55—discuss potential benefits and harms with a doctor (see chapter 3)

☐ BRCA genetic counseling and evaluation referral for women with certain family history patterns of breast and ovarian cancer (See chapter 5 for a list of applicable family history patterns.)

☐ Breast cancer chemoprevention: considered in women at high risk of breast cancer and at low risk of adverse effects from therapy (see chapter 5)

☐ Breast cancer screening mammograms every two years (see chapter 5)

☐ Cervical cancer screening at least every three years except for women who have had a total hysterectomy for benign disease (see chapter 6)

☐ Chlamydia screening in women at risk for infection
(see chapter 7):
- ▸ new or multiple partners
- ▸ history of sexually transmitted infection
- ▸ inconsistent condom use
- ▸ exchange of sex for drugs or money

☐ Cholesterol screening in women at risk for cardiovascular disease
(see chapter 8):
- ▸ diabetes
- ▸ tobacco use
- ▸ high blood pressure
- ▸ obesity (body mass index [BMI] ≥30 kg/m²)
- ▸ family history of early heart disease (before age 50 in first-degree male relatives or before age 60 in first-degree female relatives)
- ▸ personal history of cardiovascular disease

☐ Gonorrhea screening in women at risk for infection
(see chapter 13):
- ▸ new or multiple partners
- ▸ history of sexually transmitted infection
- ▸ inconsistent condom use
- ▸ exchange of sex for drugs or money

☐ Osteoporosis screening for women ages 60 to 64 at increased risk
(see chapter 18):
- ▸ low weight (under 154 lb)
- ▸ not currently using hormone (estrogen) replacement therapy

Additional Measures for Men

☐ Aspirin to prevent cardiovascular disease in men—discuss potential benefits and harms with a doctor (see chapter 3)

☐ Cholesterol screening (see chapter 8)

Additional Measures for At-Risk People

☐ Alcohol misuse screening for people who consume alcohol
(see chapter 2)

☐ Diabetes screening if sustained blood pressure ≥135/80 mmHg
(see chapter 11)

(continues)

(Ages 50–64, Additional Measures for At-Risk People, continued)

☐ Healthy eating counseling if at risk for cardiovascular and diet-related chronic disease (see chapter 14):
  ‣ cholesterol disorder
  ‣ high blood pressure
  ‣ diabetes
  ‣ obesity (BMI ≥30 kg/m^2)
  ‣ overweight (BMI 25–29.9 kg/m^2)
  ‣ abdominal obesity (weight circumference ≥40 inches in men or ≥35 inches in women)

☐ HIV screening if at risk for infection (see chapter 16):
  ‣ men and women who have unprotected sex with multiple partners
  ‣ men who have sex with men
  ‣ people being treated for a sexually transmitted infection (e.g., syphilis, gonorrhea, or chlamydia)
  ‣ injection drug users
  ‣ people who exchange sex for drugs or money
  ‣ sexual partners of anyone with one or more of the above risk factors

☐ Sexually transmitted infection (STI) counseling if at risk for STI (chapter 20):
  ‣ multiple current sexual partners
  ‣ current STI or history of infection in past year

☐ Syphilis screening if at risk for infection (see chapter 21):
  ‣ men who have sex with men
  ‣ people who exchange sex for drugs or money
  ‣ people in adult correctional facilities

☐ Tobacco use counseling for people who smoke or use tobacco products (see chapter 22)

HEALTHY CHECKS: AGE 65 OR OLDER

Everyone Age 65 or Older

- ☐ Aspirin for the prevention of cardiovascular events in people 79 and younger—discuss potential benefits and harms with a doctor (see chapter 3)

- ☐ Blood pressure screening (see chapter 4)

- ☐ Colon cancer screening until age 75, with one of the three following options (see chapter 9):
  - ▸ high-sensitivity fecal occult blood testing (FOBT) every year
  - ▸ flexible sigmoidoscopy every five years, with high-sensitivity FOBT every three years
  - ▸ colonoscopy every ten years

- ☐ Depression screening (see chapter 10)

- ☐ Obesity screening and counseling (see chapter 17)

- ☐ Pneumococcal polysaccharide (PPV23) vaccine once after age 65 if not received earlier (see appendix and chapter 23)

- ☐ Seasonal influenza vaccine every year (November through March; see appendix and chapter 23)

- ☐ Shingles vaccine once after age 60 if not received earlier (see appendix and chapter 23)

- ☐ Tetanus vaccine every ten years (see appendix and chapter 23)

- ☐ Vaccinations as recommended by the latest CDC guidelines (see appendix and chapter 23)

Additional Measures for Women

- ☐ Breast cancer chemoprevention: considered in women at high risk of breast cancer and at low risk of adverse effects from therapy (see chapter 5)

- ☐ Breast cancer screening mammograms every two years until age 75 (see chapter 5)

(continues)

(Everyone Age 65 or Older, continued)

☐ Cervical cancer screening at least every three years (see chapter 6); may discontinue in women over age 65 with a recent history of normal Pap smears and who are otherwise not at high risk for cervical cancer and in women who have had a total hysterectomy for benign disease

☐ Chlamydia screening in women at risk for infection (see chapter 7):
  ‣ new or multiple partners
  ‣ history of sexually transmitted infection
  ‣ inconsistent condom use
  ‣ exchange of sex for drugs or money

☐ Cholesterol screening in women at risk for cardiovascular disease (see chapter 8):
  ‣ diabetes
  ‣ tobacco use
  ‣ high blood pressure
  ‣ obesity (body mass index [BMI] ≥30 kg/m^2)
  ‣ family history of early heart disease (before age 50 in first-degree male relatives or before age 60 in first-degree female relatives)
  ‣ personal history of cardiovascular disease

☐ Gonorrhea screening in women at risk for infection (see chapter 13):
  ‣ new or multiple partners
  ‣ history of sexually transmitted infection
  ‣ inconsistent condom use
  ‣ exchange of sex for drugs or money

☐ Osteoporosis screening (see chapter 18)

Additional Measures for Men

☐ Abdominal aortic aneurysm screening (see chapter 1): one-time screening in men ages 65 to 75 who have ever smoked

☐ Cholesterol screening (see chapter 8)

Additional Measures for At-Risk People

☐ Alcohol misuse screening for people who consume alcohol (see chapter 2)

☐ Diabetes screening if sustained blood pressure ≥135/80 mmHg (see chapter 11)

☐ Healthy eating counseling for people at risk of cardiovascular and diet-related chronic disease (see chapter 14):
  ‣ cholesterol disorder
  ‣ high blood pressure
  ‣ diabetes
  ‣ obesity (BMI ≥30 kg/m^2)
  ‣ overweight (BMI 25–29.9 kg/m^2)
  ‣ abdominal obesity (weight circumference ≥40 inches in men or ≥35 inches in women)

☐ HIV screening if at risk for infection (see chapter 16):
  ‣ men and women who have unprotected sex with multiple partners
  ‣ men who have sex with men
  ‣ people being treated for a sexually transmitted infection (e.g., syphilis, gonorrhea, or chlamydia)
  ‣ injection drug users
  ‣ people who exchange sex for drugs or money
  ‣ sexual partners of anyone with one or more of the above risk factors

☐ Sexually transmitted infection (STI) counseling if at risk for STI (chapter 20):
  ‣ multiple current sexual partners
  ‣ current STI or history of infection in past year

☐ Syphilis screening if at risk for infection (see chapter 21):
  ‣ men who have sex with men
  ‣ people who exchange sex for drugs or money
  ‣ people in adult correctional facilities

☐ Tobacco use counseling for people who smoke or use tobacco products (see chapter 22)

HEALTHY CHECKS: PREGNANCY

All Pregnant Women

☐ Asymptomatic bacteriuria screening at the end of the first trimester (see chapter 19)

☐ Breastfeeding education and counseling (see chapter 19)

☐ Folic acid supplements for all women planning or capable of pregnancy (see chapter 19)

☐ Hepatitis B screening at the first prenatal visit (see chapters 15 and 19)

☐ HIV screening at the first prenatal visit (see chapters 16 and 19)*

☐ Influenza vaccine (see appendix and chapter 23)

☐ Iron deficiency anemia screening (see chapter 19)

☐ Rh(D) blood typing at the first prenatal visit (see chapter 19)

☐ Syphilis screening at the first prenatal visit (see chapters 19 and 21)

Pregnant Women at Increased Risk

☐ Alcohol misuse counseling for pregnant women who drink alcohol (see chapters 2 and 19)

☐ Chlamydia screening at the first prenatal visit if at increased risk (see chapters 7 and 19):
  ‣ new or multiple partners
  ‣ history of sexually transmitted infection
  ‣ inconsistent condom use
  ‣ exchange of sex for drugs or money

☐ Gonorrhea screening at the first prenatal visit if at increased risk (see chapters 13 and 19):
  ‣ new or multiple partners
  ‣ history of sexually transmitted infection
  ‣ inconsistent condom use
  ‣ exchange of sex for drugs or money

☐ Tobacco use counseling for pregnant women who smoke or use tobacco products (see chapters 19 and 22)

* The USPSTF does not specify when HIV screening should be performed in pregnant women, but the first prenatal visit is a reasonable choice.

PART III

Preventive Services Explained

This part of the book describes preventive health for different diseases and conditions. Each chapter explains the specific disease or condition, the rationale behind the checklist of preventive services for this disease or condition, and what's involved—including details of the preventive service as well as its risks and benefits. The chapters are organized alphabetically. Check the table of contents for a complete list of the diseases and conditions discussed in these pages.

Abdominal Aortic Aneurysm Screening

A n *aneurysm* (AN-yur-ism) is a localized widening, or "ballooning," of an artery. The greatest health risk of an aneurysm is that the artery can rupture, or burst, because the artery wall is weakened. An aneurysm that occurs in the abdominal portion of the *aorta* (ay-OR-ta), the main artery leading from the heart, is called an *abdominal aortic aneurysm,* or AAA (sometimes pronounced "triple A").

An estimated 5 to 10 percent of men between 65 and 79 years old have an AAA. Although the presence of an AAA usually does not cause any health problems, its rupture is a surgical emergency. Only 40 percent of people with ruptured AAAs survive long enough to make it to the hospital, and of those people, only 50 percent live. Ruptured AAA is the tenth leading cause of death in men over age 50 in the United States and accounts for nearly 15,000 deaths per year.

Screening for aortic aneurysms in at-risk men reduces the death rate from AAAs by over 40 percent. Because these aneurysms usually do not cause symptoms, they often remain undiagnosed until rupture. Men with large AAAs may undergo surgery or endovascular repair to mend the aorta and prevent rupture. Through early diagnosis and treatment, many cases of rupture could be prevented.

The United States Preventive Services Task Force (USPSTF) recommends one-time screening for AAA with ultrasound in men ages 65 to 75 who have ever smoked.[1] The following sections provide an overview of AAAs and detail the guidelines for screening.

SECTION I: ABDOMINAL AORTIC ANEURYSM 101

The aorta is our main artery, which carries blood from the heart to the rest of the body. This long blood vessel starts in the chest and ends in the abdomen, around the level of the navel. The part of the aorta in the abdomen is

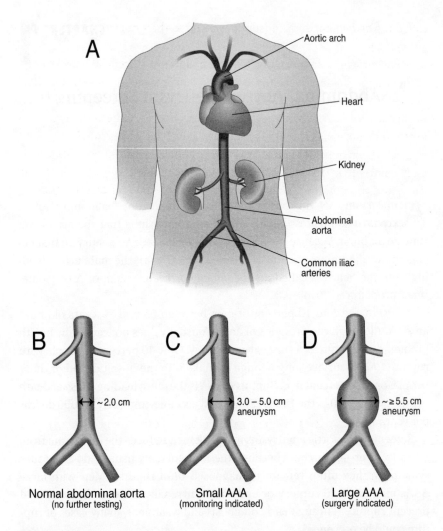

Figure 1.1. (A) The aorta, the largest artery in the body, carries blood directly from the heart. The abdominal aorta is the portion of the aorta that courses through the abdomen before it divides into the common iliac arteries. An abdominal aortic aneurysm, or AAA, is a ballooning of the aorta, which carries a risk of rupture. This risk is directly related to the size of the aneurysm. (B) People with normal-sized aortas do not require further testing beyond the initial screening for AAAs. (C) AAAs between 3 and 5 cm are generally monitored with regular abdominal ultrasounds. (D) Surgery is recommended for AAAs over 5.5 cm.

called the *abdominal aorta*. It supplies blood to the stomach, intestines, pelvis, and legs.

An aneurysm, an abnormal widening of an artery, occurs when the walls of the artery weaken. Over time, the aneurysm tends to increase in size. If an aneurysm grows too large, it may rupture or burst, causing dangerous bleeding inside the body. Most aneurysms, like AAAs, occur in the aorta. Figure 1.1 illustrates a normal abdominal aorta and a small and large AAA.

Doctors can prevent many AAAs from bursting if they find and repair them early using surgery or endovascular techniques. Because most AAAs do not cause any symptoms, screening is the preferred method for early diagnosis.

What causes an AAA?

Although scientists do not fully understand why AAAs develop, the major risk factors are

- male gender
- older age
- smoking
- high blood pressure
- a family history of aneurysms in parents, siblings, or children

AAAs are rare before age 55. Furthermore, most AAA-related deaths occur in men older than age 65. These aneurysms are about five times more common in men than in women, and because women tend to get AAAs at an older age than men, the risks of repair are usually too great. Tobacco users are eight times more likely than nonusers to develop aneurysms. Other associated conditions include coronary heart disease, stroke, and peripheral vascular disease.

How can I prevent AAA?

Given the risk factors for AAA, the best way to prevent aneurysms is to adopt a healthy lifestyle: abstain from smoking, maintain a healthy weight, eat a balanced diet, get regular physical activity, and control high blood pressure and cholesterol. Appropriate screening is also important to prevent AAA rupture and other complications.

What are the symptoms of an AAA?

Aneurysms can develop and grow for years without causing any signs or symptoms. Most people with AAAs have no symptoms until an aneurysm ruptures or grows large enough to press on nearby parts of the body. When symptoms are present, they may include

- deep, penetrating pain in the back or flank
- steady gnawing pain in the abdomen that lasts for hours or days at a time
- coldness, numbness, or tingling in the feet

Unfortunately, the first time many people experience symptoms from their aneurysm is when it ruptures. Symptoms of aneurysm rupture include

- sudden, severe pain in the lower abdomen and back
- a pulsating sensation in the abdomen
- abdominal wall stiffness
- nausea and vomiting
- clammy, sweaty skin
- lightheadedness

A ruptured aneurysm is a surgical emergency and requires immediate medical attention. But keep in mind that some of the symptoms listed above, such as lightheadedness, are common to other, much less serious health problems and are not necessarily cause for concern.

If you have any symptoms of AAA or ruptured aneurysm, please see your doctor.

How are AAAs diagnosed?

Because AAAs usually do not cause symptoms, three-quarters of aneurysms in the past were detected accidentally during a diagnostic test (e.g., CT scan) performed for another health reason. Increasingly, aneurysms are being diagnosed through screening, which is performed with ultrasound. Abdominal ultrasounds detect 95 percent of aneurysms and can be used to accurately measure the width of the aorta. (Section II of this chapter covers screening for AAAs in greater depth.)

People who come to the hospital with symptoms of an AAA are often suspected of having a leaking or ruptured aneurysm. In these individuals, the diagnosis is often made using CT or, less commonly, MRI.

How are AAAs treated?

Because of the risks associated with surgery, not all aneurysms are repaired. Surgery is best reserved for those AAAs most likely to rupture.

The most important risk factor for an aneurysm rupturing is its size. The larger the aneurysm, the greater its chance of rupturing. The normal diameter of the aorta is about 2.0 cm. By definition, an AAA is present when the diameter of the aorta in the abdomen exceeds 3.0 cm. Studies show that aneurysms smaller than 4.0 cm have a 2 percent chance of rupture over five years, compared with aneurysms larger than 5.0 cm, which have a 25 percent chance of rupture. In general, people with aneurysms over 5.5 cm or that grow quickly—over 1.0 cm per year—are recommended to have surgery. Smaller aneurysms are not usually operated on because the risk for rupture is low, but they are generally monitored closely to look for changes in size. Additional imaging such as a CT scan is often ordered when the aneurysm is approaching the need for repair because this scan is slightly more accurate than an ultrasound and helps with procedural planning.

The risk of death from surgical repair of an AAA is about 5 percent. This means that one in every twenty people who have surgery for an AAA dies. Additionally, about 30 percent of people who undergo surgery have serious complications, such as heart attack, stroke, kidney failure, or blood clots in the lung. As with any surgery, the risk of AAA repair increases with the age and poor health of the patient. At a certain point, the risks of surgery in older people or those with other major medical illness exceed the potential benefits.

There are two approaches to AAA repair. In a traditional, or open, surgical repair, a large cut is made in the abdomen and the diseased aorta (aneurysm) is removed and replaced with a graft made of synthetic material. An alternative approach is called *endovascular stent grafting*. With the endovascular approach, a small incision is made in the groin to reach a smaller artery that comes off the aorta. The stent graft is then snaked up the artery to the abdominal aorta, where it is permanently placed to support blood flow.

Do women get AAAs?

Women can develop AAAs, but they are five times less common than in men and tend to occur at an older age, when the risks of surgery or endovascular repair are greater. In addition, for unclear reasons, women also have more complications from surgery than men do and so may benefit less from AAA repair.

SECTION II: SCREENING FOR ABDOMINAL AORTIC ANEURYSM

The USPSTF recommends one-time screening for AAAs with ultrasound in men ages 65 to 75 who have ever smoked. This recommendation is based on evidence that ultrasound is an accurate screening test for these aneurysms and that screening and elective surgical repair of large AAAs leads to a decrease in AAA-related death. Most studies show a 40 to 45 percent reduction in death from AAAs in men at risk who were screened for AAAs compared with those who were not.

What does "ever smoked" mean?

Experts define a history of ever smoking as smoking at least one hundred cigarettes in a lifetime.

Why stop at age 75?

For most men, the benefits of screening and subsequent surgery are lower in men over 75, in part because they are more likely to die of other causes. In addition, the potential harms of surgery are greater in older men and in those with poor health.

What about men who have never smoked?

The USPSTF makes no recommendation for or against AAA screening in men who have never smoked. Because these men are at lower risk of AAA, the potential benefits of screening in this population are likely to be lower than in men who have smoked. The USPSTF concludes that the balance between benefit and harm is too close to make a general recommendation.

Decisions about screening in this population are best made on a case-by-case basis. The presence or absence of other risk factors, such as a family history of AAA, may help guide decision making. If you are a male between the ages of 65 and 75 who has never smoked, talk to your doctor about whether screening for AAA is right for you.

Should women be screened?

The USPSTF recommends against routine screening for AAA in women. A large medical study comparing the health benefits of screening in women ages 65 to 75 found no difference between the death rates of women who were screened for AAAs and those of women who were not screened. Individualized decision making, however, is still required, and women with multiple risk factors may be good candidates for screening. If you are an older female and have one or more risk factors for AAA, talk to your doctor about whether screening is right for you.

How is screening done?

Screening for AAAs is done with ultrasound, the same technology used to see the fetus during pregnancy. Ultrasound works by using high-frequency sound waves to create images of the inside of the body. In AAA screening, an ultrasound of the abdomen is done to see the abdominal aorta and measure its size. If the aorta is wider than 3.0 cm, an AAA is diagnosed.

The ultrasound test is quick, inexpensive, and carries no risk of radiation exposure. In addition, ultrasound is highly accurate and detects 95 percent of AAAs. Note, however, that the accuracy of ultrasound can vary with the quality of the testing center. Be sure to have your screening done in a specialized center by a technologist experienced in screening for AAAs.

What happens during the test?

The test is usually done in a vascular laboratory. You will be advised not to eat, smoke, or chew gum for six to eight hours prior to your appointment. During the test, you will be lying down on your back. A technologist will begin by applying a clear water-based gel to the skin around your navel. Then the ultrasound transducer (a handheld probe) is moved around the abdomen until a clear view of the abdominal aorta is obtained. At times, you may be asked to hold your breath for short periods or to shift positions to help get the clearest pictures possible. The procedure usually takes fifteen minutes.

What if my aorta measures less than 3.0 cm?

An aorta measuring less than 3.0 cm is considered normal. You do not have an AAA, and no further testing is required. Studies show that normal results on a single ultrasound test around age 65 virtually exclude the risk for future AAA rupture. Because AAA screening is recommended as a one-time screening, you do not need to be rescreened for it.

What if my aorta measures greater than 3.0 cm?

By definition you have an AAA if your aorta is wider than 3.0 cm. Because ultrasound is diagnostic for AAA, no further testing is required to establish the diagnosis. The next step depends on the size of the aneurysm. Although individual doctors vary in their practice, the following measures are generally taken:

▸ If the aorta measures between 3.0 and 4.5 cm, you will be monitored with regular ultrasounds every six to twelve months to look for a change in the size of the aneurysm. Additional imaging such as a CT scan may be helpful if the AAA is approaching 4.5 to 5.0 cm. If the aneurysm grows to 5.5 cm or grows at a rate greater than 1.0 cm per year, you will be recommended for surgery.

‣ If the aorta measures above 5.5 cm, you will be referred to a vascular specialist or surgeon for AAA repair.

In women who undergo screening, AAA repair may be considered at a smaller size because women's aortas are smaller and because AAAs in women tend to rupture at smaller sizes.

In addition, people with AAAs are at increased risk of coronary heart disease (CHD). An AAA is considered to be a CHD risk equivalent, meaning doctors consider it to be as significant a risk factor for future CHD as having a history of heart attack. The diagnosis of AAA therefore has important implications for overall medical management, including decisions about cholesterol management and the use of aspirin therapy for the prevention of CHD. If you are diagnosed with an AAA, be sure to talk to your doctor about what steps you can take to lower your risk of heart disease.

What are the risks of screening?

Although the ultrasound test carries no health risks, a positive screening result (wider than 3.0 cm) has important risks. A small aneurysm will not require surgical intervention but may lead to unnecessary anxiety. Large aneurysms requiring surgical repair may not necessarily rupture without treatment and often do not cause any pain or troublesome symptoms. Not all people with large aneurysms are necessarily going to die from them. In addition, most people with large aneurysms do not have any pain or troubling symptoms from their condition. As a result, some people with large AAAs will not benefit from surgery. At the same time, the risks of aneurysm repair are not small. As noted earlier, one in twenty people who undergo the surgery will die from the operation, and one in three will have serious complications.

Taking these risks into consideration, the USPSTF still found that in the right population—namely, men between 65 and 75 years old who have ever smoked—the benefits outweigh these harms. However, in the end, it is up to you to weigh the potential risks and benefits of AAA screening and decide whether screening is right for you.

REFERENCES

National Heart, Lung, and Blood Institute (NHLBI). U.S. Department of Health and Human Services. National Institutes of Health. www.nhlbi.nih.gov.
Vascular Disease Foundation. www.vdf.org.

CHAPTER 2

Alcohol Misuse Counseling

Drinking alcohol is associated with multiple adverse health consequences. Each year nearly 100,000 Americans die from alcohol-related causes, making it the third leading preventable cause of death in the United States. Many more people are affected by alcohol daily—through strained personal relationships, poor job performance, and chronic medical conditions such as liver disease, cardiovascular disease, cancer, depression, and sexual dysfunction.

It is not only alcoholics who are at increased risk for these problems. A growing body of data shows that less severe forms of drinking also carry significant health risks. Three out of every ten adults drink enough alcohol to increase their chances of having problems with their physical and mental health as well as troubles with work and personal relationships. Of these people, one in four suffers from *alcohol abuse* or *alcohol dependence* (also called *alcoholism*). The remainder are said to have *alcohol misuse.*

Most people who misuse alcohol are unaware of the risks they are taking. By identifying people with at-risk drinking, doctors can effectively counsel them to reduce consumption, sometimes to levels no longer considered harmful. But because alcohol misuse often goes unrecognized, many people continue to drink alcohol at levels that put them at serious health risk without realizing the harm.

The United States Preventive Services Task Force (USPSTF) recommends screening and behavioral counseling interventions to reduce alcohol misuse in adults, including pregnant women.[1] The following sections provide an introduction to alcohol misuse and detail the guidelines for screening and counseling.

SECTION I: ALCOHOL MISUSE 101

Alcohol misuse refers to drinking in amounts or patterns that place individuals at risk for health problems.[2] Alcohol misuse is not a disease, and people who misuse alcohol are not "alcoholics." Alcohol misuse is simply a term that identifies at-risk drinking. In this chapter, the terms *alcohol misuse* and *at-risk drinking* are used interchangeably.

In practice, alcohol use represents a spectrum from abstinence to alcoholism (also called *alcohol dependence*). Table 2.1 presents working definitions of alcohol use terms.

This section, however, is not about defining terms. It is about giving you the tools you need to assess your drinking levels. Consider the analogy to fatty foods. For you to make healthier food choices, it is important to know how much fat is too much and how to read nutrition labels for fat content. Likewise, with alcohol, the first steps are to know how much drinking is too much and how much alcohol there is in various alcoholic beverages.

Does alcohol misuse depend on the number or type of drinks?

The term *drink* does not necessarily refer to one can of beer or one glass of alcohol. Rather, drink refers to a *standard drink,* which is defined as the amount of an alcoholic beverage equal to half an ounce (or 14 grams) of pure alcohol. Figure 2.1 illustrates U.S. standard drink equivalents. Note that these are approximate, since different brands and types of beverages vary in their alcohol content.

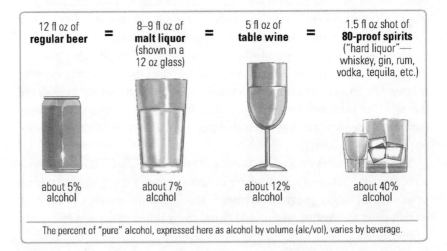

Figure 2.1. Standard drink equivalents. From *Helping Patients Who Drink Too Much: A Clinician's Guide*, U.S. Department of Health and Human Services, National Institutes of Health, National Institute of Alcohol Abuse and Alcoholism. NIH Publication No. 07-3769. May 2007. Reprinted by permission.

Table 2.1: Classification of alcohol use

No health risks*	Abstinence: complete avoidance of alcohol
	Moderate drinking: 2 drinks per day or less in men under age 65; 1 drink per day or less in women of any age and men over age 65
Unclear health risks	Heavy drinking: quantity or pattern of use that exceeds moderation but is not associated with known health risks
Moderate health risks	Alcohol misuse: quantity or pattern of use that is associated with health risks, defined as more than 4 drinks per day in men (or more than 14 drinks per week) and more than 3 drinks per day in women (or more than 7 drinks per week)
Severe health risks (alcohol disease)	Alcohol abuse: pattern of drinking that is accompanied by one or more of the following problems: (1) failure to fulfill major work, school, or home responsibilities because of drinking; (2) drinking in situations that are physically dangerous; (3) recurring alcohol-related legal problems; and (4) having social or relationship problems that are caused by or worsened by the effects of alcohol.[†]
	Alcoholism (alcohol dependence): severe pattern of drinking that includes the problems of alcohol abuse plus persistent drinking despite obvious physical, mental, and social problems caused by alcohol. Also typical are (1) loss of control —inability to stop drinking once begun; (2) withdrawal symptoms (symptoms associated with stopping drinking such as nausea, sweating, shakiness, and anxiety); and (3) tolerance (needing increased amounts of alcohol in order to feel drunk).[†]

*This is true for the general population, but in pregnant women, adolescents, and people with certain medical conditions or taking certain medications, there are risks to even moderate levels of alcohol consumption.

[†]Adapted from http://jama.ama-assn.org/cgi/content/full/295/17/2100.

The number of standard drinks an alcoholic beverage is equivalent to depends on the size of the beverage and the type of alcohol. For example, 40 ounces of beer is equivalent to 3.3 standard drinks (40 ounces / 12 ounces of beer in a standard drink); half a bottle of wine is equivalent to 2.5 standard drinks (12.5 ounces / 5 ounces of wine in a standard drink). From these calculations, it is easy to see how the drinks can quickly add up.

It is a common misconception that beer and wine are in some way "safer" than hard alcohol. In clinics, people often say, "I don't drink alcohol; I just drink beer." But beer and wine are not safer than other forms of alcohol. Although you need to drink a full beer to get the same amount of alcohol found in a shot of hard liquor, the alcohol in that beer has the potential to be just as harmful.

How much is too much?

For men under age 65, drinking more than four standard drinks in a day or more than fourteen drinks in a week increases the risk of alcohol-related problems. For men over 65 and for women, drinking more than three standard drinks in a day or more than seven drinks per week is considered at-risk drinking. To be on the safe side, avoid drinking more than the maximum recommended consumption of alcohol: two standard drinks per day for adult men under age 65 and one standard drink per day for men over age 65 and for women. For many people, however, even these levels of drinking are too much. This includes people taking medications that may interact with alcohol; those with a family history of alcohol dependence; people with physical or psychiatric conditions that are caused by or exacerbated by alcohol; and anyone who is planning to drive or operate heavy machinery. Because it isn't known whether any amount of alcohol is safe during pregnancy, complete abstinence is recommended for women who are or may become pregnant.

Why are the limits lower for women and older adults?

Research shows that women and older adults start to have alcohol-related problems at lower drinking levels than younger men do. One reason for this may be that women and older adults have proportionally less body water than men do and therefore have higher blood alcohol concentrations after drinking the same amount of alcohol.

What if I just have a high tolerance to alcohol?

Surprisingly, people who have a high tolerance to alcohol, or who can "hold their drinks" better, are actually at a higher risk of alcohol-related problems. Think of it this way—the "buzz" you get when you drink alcohol is your body's way of telling you that you've had enough to drink. People who need more alcohol to get a buzz or to feel relaxed drink more than people who have a lower tolerance and as a result are more likely to misuse alcohol.

What if I consume more than four standard drinks only once a year?

People who consume more than four standard drinks even once a year are considered to be misusing alcohol. Clearly, the greater the number of heavy drinking days, the greater the risk of alcohol-related problems. Therefore, compared with someone who drinks more than four standard drinks once a week, your risk of alcohol-related problems is lower. However, you are still at increased health risk because for some problems, such as driving while intoxicated or alcohol-related accidents, a single occasion of heavy drinking is enough to cause serious health consequences.

Despite the apparent strictness of this definition, a large national survey by the National Institutes on Alcohol Abuse and Alcoholism showed that nearly three-fourths of U.S. adults never exceed the maximum recommended daily consumption of alcohol. If they can do it, so can you.

What's the harm in alcohol?

Excessive alcohol use has immediate and long-term health risks. Some of these risks are related to the harmful effects of alcohol on the body. Others are related to the psychological effects of alcohol on thinking and decision making. And still others are related to the social effects of alcohol. In general, the harms of alcohol are dose dependent, meaning that the greater the alcohol consumption, the greater the risk of problems.[3]

Immediate Health Risks

- *Accidents:* traffic injuries, falls, drownings, burns, and unintentional firearm injuries increase with alcohol use.
- *Violence:* one-third of victims of violence report that offenders are under the influence of alcohol. This fraction increases to two-thirds when considering intimate partner violence and domestic abuse. Alcohol is also a leading factor in child maltreatment and neglect, and it can increase the risk of sexual assault.
- *Risky sexual behaviors:* unprotected sex and sex with multiple partners can increase with alcohol misuse. These behaviors can result in unintended pregnancy and sexually transmitted infections.

‣ *Pregnancy complications:* the incidence of miscarriage and stillbirth increases with alcohol use by pregnant women.
‣ *Birth defects:* drinking alcohol while pregnant is the number one preventable cause of mental disability and can lead to fetal alcohol syndrome.
‣ *Sexual dysfunction:* erectile dysfunction in men and loss of libido in women can stem from alcohol use.
‣ *Alcohol poisoning:* this medical emergency results from high blood alcohol levels and may cause loss of consciousness, respiratory depression, coma, and death.

Long-Term Health Risks

‣ *Brain and nerve problems:* dementia, stroke, numbness of the hands or feet.
‣ *Heart and blood vessel problems:* damage to the heart, high blood pressure.
‣ *Psychiatric problems:* depression, suicide, anxiety.
‣ *Social problems:* unemployment, lost productivity, family problems.
‣ *Increased risk of cancer:* cancers of the mouth, throat, esophagus, liver, and colon, as well as of the breast in women.
‣ *Liver disorders:* alcoholic hepatitis, or inflammation of the liver. Over years, this may lead to cirrhosis (or scarring) of the liver, liver failure, or liver cancer.
‣ *Bone loss:* decreased production of new bone leading to osteoporosis, or thinning of the bones, and increased risk of fracture.
‣ *Intestinal complications:* inflammation of the pancreas and stomach.
‣ *Nutritional deficiencies:* folate and thiamine deficiency.

I heard that alcohol is actually good for the heart. Is that true?

Light to moderate alcohol consumption in middle-aged and older adults has been associated with a lower risk of coronary heart disease. For higher levels of alcohol consumption, these benefits are likely offset by an increased risk of high blood pressure and other cardiovascular diseases. In addition, even at moderate levels of alcohol consumption, the benefits to cardiovascular health must be balanced by the potential risks to other aspects of health.

How much is okay to drink during pregnancy?

Each year in the United States, between 2,000 and 8,000 infants are born with fetal alcohol syndrome, a lifelong condition that causes physical and mental disabilities. Thousands more are born with milder impairments related to their mothers' drinking in pregnancy. In addition, women who drink alcohol during pregnancy are at greater risk of miscarriage and stillbirth.

There is no known safe amount of alcohol to drink during pregnancy. Therefore, it is recommended that pregnant women abstain from drinking alcohol. In addition, abstinence is recommended for women who may become pregnant, such as those who are sexually active and do not use birth control.

How is alcohol misuse treated?

Alcohol misuse is not a disease and therefore does not warrant treatment per se. For many people, simply being made aware of the potential harms of their drinking is sufficient to change their habits. Other people benefit from brief counseling sessions. Counseling focuses on helping people change specific behaviors related to alcohol misuse and often includes feedback, advice, and goal setting. Examples of techniques taught in counseling include recording alcohol consumption; calculating standard drink equivalents; planning ahead for drinking; identifying people or places that trigger urges to drink; and learning how to pace drinking.

These counseling sessions effectively reduce alcohol consumption for sustained periods and often to levels no longer considered harmful to health. Studies show that through behavioral counseling interventions, doctors can help people who misuse alcohol to reduce alcohol consumption by three to nine drinks per week (a 13 to 34 percent net reduction), with effects lasting up to six to twelve months. Compared with people who do not receive any counseling, up to 20 percent more people who receive counseling reduce their alcohol consumption to levels no longer considered harmful.

While medications and other more intensive interventions to reduce alcohol use are available, these are reserved for people with more severe alcohol disorders, such as alcohol dependence and alcohol abuse.

SECTION II: ALCOHOL MISUSE SCREENING AND COUNSELING

The USPSTF recommends screening and behavioral counseling interventions to reduce alcohol misuse in adults, including pregnant women. This recommendation is based on evidence that screening can accurately identify people whose patterns of alcohol consumption place them at increased health risks and on evidence that counseling produces sustained reductions in alcohol consumption and therefore an increase in associated health benefits.

Although this recommendation is written for doctors, if you drink alcohol, you should talk to your doctor about your alcohol use. If your levels of alcohol consumption are unhealthy, you should work with your doctor to lessen how much you drink.

How is talking to my doctor going to help?

Many people do not see alcohol use as a medical issue. But as this chapter stresses, alcohol consumption can lead to short- and long-term health problems. Because your alcohol intake may affect your health, talking to your doctor about it is important, even if you drink only moderate amounts.

If your alcohol consumption puts you at risk for health problems, counseling can help you lower your intake and decrease your risk of alcohol-related illness. Studies show that even brief behavioral counseling sessions can help you reduce your alcohol consumption by up to a third and often to levels no longer considered harmful to your health.

How do I get screened for alcohol misuse or abuse?

Screening is designed to identify people whose drinking habits put them at risk, draw their attention to the risks, and encourage them to reduce their drinking. The process involves a series of questions aimed at determining your levels and patterns of alcohol consumption (e.g., number of standard drinks per week and per day) and the presence of any red flags (e.g., physical, psychological, or social problems related to alcohol use; characteristics of dependence or tolerance). Sometimes doctors administer these questions through surveys or checklists that you fill out in the waiting room; other times, doctors screen informally through questions they ask during your clinic appointment.

The same screening questions used to screen for alcohol misuse can be used to screen for alcohol abuse and dependence. Therefore, after talking to your doctor about your alcohol use, you may be diagnosed with one of those alcohol disorders.

What if I misuse alcohol?

Not all doctors feel comfortable counseling patients about alcohol misuse. Talk to your doctor about whether he or she has experience counseling people about alcohol. If your doctor is willing to counsel you, talk to him or her about scheduling one or more sessions to focus on your alcohol use and on teaching you techniques for decreasing your consumption to healthy levels. Your doctor may refer you to another doctor or health care professional. The USPSTF concluded that the best interventions do not necessarily have to be intensive or long term. Rather, a ten- to fifteen-minute initial session focusing on feedback, advice, and goal setting followed by multiple shorter sessions can be effective.

What if I have alcohol abuse or alcohol dependence?

Alcohol abuse and alcohol dependence are more serious diagnoses than alcohol misuse, but effective treatments are available. As with alcohol misuse, counseling is an important component to treatment, but it is more intensive and is usually supplemented by other interventions, such as referrals to specialists, medications, and enrollment in peer support groups (such as Alcoholics Anonymous, or AA).

REFERENCES

National Institute of Alcohol Abuse and Alcoholism (NIAAA). *Helping Patients Who Drink Too Much: A Clinician's Guide*. NIH Publication No. 07-3769. U.S. Bethesda, Md.: Department of Health and Human Services, National Institutes of Health, May 2007.
———. *Rethinking Drinking—Alcohol and Your Health*. NIH Publication No. 09-3770. Bethesda, Md.: Department of Health and Human Services, National Institutes of Health, January 2009.

CHAPTER 3

Aspirin to Prevent Cardiovascular Disease

In addition to its uses as a pain reliever, aspirin reduces the risk of heart attack and stroke. It has long been part of the standard regimen of medications prescribed to people with a history of heart attack or stroke. More recently, studies have shown that aspirin is also beneficial in people without any existing cardiovascular disease but who are at increased risk. In men at increased risk for cardiovascular disease, daily aspirin therapy reduces the chance of a heart attack by 30 percent. In at-risk women, aspirin reduces the risk of stroke by 25 percent.*

Aspirin therapy is not without potential harm, however. The major risk is bleeding, particularly from the gastrointestinal system. Thus, the beneficial effects of aspirin must be weighed against its potential harms.

The United States Preventive Services Task Force (USPSTF) recommends the use of aspirin for men ages 45 to 79 years and for women ages 55 to 79 years for whom the benefits of aspirin outweigh the potential harm.[1] Currently, about 40 percent of men age 40 or older and women age 50 or older are on aspirin therapy. The following sections introduce tools for assessing risk of cardiovascular disease and detail the recommendations about aspirin.

If you have not read the "Special Section on Cardiovascular Disease" in part I, you may want to read it now to gain a better understanding of that disease.

SECTION I: ESTIMATING YOUR RISK OF HEART ATTACK OR STROKE

Risk factors for cardiovascular disease can be categorized into *nonmodifiable risk factors*—those you can't change through lifestyle modifications or medications—and *modifiable risk factors*. Nonmodifiable risk factors include

---

* Although some controversy remains, the most recent data suggest that aspirin does not reduce the risk of heart attacks in women and does not reduce the risk of strokes in men.

age, gender, and family history of cardiovascular disease. Modifiable risk factors include smoking, cholesterol disorders, high blood pressure, diabetes, inactive lifestyle, unhealthy eating, and obesity. However, simply listing risk factors does not help us assess our overall risk. We know that smoking and high blood pressure are dangerous, but exactly how dangerous are they?

Doctors have developed risk calculators to estimate an individual's risk of cardiovascular disease. The best known of these calculators is based on the Framingham Heart Study. Using information about your health today, the Framingham calculator estimates your risk of developing coronary heart disease (CHD) over the next ten years. The calculator takes into account age, gender, cholesterol, blood pressure, and smoking status. In return, it estimates the chances of developing CHD, including heart attack or death from the disease, over the next ten years.

The Framingham risk calculator is not perfect. It is designed for people without any history of CHD—people who have never had a heart attack and who don't suffer from chest pain. It does not take into account important risk factors such as diabetes, obesity, and family history. And it includes only CHD and not other cardiovascular diseases, such as heart failure or stroke.

What about estimating someone's risk of stroke?

Although less established, there are separate risk calculators for stroke. Stroke risk calculators take into account age, blood pressure, diabetes, smoking, history of cardiovascular disease, atrial fibrillation (a rhythm disorder), and left ventricular hypertrophy (enlargement of the heart). Similar to the Framingham risk calculator, stroke risk calculators estimate the chances of developing a stroke over the next ten years.

How do I determine my risk of heart attack?

To estimate your ten-year risk of CHD, you can use online risk calculators or risk calculator worksheets. You need to know your total cholesterol, HDL cholesterol ("good" cholesterol), and systolic blood pressure. If you don't know these numbers or have not recently had them checked, talk to your doctor.

A typical risk calculator worksheet is presented in table 3.1. Here are instructions on how to use it.

Step 1: Using the tables provided within the worksheet, determine the point equivalents for your age, total cholesterol, smoking status, HDL cholesterol, and systolic blood pressure. Keep in mind the following: First, the tables on the left side of the worksheet are for men, and those on the right are for women. Second, the point values for your total cholesterol and smoking status also depend on your age, so find the row *and column* that apply to you. Finally, the point value for your systolic blood pressure depends on whether you are being treated for high blood pressure. If you are taking blood pressure medications, use the "if treated" column.

Step 2: Next, add all your points. Then use the table at the bottom to determine your estimated ten-year risk. For example, if you are a man with a total point score of 9, you have a 5 percent risk of developing CHD over the next ten years.

If you prefer an electronic risk calculator, you can find one online at http://hp2010.nhlbihin.net/atpiii/calculator.asp, hosted by the National Institutes of Health. Note that the online calculator and the worksheet provided here may give you slightly different estimates. Alternatively, you could talk to your doctor about helping you estimate your risk of coronary heart disease.

How do I determine my risk of stroke?

To date, there are not any publicly supported risk calculator worksheets or online risk calculators for stroke. The USPSTF recommends a stroke risk calculator developed by the Western States Stroke Consortium, which can be found online at www.westernstroke.org. This address provides a link (WSSC Stroke Tools) to an Excel-based spreadsheet that you can download to estimate your stroke risk. To use the spreadsheet, you will need to know your systolic blood pressure and whether or not you have diabetes, cardiovascular disease, atrial fibrillation, or left ventricular hypertrophy. Until easy-to-use stroke risk calculators become available, however, it may be best to talk to your doctor about estimating your stroke risk.

SECTION II: ASPIRIN RECOMMENDATION

The USPSTF recommendations for aspirin take into account potential benefits and harms as shown by the evidence:

- Men ages 45 to 79 years should use aspirin when the potential reduction in heart attacks outweighs the potential increase in gastrointestinal bleeding.
- Women ages 55 to 79 years should use aspirin when the potential reduction in strokes outweighs the potential increase in gastrointestinal bleeding.
- Women younger than 55 years and men younger than 45 years should not use aspirin for cardiovascular disease prevention.

Table 3.1: Framingham risk assessment worksheet

Estimate of 10-Year Risk for Men
(Framingham Point Scores)

Age	Points
20–34	−9
35–39	−4
40–44	0
45–49	3
50–54	6
55–59	8
60–64	10
65–69	11
70–74	12
75–79	13

Total Cholesterol	Points				
	Age 20–39	Age 40–49	Age 50–59	Age 60–69	Age 70–79
<160	0	0	0	0	0
160–199	4	3	2	1	0
200–239	7	5	3	1	0
240–279	9	6	4	2	1
≥ 280	11	8	5	3	1

	Points				
	Age 20–39	Age 40–49	Age 50–59	Age 60–69	Age 70–79
Nonsmoker	0	0	0	0	0
Smoker	8	5	3	1	1

HDL (mg/dL)	Points
≥60	−1
50–59	0
40–49	1
<40	2

Systolic BP (mmHG)	If Untreated	If Treated
<120	0	0
120–129	0	1
130–139	1	2
140–159	1	2
≥ 160	2	3

Point Total	10-Year Risk %
<0	<1
0	1
1	1
2	1
3	1
4	1
5	2
6	2
7	3
8	4
9	5
10	6
11	8
12	10
13	12
14	16
15	20
16	25
≥17	≥30

10-Year Risk _____%

Estimate of 10-Year Risk for Women
(Framingham Point Scores)

Age	Points
20–34	−7
35–39	−3
40–44	0
45–49	3
50–54	6
55–59	8
60–64	10
65–69	12
70–74	14
75–79	16

Total Cholesterol	Points				
	Age 20–39	Age 40–49	Age 50–59	Age 60–69	Age 70–79
<160	0	0	0	0	0
160–199	4	3	2	1	1
200–239	8	6	4	2	1
240–279	11	8	5	3	2
≥ 280	13	10	7	4	2

	Points				
	Age 20–39	Age 40–49	Age 50–59	Age 60–69	Age 70–79
Nonsmoker	0	0	0	0	0
Smoker	9	7	4	2	1

HDL (mg/dL)	Points
≥60	−1
50–59	0
40–49	1
<40	2

Systolic BP (mmHG)	If Untreated	If Treated
<120	0	0
120–129	1	3
130–139	2	4
140–159	3	5
≥ 160	4	6

Point Total	10-Year Risk %
<9	<1
9	1
10	1
11	1
12	1
13	2
14	2
15	3
16	4
17	5
18	6
19	8
20	11
21	14
22	17
23	22
24	27
≥25	≥30

10-Year Risk _____%

Source: Adapted from "ATP III Guidelines At-A-Glance Quick Desk Reference," National Heart, Lung, and Blood Institute, U.S. Department of Health and Human Services, National Institutes of Health. NIH Publication No. 01-3305. May 2001.

▸ Evidence is insufficient to assess the balance of benefits and harms of aspirin for cardiovascular disease prevention in men and women 80 years or older.

These guidelines are based on evidence that aspirin is effective in preventing heart attacks in men and in preventing strokes in women but also that it increases the risk of serious gastrointestinal bleeding.

Whether the benefits of aspirin exceed the harms depends on an individual's risk of cardiovascular disease and gastrointestinal bleeding. A greater risk of cardiovascular disease increases the benefits of aspirin. That means that the older you are and the more risk factors for cardiovascular disease you have, the more likely you are to benefit from aspirin. Risk of gastrointestinal bleeding also increases with age as well as with a history of gastrointestinal pain or stomach ulcers and chronic nonsteroidal anti-inflammatory drug (NSAID) use.

Figuring out whether your risk of cardiovascular disease exceeds the risk of gastrointestinal bleeding can be difficult and is best done with the help of your doctor. If you are a man between 45 and 79 or a woman age 55 to 79, talk to your doctor about whether aspirin is right for you.

Can aspirin prevent cardiovascular disease? Isn't it for headaches?

Yes and yes. Aspirin can prevent heart attacks and strokes. And aspirin can treat headaches. Most people know aspirin as a pain reliever, but it has been used for years to treat cardiovascular disease. It is one of the first medications doctors give to patients having a heart attack, and it is part of the standard medication regimen for people who have had a heart attack or stroke to prevent them from having another one. Recent studies have shown that giving aspirin to people who have never had a cardiovascular event but who are at increased risk for one is also beneficial.

How does aspirin prevent heart attacks and strokes?

People at risk for cardiovascular disease have *atherosclerosis* (ath-er-o-skle-RO-sis), or fatty buildup and plaque inside their blood vessels. Under certain conditions, this plaque can rupture suddenly, putting the blood vessel at risk of being completely blocked off. Aspirin works by blocking the action of platelets, key players in the blood-clotting cascade that ensues during plaque rupture. By preventing the formation of blood clots, aspirin keeps atherosclerotic blood vessels open (see figure 3.1). In blood vessels in the brain, this helps prevent strokes; in blood vessels in the heart, this helps prevent heart attacks.

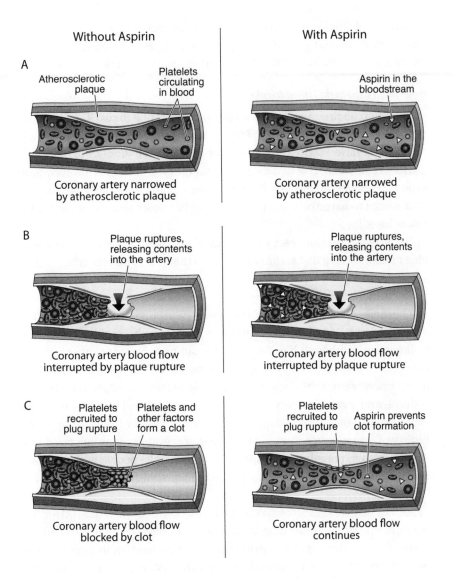

| Without Aspirin | With Aspirin |

A

Atherosclerotic plaque

Platelets circulating in blood

Aspirin in the bloodstream

Coronary artery narrowed
by atherosclerotic plaque

Coronary artery narrowed
by atherosclerotic plaque

B

Plaque ruptures,
releasing contents
into the artery

Plaque ruptures,
releasing contents
into the artery

Coronary artery blood flow
interrupted by plaque rupture

Coronary artery blood flow
interrupted by plaque rupture

C

Platelets
recruited to
plug rupture

Platelets and
other factors
form a clot

Platelets
recruited to
plug rupture

Aspirin prevents
clot formation

Coronary artery blood flow
blocked by clot

Coronary artery blood flow
continues

Figure 3.1. (A) Atherosclerosis leads to fatty buildup and plaque deposition. (B) Over time, these plaques are at risk for rupture. In the arteries of the heart, plaque rupture leads to a heart attack. (C) Aspirin works by preventing plaque rupture from leading to clot formation. By blocking platelet activation, aspirin prevents clots from forming at the rupture site and allows blood flow to continue.

Studies of high-risk individuals show a 30 percent reduction in heart attacks in men taking aspirin compared with those not taking aspirin. In women, similar studies show a 25 percent reduction in strokes.

How much aspirin do I need to take?

To treat pain or fever, a standard aspirin dose is one to two 325-milligram tablets every four to six hours. Studies of aspirin to prevent heart attacks and strokes have used varying doses of aspirin, including 75 to 100 milligrams per day and 100 to 325 milligrams every other day. However, most experts recommend one 81 milligram tablet—one baby aspirin—a day. This dose seems to have the same benefits as higher doses while minimizing the risk of bleeding.

Because aspirin can upset your stomach, take it with food. It's also a good idea to take it every day at the same time so that it becomes routine.

What are the potential harms?

The major side effect of aspirin therapy is gastrointestinal bleeding, which is bleeding from anywhere in the digestive tract (mouth, esophagus, stomach, or intestines), although bleeding from the stomach is most common. Minor cases can often be treated by simply stopping the offending medication, such as aspirin. More serious cases may require blood transfusion, endoscopic procedures, and, rarely, surgery. The risk of gastrointestinal bleeding is not the same for everyone. Older people and men are at greater risk. Anyone with a history of upper gastrointestinal pain or stomach ulcers is at increased risk. And people who regularly use NSAIDS—for example, people who take daily ibuprofen for arthritis—are at significantly increased risk of gastrointestinal bleeding.

Aspirin also increases the risk of *hemorrhagic strokes* (heh-ma-RAH-jik). A hemorrhagic stroke is bleeding in the brain that causes damage to the brain tissue. Studies show that it is primarily men who have an increased risk of hemorrhagic strokes with aspirin and that this risk is small compared with the risk of gastrointestinal bleeding. However, hemorrhagic strokes are serious and can result in disability or death.

What about people 80 and older?

The USPSTF has not found enough evidence to make a recommendation for or against aspirin use in people age 80 or older. On one hand, people in this age group have the highest risk of heart attacks and strokes, so the benefit of aspirin, at least theoretically, seems large. On the other hand, they are also at greater risk of gastrointestinal bleeding due to their age and coexisting medical conditions. Because people age 80 or older may have a range of health conditions, a one-size-fits-all approach is unlikely to work. Instead, a careful discussion of the benefits and harms of aspirin that takes into account individual circumstances and preferences is recommended.

How should I decide?

Although aspirin is readily available as an over-the-counter medication, under no circumstances should you begin daily aspirin therapy without the direct consultation of a physician.

Discussions about aspirin therapy should address the potential benefits and harms of aspirin therapy and take into account your individual risk factors and concerns about heart attack, stroke, and gastrointestinal bleeding. The higher your risk of cardiovascular disease and the lower your risk of gastrointestinal bleeding, the more likely aspirin is to benefit you, but ultimately the decision depends on how you personally weigh the benefits and harms of aspirin therapy. For example, some women may feel that a stroke is more concerning to them than gastrointestinal bleeding (e.g., a woman who had a close family member suffer from a stroke). These women would probably be more agreeable to taking aspirin than those for whom gastrointestinal bleeding is considered more dangerous (e.g., someone who, for personal reasons, cannot accept blood transfusions). An open discussion between you and your doctor is the best way to weigh these factors and arrive at a shared decision.

Once a decision is made, it can be changed. If you start aspirin but later experience side effects, you can stop the medication. Likewise, if you do not start aspirin therapy, you can revisit this decision later. Regardless of what you decide, revisit it periodically to make sure it continues to be the right choice for you.

REFERENCES

American Heart Association (AHA). www.americanheart.org.
National Heart, Lung, and Blood Institute (NHLBI). U.S. Department of Health and Human Services. National Institutes of Health. www.nhlbi.nih.gov.

Blood Pressure Screening

High blood pressure, or *hypertension,* affects more than 65 million Americans—or one in three adults. An additional 59 million Americans—another one in three adults—have *prehypertension,* a condition that if untreated often leads to high blood pressure. In the United States, high blood pressure is responsible for half the episodes of heart failure; one-third of all cardiovascular events, including heart attacks and strokes; and one-quarter of all premature deaths. People with high blood pressure have between two and four times greater risk of stroke, heart attack, heart failure, and peripheral vascular disease than those without high blood pressure. Additionally, hypertension is the second most common cause of end-stage kidney disease and is a major cause of retinopathy (a condition that can lead to blindness) and aortic aneurysm (a life-threatening condition of the aorta).

The good news is that high blood pressure is very treatable. Combination therapy with lifestyle modifications—including healthier eating, reducing dietary salt, increasing physical activity, losing weight, and smoking cessation—and blood pressure–lowering medications can safely and effectively bring high blood pressure under control. In addition, combination therapy has been shown to lower the risk of heart attack by 20 to 25 percent, the risk of stroke by 35 to 40 percent, and the risk of heart failure by over 50 percent.

The bad news is that despite the widespread appreciation of the dangers of high blood pressure and the availability of effective medications to treat the disease, Americans are generally underaware, undertreated, and undercontrolled for the condition. The most recent data suggest that 30 percent of people with high blood pressure are unaware of their condition; 40 percent are not on treatment; and 66 percent do not have their blood pressure under control.

Getting informed and getting serious about high blood pressure is the first step to keeping your blood pressure under control and minimizing your risks of cardiovascular disease. The United States Preventive Services Task Force (USPSTF) recommends screening for high blood pressure in all adults age 18 or older.[1] Screening is generally recommended at least every two years in individuals with previously normal blood pressures, and at least every year in individuals with elevated blood pressures (called *prehypertension*).

The following sections provide a brief introduction to high blood pressure and detail how routine screening can help you lower your risk of cardiovascular disease. *If you have not read the "Special Section on Cardiovascular Disease" in part I, you may want to read it now to gain a better understanding of that disease and to learn basic terminology relevant to this chapter.*

SECTION I: HIGH BLOOD PRESSURE 101

When the heart beats, it pumps blood to the arteries that supply the tissues in the body. The force of the blood through the arteries is called *blood pressure*. Blood pressure is highest when the heart beats and is lowest between beats, when the heart relaxes. The highest blood pressure recorded is the *systolic blood pressure,* and the lowest is the *diastolic blood pressure*. Blood pressure is measured in millimeters of mercury (abbreviated as mmHg) and is reported as systolic over diastolic (e.g., 120 over 80, or 120/80).

Although blood pressure can increase with stress, exertion, pain, and other factors, at rest it should normally be below 120 mmHg systolic and 80 mmHg diastolic. When blood pressure stays elevated above this level, the heart is overworked and the blood vessels are at greater risk of damage from *atherosclerosis* (ath-er-o-skle-RO-sis). Over time, this can lead to complications in the vital organs, including the heart, kidneys, brain, and eyes. Risk for heart disease and stroke doubles for every 20 mmHg increase in systolic pressure or 10 mmHg increase in diastolic pressure.

The classification of blood pressure is presented in table 4.1. Normal blood pressure means that *both* the systolic blood pressure and the diastolic blood pressure must be below certain levels: 120 mmHg and 80 mmHg, respectively. People with elevated blood pressure fall into two broad groups: prehypertension and hypertension. *Prehypertension* is a condition that often precedes hypertension. It is not considered a disease state and is not typically treated with blood pressure–lowering medications. However, everyone with prehypertension is strongly encouraged to undergo lifestyle modifications to lower their risk of developing hypertension. *Hypertension* is a disease state

Table 4.1: Classification of blood pressure

Blood pressure classification	SBP (mmHg)	DBP (mmHg)
Normal	<120	and <80
Prehypertension	120–139	or 80–89
Stage 1 hypertension	140–159	or 90–99
Stage 2 hypertension	≥160	or ≥100

Source: Seventh Report on the Joint National Committee on Prevention, Detection, Evaluation, and Treatment of High Blood Pressure (JNC VII), U.S. Department of Health and Human Services, National Institutes of Health, National Heart, Lung, and Blood Institute. NIH Publication No. 04-5230, August 2004.

Note: SBP=systolic blood pressure; DBP=diastolic blood pressure

that often requires medical therapy. It is further divided into stage 1 and stage 2 hypertension, depending on the degree of elevation in blood pressure.

People often ask, "Doc, which of the two numbers is more important?" The answer is both. Blood pressure classification is determined by which of the two blood pressure measurements is worse. For example, if your blood pressure is 150/75 mmHg, you have stage 1 hypertension, despite the fact that your diastolic blood pressure is in the normal range.

What symptoms does high blood pressure cause?

High blood pressure usually causes no symptoms. Therefore, the only way to truly know your blood pressure is to have it checked regularly. Rarely, if blood pressure becomes extremely high over a short period, symptoms of a life-threatening condition called *hypertensive emergency* can develop. Symptoms of hypertensive emergency include severe headache, vision problems, chest pain, difficulty breathing, and blood in the urine. If you develop any of these symptoms, you should immediately consult a doctor.

What causes high blood pressure?

High blood pressure can be either primary or secondary. Usually when people talk about high blood pressure, they are referring to primary (or essential) hypertension. *Essential hypertension* is high blood pressure that cannot be attributed to a specific medical cause. In contrast, secondary hypertension is caused by another disease or medical condition—such as kidney disease, blood vessel abnormalities, or thyroid disorders—and normally resolves once the underlying condition is treated. Most cases of high blood pressure are due to essential hypertension. In this chapter, the term high blood pressure loosely refers to essential hypertension.

Who is at risk for high blood pressure?

The most important risk factor for developing high blood pressure is older age. The risk increases with every year of life, and over time, high blood pressure becomes more the norm than the exception. After age 60, one in two adults has high blood pressure, and after age 70, this increases to three in four adults. Remarkably, 90 percent of people with normal blood pressure at age 55 can expect to develop high blood pressure in their lifetime. Other important risk factors for high blood pressure include

- alcohol consumption
- excess salt in the diet
- family history of high blood pressure
- inadequate intake of fruits and vegetables
- lack of physical activity
- lack of potassium in the diet
- overweight or obesity
- smoking

Staying away from cigarettes; maintaining a healthy weight; exercising regularly; adhering to a well-balanced, low-salt diet; and drinking alcohol in moderation have all been shown to lower blood pressure. For people diagnosed with prehypertension or hypertension, developing these healthy habits is an essential component of any treatment regimen.

However, even if you do "all the right things," you may still develop high blood pressure. After all, one in three adults has it. This underscores the importance of screening for high blood pressure in everyone age 18 or older, regardless of risk factors.

How is high blood pressure treated?

High blood pressure is a very treatable condition. In all people with prehypertension and hypertension, lifestyle modifications are an integral component to the treatment regimen. In those with hypertension, combination therapy with lifestyle modifications and blood pressure–lowering medications is often recommended to maximize blood pressure control.

What are "lifestyle modifications"? How good are they?

Lifestyle modifications are behavioral changes that lead to sustained improvements in blood pressure and other cardiovascular risk factors. They include healthy eating, reduced salt intake, increased physical activity, moderate alcohol consumption, and weight loss. Remarkable reductions in blood pressure can be achieved through lifestyle modifications alone, as illustrated in table 4.2. For example, reducing the amount of sodium in the diet to no more than 2.4 grams per day can reduce systolic blood pressure by up to 8 mmHg. If you add up the changes in blood pressure from the table, you can clearly see that through lifestyle modifications alone, you can keep your blood pressure under control. The best part is that these recommendations will not only improve your blood pressure but also help you improve your cholesterol levels, maintain a healthier weight, and get more energy.

Diet

Table 4.2 recommends adopting the DASH diet as a lifestyle modification. DASH stands for Dietary Approaches to Stop Hypertension. It is an eating plan developed by scientists at the National Heart, Lung, and Blood Institute (NHLBI) that is low in saturated fat, cholesterol, and total fat, and that emphasizes fruits, vegetables, and fat-free or low-fat dairy products. Through a series of clinical trials, NHLBI scientists showed not only that people who followed the DASH diet reduced their blood pressure compared with those who followed a regular American diet, but also that those reductions came within *two weeks* of starting the diet. Table 4.3 outlines characteristics of the DASH diet.

Salt

Reducing salt intake is also helpful in controlling blood pressure. There is a direct physiological relationship between the two: the lower your salt intake, the lower your blood pressure. The average American man consumes 4,200 milligrams of sodium per day; the average American woman, 3,300 milligrams. Some experts recommend a maximum intake of 2,300 milligrams per day, and others recommend going even lower—1,500 milligrams. The key to reducing salt intake is making better food choices. Only a small amount of the salt that we consume comes from salt added at the table. Most of the salt we eat comes from processed and packaged foods, such as canned soups, deli meats, and frozen dinners. So be sure to read food labels and choose products lower in sodium.

Table 4.2: Lifestyle modifications to prevent and manage hypertension

Modification	Recommendation	Approximate SBP reduction (range)*
Weight reduction	Maintain normal body weight (body mass index 18.5–24.9 kg/m²).	5–20 mmHg/10kg
DASH eating plan adoption	Consume a diet rich in fruits, vegetables, and low-fat dairy products with a reduced content of saturated and total fat.	8–14 mmHg
Dietary sodium reduction	Reduce dietary sodium intake to no more than 100 mmol per day (2.4 g sodium or 6 g sodium chloride).	2–8 mmHg
Physical activity	Engage in regular aerobic physical activity, such as brisk walking (at least 30 min. per day, most days of the week).	4–9 mmHg
Moderation of alcohol consumption	Limit consumption to no more than 2 standard drinks (e.g., 24-oz beer, 10-oz wine, or 3-oz 80-proof whiskey) per day in most men, and to no more than 1 standard drink per day in women and lighter-weight persons.	2–4 mmHg

Source: Seventh Report on the Joint National Committee on Prevention, Detection, Evaluation, and Treatment of High Blood Pressure (JNC VII), U.S. Department of Health and Human Services, National Institutes of Health, National Heart, Lung, and Blood Institute. NIH Publication No. 04-5230, August 2004.

Note: DASH=Dietary Approaches to Stop Hypertension; SBP=systolic blood pressure

* The effects of implementing these modifications are dose and time dependent and could be greater for some individuals.

SECTION II: HIGH BLOOD PRESSURE SCREENING

The USPSTF recommends screening for high blood pressure in adults age 18 or older. Although the task force does not specify the optimal interval for screening, the following approach is generally accepted:

‣ screening at least every two years in people with previously normal blood pressures (under 120 mmHg systolic and 80 mmHg diastolic)
‣ screening at least every year in people with prehypertension (120–139 mmHg systolic or 80–90 mmHg diastolic)

Table 4.3: General characteristics of the DASH Eating Plan

Food group	Daily servings	Serving sizes
Grains*	6–8	1 slice bread 1 oz dry cereal[†] ½ cup cooked rice, pasta, or cereal
Vegetables	4–5	1 cup raw leafy vegetable ½ cup cut-up raw or cooked vegetable ½ cup vegetable juice
Fruits	4–5	1 medium fruit ¼ cup dried fruit ½ cup fresh, frozen, or canned fruit ½ cup fruit juice
Fat-free or low-fat milk and milk products	2–3	1 cup milk or yogurt 1½ oz cheese
Lean meats, poultry, and fish	6 or fewer	1 oz cooked meats, poultry, or fish 1 egg
Nuts, seeds, and legumes	4–5 per week	⅓ cup or 1½ oz nuts 2 tbsp peanut butter 2 tbsp or ½ oz seeds ½ cup cooked legumes (dry beans and peas)
Fats and oils	2–3	1 tsp soft margarine 1 tsp vegetable oil 1 tbsp mayonnaise 2 tbsp salad dressing
Sweets and added sugars	5 or fewer per week	1 tbsp sugar 1 tbsp jelly or jam ½ cup sorbet, gelatin 1 cup lemonade

Source: Your Guide to Lowering Your Blood Pressure with DASH, U.S. Department of Health and Human Services, National Institutes of Health, National Heart, Lung, and Blood Institute. NIH Publication No. 06-4082, originally printed 1998; revised April 2006.

* Whole grains are recommended for most grain servings as a good source of fiber and nutrients.

[†] Serving sizes vary between ½ cup and 1¼ cups, depending on cereal type. Check the product's Nutrition Facts label.

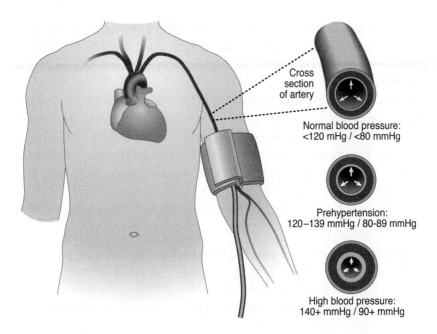

Cross
section
of artery

Normal blood pressure:
<120 mHg / <80 mmHg

Prehypertension:
120–139 mmHg / 80-89 mmHg

High blood pressure:
140+ mmHg / 90+ mmHg

Figure 4.1. Blood pressure screening measures the pressure through the arteries in systole (when the heart contracts) and diastole (when the heart relaxes). Blood pressure is reported as systolic blood pressure over diastolic blood pressure (e.g., 135 over 75, or 135/75 mmHg). Blood pressure correlates with the degree of atherosclerosis in the arteries. A healthy blood pressure is a systolic pressure under 120 mmHg and a diastolic pressure under 80 mmHg. People with a systolic pressure over 140 mmHg or a diastolic pressure over 90 mmHg have high blood pressure, or hypertension. Those with blood pressures in between have prehypertension, which places them at risk of developing high blood pressure.

Screening is most often performed with an in-office measurement using a blood pressure cuff (or sphygmomanometer; see figure 4.1). A diagnosis of high blood pressure is typically made based on two or more elevated readings taken on separate visits.

How does screening work?

Screening for high blood pressure involves getting your blood pressure checked by a health care professional. It usually takes a few minutes to perform, and it carries no risks.

However, blood pressure measurement is often not as straightforward as it appears. Blood pressure can vary with meals, stress, exertion, pain, and a host of other factors. In addition, the USPSTF notes that measurements vary between health care professionals, blood pressure instruments, and measuring techniques. Even readings a few hours apart can differ. These factors can cause differences in blood pressure readings of up to 12 mmHg systolic and 8 mmHg diastolic.

But this variation should not lead you to discredit blood pressure readings. Sometimes people say, "Doctor, what good is measuring my blood pressure? Every time I get it checked, it comes out differently." Like every test we use in medicine, blood pressure measurement is not perfect. However, when done correctly, studies show that blood pressure measurements are 94 to 98 percent accurate.

Below are three steps you can take to improve the accuracy of your blood pressure measurement:

▸ Avoid caffeine, exercise, and smoking for at least thirty minutes prior to measurement.
▸ Insist on being seated quietly for at least five minutes, with feet on the floor and arm supported at heart level, before having your blood pressure taken.
▸ Ask that at least two measurements be taken, for example, once on each arm, and the average recorded.

What happens if my blood pressure is within the normal range?

This means you do not have high blood pressure. Be sure to document the date of the screening for your records. Find out when your next blood pressure test should be and document this date as well. Your next screening should not be more than two years from the last one.

What happens if my blood pressure is elevated?

An elevated blood pressure measurement should generally be confirmed with at least one repeat screening during a separate office visit. The results from both measurements are then averaged. It is easy to forget to follow up on an abnormal blood pressure measurement. Schedule the appointment before you leave the clinic, and make it a priority.

What happens if the repeat measurement is also elevated?

Having two elevated blood pressure measurements is sufficient to diagnose you with prehypertension or hypertension. It is important to understand what this means and what this does not mean. It doesn't mean that something bad is necessarily going to happen to you. It also doesn't necessarily mean you have to take blood pressure–lowering medicines for the rest of your life. It simply means that you are at increased risk for cardiovascular disease and need to take measures to control your blood pressure.

Unfortunately, many people do not take the critical next step of addressing their condition. Only one-third of people with hypertension have their blood pressure under control. Controlling your blood pressure is possible —thousands of Americans do it every year. The key is to partner with your doctor and take action.

One of the reasons high blood pressure is not taken seriously is that people assume their blood pressure will return to normal in a few months or years. In reality, the opposite is more likely to happen. Without intervention, hypertension tends to worsen with age and as the arteries continue to stiffen. Furthermore, the harmful effects of high blood pressure are cumulative. The longer you have high blood pressure, the greater your risk of complications.

Prehypertension

If your systolic blood pressure is between 120 and 139 mmHg or your diastolic blood pressure is between 80 and 90 mmHg, you have prehypertension. As discussed earlier, prehypertension is not a disease, and medications are usually not recommended unless you have other medical conditions like diabetes. Still, prehypertension should be taken seriously as a warning that unless you act, you will probably develop hypertension in the next few years. Fortunately, through intensive lifestyle modifications, people with prehypertension can successfully reduce their risk of developing hypertension and can even get their blood pressure down into the normal range.

Hypertension

If your systolic blood pressure is greater than 140 mmHg or your diastolic blood pressure is greater than 90 mmHg, you have high blood pressure (or hypertension). Before initiating treatment, your doctor may order additional tests, including blood work, urine studies, and an electrocardiogram (EKG). The purpose of these tests is to better determine the stage of your condition and exclude other potential causes of high blood pressure before determining that you have essential hypertension.

For stage 1 hypertension, your doctor will typically recommend that you try two to three months of intensive lifestyle modifications before starting blood pressure–lowering medications. Studies show that some people with stage 1 hypertension can lower their blood pressure without medication. In other cases, you and your doctor may choose to initiate combination therapy with lifestyle modifications and medications at diagnosis. For stage 2 hypertension, your doctor will most likely recommend starting blood pressure–lowering medications right away along with lifestyle modifications.

As recommended elsewhere in this book, your doctor should also order additional blood work to screen for cholesterol disorders (see chapter 8) and diabetes (chapter 11). If you have other risk factors for cardiovascular disease, you and your doctor may also want to discuss starting you on aspirin (chapter 3).

How can I lower my blood pressure?

Changing your diet to reduce salt intake and increase servings of fruits and vegetables; getting regular aerobic exercise; managing your weight; moderating your alcohol consumption; and stopping smoking will lower your blood pressure, but changing habits is never easy. Talk to your doctor about behavior-modification techniques and possible referrals to nutritionists and other specialists. As discussed elsewhere in the book, healthy eating counseling (chapter 14) is recommended for people with hypertension.

Everyone with high blood pressure should undergo lifestyle modifications; however, the decision to start blood pressure–lowering medications is better left between you and your doctor. Several classes of drugs are available, including diuretics, ACE inhibitors, calcium channel blockers, and beta blockers. Most of these medicines have excellent side effect profiles and are most effective when used with lifestyle modifications.

Although effective blood pressure control can be achieved in most patients who have high blood pressure, the majority will require two or more medications. The most common reasons for unsuccessful blood pressure control include failure to make lifestyle modifications, reluctance to increase medication dosage or take additional blood pressure–lowering medications, and low patient follow-through with the treatment plan. Be open with your doctor about your goals and preferences. By partnering with your doctor, you have the best chance of finding a treatment regimen that works for you.

REFERENCES

National Heart, Lung, and Blood Institute (NHLBI). *The Seventh Report of the Joint National Committee on Prevention, Detection, Evaluation, and Treatment of High Blood Pressure.* NIH Publication No. 04-5230. Bethesda, Md.: Department of Health and Human Services, National Institutes of Health, August 2004.

——. U.S. Department of Health and Human Services. National Institutes of Health (NIH). www.nhlbi.nih.gov.

——. *Your Guide to Lowering Your Blood Pressure with DASH.* NIH Publication No. 06-4082. Bethesda, Md.: Department of Health and Human Services, National Institutes of Health, 1998. Revised April 2006. http://hp2010.nhlbihin.net/yourguide.

CHAPTER 5

Breast Cancer Preventive Services

B reast cancer is the most common cancer in women in the United States.*
The National Cancer Institute (NCI) estimates that over 190,000 women
will have been diagnosed with invasive breast cancer in 2009. This means
that one in every eight women born today will develop invasive breast cancer in her lifetime. Despite major advancements in treatment, breast cancer
is still the second most common cause of cancer-related death in women.
However, there is greater hope than ever today because of three different
approaches to preventing it: screening, genetic counseling and testing, and
preventive medications (called *chemoprevention*).

Mammography is the most reliable method for breast cancer screening in
older women and reduces death from breast cancer by as much as 34 percent.
Screening can detect breast cancers earlier than they would be found otherwise and offers the best hope of early diagnosis and treatment—even cure.
And yet, 30 percent of women eligible for screening do not get mammograms
regularly.

Through genetic testing, women with strong family histories of breast cancer can find out if they are carriers of mutations, or changes, in certain genes—
named BRCA1 and BRCA2—that make women susceptible to developing
breast cancer. Women who carry these mutations may benefit from preventive measures aimed at reducing their high risk of breast cancer—intensive
screening, chemoprevention, or surgery (called *prophylactic mastectomy*).

For women at increased risk for breast cancer, chemoprevention can reduce the risk of disease. When taken regularly, certain medications, including tamoxifen and raloxifene, prevent up to 50 percent of invasive breast cancers in these women.

---

* Excluding nonmelanoma skin cancer (e.g., basal cell carcinoma, squamous cell
  carcinoma).

The United States Preventive Services Task Force (USPSTF) makes the following recommendations regarding breast cancer preventive services:

- screening for breast cancer with screening mammography every two years in women ages 50 to 74 years
- referral to genetic counseling and evaluation for women with higher-risk family history patterns of breast and ovarian cancer
- discussion of chemoprevention with women at high risk for breast cancer and at low risk for adverse events[1]

Section I provides a basic introduction to breast cancer. Section II discusses breast cancer risk assessment, an important tool in making decisions about breast cancer prevention. Sections III, IV, and V detail the USPSTF recommendations for screening, genetic counseling and testing, and chemoprevention.*

SECTION I: BREAST CANCER 101

Breast cancer is a disease in which cancer cells form in the tissues of the breast, including the *ducts* and *lobules*. The lobules contain the tiny glands that produce milk during lactation; the ducts are the tubes that deliver milk from the glands to the nipple. In addition to the structures readily identified as breasts, breast tissue is present around the collar bone and *axilla,* or underarm.

What is breast cancer?

If you have not read the "Special Section on Cancer" in part I, you may want to read it now to gain a better understanding of cancer.

A *cancer,* or a *malignant tumor,* can be understood as a mass of abnormal cells that developed from normal tissue. Cancer cells are abnormal because they do not stop growing and die as normal cells do—instead they continue to grow larger and multiply. What differentiates breast cancer from other cancers is that it develops from breast tissue.

Breast cancer is a progressive disease that takes years to develop. The disease begins with a mass of abnormal cells so small it cannot be felt or even seen with x-rays. Over time, the cells multiply and become more abnormal.

---

* Breast cancer also develops in men, although much less commonly. Because there are no preventive health measures for breast cancer in men, the focus of this chapter is on breast cancer in women.

Eventually, the abnormal cells take on some characteristics of cancer and are called *noninvasive cancer,* or *precancers.* Noninvasive cancer is still cancer, meaning it is an uncontrolled growth of cells, but it differs from invasive cancer because it cannot invade surrounding tissues and cannot spread to other parts of the body. These precancers are named for the type of tissue from which they develop. If they develop in the ducts, they are called *ductal carcinoma in situ* (DCIS); if they develop in the lobules, they are called *lobular carcinoma in situ* (LCIS). Sometimes these noninvasive breast cancers can be detected by a mammogram, which is a special type of x-ray.

If untreated, some but not all of these noninvasive cancers will progress to become invasive breast cancer. Invasive cancer can spread to adjacent breast tissue and, over time, to other parts of the body. Cancer that spreads like this is called *metastatic cancer.* Mammography can detect most invasive breast cancers. In addition, some of these cancers can be detected through routine breast examination.

The earlier the cancer is found, the more easily and effectively it can be treated. Women with localized breast cancer have a greater than 95 percent survival rate over five years. Women with breast cancer that has regional spread, for example to lymph nodes in the underarm, have a 75 percent survival rate over five years. Women with distant metastases have a 20 percent survival rate over five years. Currently, only 60 percent of breast cancers are diagnosed while the cancer is still locally confined.[2]

What are the symptoms of breast cancer?

Common symptoms of breast cancer include the following:

▸ *a change in how the breast feels:* a lump or thickening in or near the breast that feels different from the surrounding tissue
▸ *a change in the how the breast looks:* breast size or shape changes; nipple inversion; a change in the skin of the breast or nipple
▸ *onset of nipple discharge:* clear, discolored, or bloody[3]

Pain is not a common symptom of breast cancer; however, breast pain that does not go away could be a sign of cancer. If you have any of these symptoms, do not be overly concerned. In most women, especially younger women, these symptoms are much more likely to be caused by something other than breast cancer. Still, please see your doctor.

By a similar token, the absence of these symptoms does not mean that you cannot have breast cancer. It is common not to have any symptoms of breast cancer before diagnosis, and detecting breast cancer before symptoms develop is often preferable because symptoms may be a sign of advanced disease (if the tumor is large enough to be felt, for example). This is why screening for breast cancer is so important.

What are the risk factors for breast cancer?

Scientists do not yet understand exactly how breast cancer develops, but they have identified several important risk factors. These factors can be divided into *modifiable* risk factors (those you can reasonably change) and *nonmodifiable* risk factors (those you cannot).

Nonmodifiable Risk Factors

- *Age:* The risk of breast cancer increases as a woman gets older, particularly after menopause. Breast cancer mostly develops in women over age 50 and is uncommon before age 40.

- *Personal history:* A woman with a history of breast cancer is at increased risk for getting cancer again.

- *Certain breast changes:* A woman with a history of precancers (e.g., DCIS, LCIS) is at increased risk.

- *Family history:* A woman with a family history of breast cancer is at greater risk. The risk increases with the number of affected relatives, their closeness (breast cancer in first-degree relatives, such as a mother or sister, suggests greater risk), and their age at diagnosis (before age 40 suggests greater risk). Maternal and paternal relatives matter equally.

- *Menstrual history:* A woman's risk of breast cancer increases with her estrogen exposure. Estrogen is a hormone produced during regular menstrual cycles. Thus, first menstrual period before age 12, menopause after age 55, not having children, and older age at first childbirth are all risk factors for breast cancer.

- *Certain gene mutations:* Mutations, or changes, in certain genes increase a woman's risk. The most commonly tested mutations are in the BRCA1 and BRCA2 genes. These mutations can be inherited from either the maternal or paternal family. An estimated 4 to 5 percent of breast cancers are attributable to these mutations. Although mutations in other genes have been identified as important in breast cancer, they have not yet received widespread clinical attention.

- *Race:* White women are at greater risk of developing breast cancer than Hispanic, Asian, or African American women. However, African

American women are more likely than white women to die of breast cancer.

Modifiable Risk Factors

▸ *Overweight or obesity after menopause:* The chance of getting breast cancer after menopause is higher in women who are overweight or obese.

▸ *Lack of physical activity:* Women who are physically inactive may have an increased risk. Being active may help reduce risk by preventing weight gain and especially obesity.

▸ *Alcohol consumption:* Studies suggest that the more alcohol a woman drinks, the greater her risk of breast cancer.

▸ *Hormone (estrogen) replacement therapy (HRT):* Women who take estrogen after menopause are at increased risk of breast cancer because of the effects of estrogen exposure.

Risk factors increase the chances of developing breast cancer but do not dictate who gets breast cancer and who does not. Most women who have known risk factors do not get breast cancer. Conversely, most women who develop breast cancer have no clear risk factors for the disease other than older age. This means that screening for breast cancer is important for every woman, even for those without major risk factors.

Understanding your individual risk for breast cancer is an important first step in making decisions about which breast cancer preventive services are right for you. This is discussed in greater detail in section II.

What can I do to prevent breast cancer?

Based on the above risk factors, there are four strategies for breast cancer prevention:

▸ *Lifestyle modification:* Maintaining a healthy weight, being physically active, reducing fat intake, and drinking alcohol in moderation are associated with a lower risk of breast cancer. Consider lowering your risk of breast cancer to be yet another reason to adopt a healthier lifestyle.*

---

* At least one study has demonstrated that women who exercised regularly had a 20 percent lower risk of invasive breast cancer. However, in general, the data are inconclusive and more studies are under way to assess the causal relationship between lifestyle and breast cancer.

▸ *Careful consideration of HRT:* HRT is used to treat perimenopausal symptoms such as hot flashes and vaginal dryness and to prevent and treat osteoporosis. However, HRT also increases a woman's risk of breast cancer. Before initiating HRT, women should carefully consider both its benefits and its risks.

▸ *Chemoprevention:* In women at high risk, tamoxifen and raloxifene prevent up to 50 percent of invasive breast cancers. However, these medications are not without harm and are known to increase the risk of blood clots and endometrial cancer. Section V discusses chemoprevention in greater detail.

▸ *Preventive mastectomy: Preventive,* or *prophylactic, mastectomy* is the removal of healthy breasts to prevent breast cancer. In certain very high-risk women, such as women who carry BRCA1 or BRCA2 mutations, prophylactic mastectomy prevents as much as 90 percent of breast cancers. However, this procedure carries the risks of major surgery and has important psychosocial consequences. Section IV discusses genetic testing for BRCA mutations and prophylactic mastectomy in greater detail.

How does breast cancer screening work?

The most common tests to screen for breast cancer are mammography, clinical breast exams, and breast self-exams. The guidelines for screening are discussed in section III. Below is a brief overview of these tests.

Mammography

Mammography, or a mammogram, is an x-ray picture of the breast used to detect breast changes in women. Mammography makes it possible to detect breast cancers too small to cause symptoms or be detected during a breast exam. Studies show that in women ages 50 to 69, routine mammograms prevent up to 34 percent—or one-third—of deaths from breast cancer. In women ages 40 to 49, mammograms prevent up to 15 percent of breast cancer–related deaths.

There are two types of mammograms: screening and diagnostic. A *screening mammogram* is used to screen for breast cancer, meaning that it is used in women who do not have any symptoms of breast cancer. It usually involves taking two x-rays of each breast from different positions. A *diagnostic mammogram* is used to test for breast cancer in women who have symptoms, such as a lump, or who have had an abnormal screening mammogram. Diagnostic mammograms involve taking x-rays of the breasts from several angles, particularly in areas that are suspicious for breast cancer.

Mammograms are the best method of screening for breast cancer in older women. In women under 40, because breast tissue is denser, mammography is less able to distinguish cancer from normal tissue.

Clinical Breast Exam

A clinical breast exam, sometimes referred to as an annual breast exam, is a physical exam of the breasts performed by a doctor or nurse to check for masses or other breast changes that may be a sign of breast cancer. Although routine clinical breast exams can effectively identify breast cancers, studies have not consistently shown that they reduce the number of deaths from the disease.

Breast Self-Exam

The breast self-exam is an exam done by a woman to check for any changes in her own breasts (see figure 5.1). The exam is usually performed routinely, often monthly, so that a woman can familiarize herself with the look and feel of her breasts and be able to readily detect changes should they occur.

Anecdotally, we may hear of many women who are diagnosed with breast cancer after detecting a mass during a routine self-exam, but studies have not shown that breast self-exams reduce the number of deaths from breast cancer.

What about using MRIs to screen for breast cancer?

MRI (*magnetic resonance imaging*) uses magnetic fields, as opposed to x-rays, to produced detailed pictures of the body. As a result, MRIs provide better soft tissue contrast than mammograms and produce clear pictures of the breast, even in younger women with dense breasts. Although MRIs are routinely used to monitor for recurrence in women with a history of breast cancer, there has recently been great interest in using MRIs to screen for breast cancer. The hope is that MRI will prove to be a better screening tool, particularly in above-average-risk women under age 40, in whom higher breast density limits the effectiveness of mammography.

How is breast cancer diagnosed?

Women who either develop symptoms consistent with breast cancer or have a positive screening test require further evaluation before a diagnosis can be made. Sometimes the next step will include additional imaging tests

A

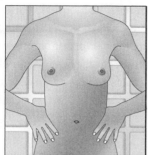

Check breasts in mirror
while pressing hands on hips

B

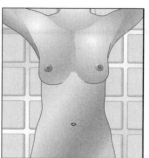

Check breasts in mirror
with arms stretched upward

C

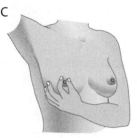

Check nipple, squeezing
gently between two fingers

D

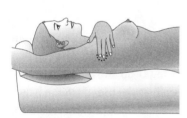
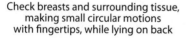

Check breasts and surrounding tissue,
making small circular motions
with fingertips, while lying on back

E

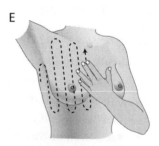

Beginning under the arm,
follow a pattern that examines
the entire area where
cancers may occur

Figure 5.1. For the breast exam, your health care provider will examine your breasts in a way that is similar to the self-examination shown in A through E. You and your health care provider must feel (also known as palpate) the breast tissue in a methodical manner. Many women find the up-and-down approach illustrated in this figure (E) most suitable. It is important to cover the entire breast tissue, and not just the breast, from the collarbone to the top of the abdomen, and from the armpit to the cleavage. Use a firm, smooth touch with the first few finger pads of the hand in a circular motion, covering areas no larger than the size of a quarter. Be sure to feel all the tissue of the breast, using varying degrees of pressure to examine the different levels of breast tissue.

such as a diagnostic mammogram, an ultrasound, or an MRI. Regardless, to make a definitive diagnosis, the area of concern must be biopsied. During a *biopsy* doctors remove a piece of breast tissue to analyze under the microscope for characteristic signs of cancer. There are many types of biopsies, including fine-needle aspiration, core biopsy, and surgical biopsy. While this procedure is not dangerous, it can be painful, anxiety provoking, and in rare cases disfiguring.

SECTION II: ESTIMATING YOUR RISK OF BREAST CANCER

Section I describes the major risk factors for breast cancer, but a simple list of risk factors won't tell you what your overall risk is. For making important decisions such as whether to start chemoprevention or to begin screening for breast cancer at an earlier age than the norm, a more precise estimate of your risk is helpful.

Doctors have developed risk calculators to estimate an individual woman's risk of breast cancer. The best known of these calculators is called the Breast Cancer Risk Assessment Tool, or BCRA. It was developed by NCI scientists and is based on a statistical model known as the Gail model, named after the lead scientist who developed it. Using information about age, medical history, family history, and menstrual history, the BCRA estimates a woman's risk of developing breast cancer in the next five years.

Can anyone use the BCRA?

The BCRA is designed for people without any history of breast cancer and should not be used to calculate risk for women who have already been diagnosed with breast cancer or precancers, including DCIS and LCIS. It also does not take into account important risk factors such as the use of HRT, a history of breast cancer in second-degree relatives, or a history of previous radiation. Finally, it is a risk assessment tool, not a prediction tool—it cannot tell you with any certainty whether you will or will not develop breast cancer.

How does the BCRA work?

Table 5.1 contains sample calculations using the BCRA tool based on a hypothetical woman: a 50-year-old white woman with no history of abnormal mammograms or biopsies. Our hypothetical woman has a family history of a mother with breast cancer. Her first menstrual period was at age 12, and her first child was born when she was 28 years old. The first row in the table shows her characteristics and her estimated risks of developing breast cancer

Table 5.1: Breast cancer risk for a hypothetical woman

Age	Race	Number of first-degree relatives with breast cancer	Age at first menstrual period	Age at first childbirth	Five-year breast cancer risk	Breast cancer risk to the age of 90
50	**White**	1	**12 to 13**	**25 to 29**	**1.9%**	**16.8%**
40	White	1	12 to 13	25 to 29	1.1%	18.8%
50	**Black**	1	12 to 13	25 to 29	1.8%	13.5%
50	White	**0**	12 to 13	25 to 29	1.1%	9.9%
50	White	1	**7 to 11**	25 to 29	2.1%	18.3%
50	White	1	12 to 13	**over 30**	2.0%	17.3%

Notes: These calculations were performed by the author on April 4, 2008. The BCRA is periodically revised, and therefore these estimates may not reflect current estimates. **Boldface** text after the first row indicates a changed risk factor.

in the next five years and over her remaining lifetime. Each subsequent row presents a different risk estimate obtained by modifying one of her risk factors (noted in bold).

Five-year breast cancer risk is the woman's estimated risk of developing invasive breast cancer over the next five years. *Breast cancer risk to the age of 90* is the woman's risk of developing invasive breast cancer over her remaining lifetime, assuming she lives to age 90.

Note how the woman's estimated risks of breast cancer change as her characteristics change. For example, as her age decreases from 50 to 40, her five-year risk decreases from 1.9 to 1.1 percent. On the other hand, her lifetime risk to the age of 90 increases from 16.8 to 18.8 percent.

How can I use the BCRA tool?

To use the risk calculator, go to www.cancer.gov/bcrisktool and follow the instructions provided. This tool will help you better understand your breast cancer risks. This understanding will help guide your decision making about which of the preventive services described in the following sections is right for you.

SECTION III: BREAST CANCER SCREENING

Screening can detect breast cancers earlier than they would be found otherwise and offers the best hope of early diagnosis, treatment, and cure. Mammography is the most reliable method for breast cancer screening in older women and reduces death from breast cancer by as much as 34 percent.

Despite these well-known benefits, many uncertainties about breast cancer screening remain. Most doctors agree that all women ages 50 to 74 should be screened for breast cancer using routine mammography. However, there is wide debate about the merits of routine mammography in women ages 40 to 49 and in women age 75 or above. In addition, there is debate about the incremental benefits of clinician breast exams, regular breast self-exams, and adjunctive imaging modalities such as ultrasound and MRI.

The USPSTF recommends screening mammography every two years in women ages 50 to 74. For women under the age of 50, the task force states that the decision to start regular screening mammography should be an individual one. The following sections discuss the guidelines for screening and detail how mammography is done.

Should I begin screening before age 50?

Although the USPSTF does not recommend routine mammography until age 50, this does not mean that women ages 40 to 49 should not be screened. Rather, the recommendations suggest that the decision about when to begin screening take into account individual risks and preferences. The USPSTF found insufficient evidence to support clinical breast exams beyond screening mammography. The greater your risk for breast cancer, the more likely screening between ages 40 and 49 will benefit you. In addition, the more concerned you are about having breast cancer and the less concerned you are about the potential harm from unnecessary testing, the more favorably you will view screening. The decision about whether to start screening at age 40 or later is best made between you and your doctor.

What about clinical breast exams?

Many physicians perform annual exams, and many professional organizations support their routine use. However, the benefits of clinical breast exams have not been borne out in clinical studies. Studies show that mammography with clinical breast exams does not further reduce deaths from breast cancer compared with mammography alone. Furthermore, women who receive clinical breast exams undergo more breast biopsies and experience more anxiety from false positives. Thus, whether to have these exams is up to you and your doctor.

What about monthly self-exams?

There is little evidence that routine breast self-exams reduce death from breast cancer. In addition, evidence suggests that breast self-exams are associated with more false-positive results, more unnecessary testing, and more anxiety. As a result, the USPSTF recommends against teaching self-exams. It is important to point out that this is not a recommendation against self-exams. Many women feel strongly about doing monthly exams and find benefit in doing them. Rather, it is a statement against doctors teaching patients about self-exams in the clinic setting.

I thought mammograms were needed every year. Why does the USPSTF recommend having them every two years?

Few data suggest that annual mammography is more effective than mammography done every other year. At the same time, the risk of false positives increases with the higher frequency of screenings, so women receiving annual mammograms are at greater risk of harm from screening.

At what age should I stop getting screened?

The USPSTF recommends routine screening until age 74; starting at age 75 the task force found the evidence insufficient to recommend for or against routine screening. Very few studies of mammography have included women older than 69 and no study has included women over 70. Women age 75 or older face a higher risk of developing breast cancer, but they also have a greater risk of dying from other causes. The health of women 75 and older varies widely, so decisions of when to discontinue screening should be made individually. It is probably reasonable for a 75-year-old woman with few health problems, who is expected to live well into her eighties, to continue screening. On the other hand, screening is unlikely to benefit a woman with a terminal condition.

How can I make all of these decisions?

These are difficult decisions to make. Many women begin annual clinical breast exams and monthly self-exams at age 20 and then annual mammograms at age 40. Others choose to get mammograms every two years beginning at age 50. And there are many options in between. All these approaches are reasonable, and there is no right answer. In your decision making, consider your overall risk for breast cancer (see section II) and your values and preferences. Include your doctor, family, and friends in an open, honest discussion about what is best for you.

Do I need additional screening if I have above-average risk of breast cancer?

Some women are considered to be at above-average risk of breast cancer. This may be because of a strong family history of breast cancer (e.g., one or more first-degree relatives with a history of breast cancer before age 40); known BRCA gene mutations or relatives with BRCA mutations; or a history of radiation exposure to the chest. For these women, additional screening for breast cancer may be warranted. While the USPSTF does not make any specific recommendations regarding screening in higher risk women, other organizations, such as the American Cancer Society, recommend annual MRI screening, in addition to routine screening mammography, in certain high-risk women.[4] If you have one or more conditions that place you at increased risk of breast cancer, talk to your doctor about whether additional screening is right for you.

I have breast implants. Do I need to get mammograms?

As long as breast tissue is present, there is a risk of breast cancer. Women with breast implants for cosmetic reasons should generally continue to have mammograms. If the implants were placed after surgery for breast cancer, you should talk to your doctor about appropriate follow-up and screening.

How is mammography done?

Mammography is performed on an outpatient basis, often in a radiology suite or hospital radiology department.

During mammography, you stand in front of a special x-ray machine. The person who takes the x-rays, called a radiology technologist, positions one breast at a time between two plastic plates. The plates compress your breast to make it flatter, which allows for a clearer x-ray picture to be taken. Most women describe a sensation of pressure on the breast for a few seconds during the compression. You might also feel momentary discomfort. Usually, two pictures are taken of the breast—one from the side, and one from above.

Screening mammograms require no preparation or follow-up and take about fifteen minutes. At least one radiologist, a doctor specializing in reading x-rays, reads the mammogram and reports the results to you and your doctor.

Does it hurt?

For most women, mammograms are mildly uncomfortable, although some women report them being painful. The discomfort usually comes from the breasts being compressed. Unfortunately, this is a necessary step in the procedure because it allows the x-ray beam to better penetrate the tissue and provide the best image possible. Often this physical discomfort is combined with some anxiety about having a test to look for cancer and being exposed in front of strangers. These are understandable and normal feelings.

Be sure to let the radiology technologist know if the procedure is overly uncomfortable so that he or she can make an adjustment. If you are still premenopausal, consider scheduling your mammogram for when you are not menstruating, because the breasts of some women become more sensitive during menstruation. Above all, do not let pain or discomfort keep you from getting regularly screened. Most women need only bear mild to moderate discomfort for a short period. If the pain is more severe, talk to your doctor about other screening options, such as MRI.

What are the risks?

The only direct risk of mammography is from radiation exposure. Although this risk is not insignificant, it is small because mammograms use low-dose x-rays and involve less radiation exposure than a standard chest x-ray. However, there are important indirect risks of screening with mammography.

False negatives: Sometimes mammograms fail to detect breast cancers and are falsely negative. Overall, one in five breast cancers present at the time of screening is missed. False negatives are more common in younger women because the increased density of their breasts makes cancers more difficult to detect using x-ray technology. False negatives cause harm by potentially delaying diagnosis and treatment of breast cancers and by creating a false sense of security.

False positives: Sometimes mammograms suggest breast cancer is present when it is not there. These false positives lead to unnecessary testing, including biopsies, which are anxiety provoking, costly, and potentially disfiguring. A 40-year-old woman who gets a mammogram every year for 10 years has a 30 percent chance of having a false positive. For women age 50 or older, the risk is 25 percent.

Overdiagnosis: Even if breast cancer is found, treating that cancer will not always lead to an improvement in health. Overdiagnosis refers to the detection of cancers that will not cause harm if left untreated. This can be because the cancer becomes dormant or regresses, or because the patient dies before the cancer becomes clinically relevant. Because it is not possible to tell which cancers will eventually cause harm and which ones will not, doctors routinely treat all cancers. The result is that some women will undergo treatment for breast cancer, including surgery and radiation, without any health benefits.

What happens if they find something on the mammogram?

First of all, remember that finding "something" does not necessarily mean finding cancer. It simply means that the radiologist has found something abnormal that requires further testing and evaluation. His or her job is to identify anything out of the ordinary; from an x-ray, it is often difficult to tell exactly what is going on. Screening mammography is not a tool for diagnosing breast cancer.

Depending on the radiologist's level of suspicion for cancer, you may be scheduled for additional imaging tests, such as a diagnostic mammogram, an ultrasound, or a breast biopsy. Only through biopsies can doctors definitively diagnose breast cancer.

What happens if the mammogram is normal?

Confirm the results of the test and be sure your primary care doctor has a copy. Record the results for your own files, including when and where you had the mammogram done. *Good documentation is the key to making sure you get your next mammogram no later than two years from the last one,* unless you and your doctor decide to discontinue screening.

While a normal result is reassuring, keep in mind that it may be a false negative. This fact underscores the importance of making sure you get your next mammogram on time.

SECTION IV: BRCA GENETIC TESTING

One in twenty women with breast cancer has mutations, or alterations, in her genes that made her susceptible to developing the cancer. The best studied of these mutations are in the BRCA1 and BRCA2 genes. These mutations increase susceptibility to breast and ovarian cancer and can be passed on from parent to child through either the maternal or the paternal side.

Not every woman who inherits a BRCA mutation develops cancer, but many do. Women with mutations in BRCA1 or BRCA2 have a lifetime breast cancer risk of 60 to 85 percent—compared with a 12 percent risk in the average woman—and a lifetime ovarian cancer risk of 15 to 40 percent.

Because BRCA mutations are inherited, families with certain patterns of breast and ovarian cancer may be carriers of a mutation. Through genetic testing, individuals in these families can find out if they carry a breast-cancer-susceptibility gene. The potential benefit of testing is that women who carry a BRCA mutation can take additional preventive measures that may reduce their risk of breast and ovarian cancer. This includes undergoing more intensive breast cancer screening, chemoprevention with tamoxifen or raloxifene, and surgery to remove the ovaries (prophylactic oopherectomy) or the breasts (prophylactic mastectomy).

Prophylactic mastectomy has been shown to reduce the risk of breast cancer by 90 percent in women with BRCA mutations. However, many preventive measures, including major surgery and preventive medication, carry significant potential for harm. Genetic testing itself has the potential for harm and may cause significant psychological distress, strain family relationships, and carry social and legal implications.

The USPSTF recommends that women with certain family history patterns of breast and ovarian cancer be referred for genetic counseling and an evaluation for BRCA genetic testing. This recommendation is based on evidence that women with these family history patterns have an increased risk for developing breast or ovarian cancer associated with BRCA1 or BRCA2 mutations and on evidence that prophylactic surgery for women with one of these genes significantly decreases their risk of breast and ovarian cancer. The USPSTF concludes that women with these family history patterns benefit from genetic counseling that allows informed decision making about testing and further prophylactic treatment.

Jewish women, especially those of Ashkenazi descent, are more likely to be BRCA carriers. Thus, the criteria for referral are related to ethnicity.

For Ashkenazi Jewish women, high-risk family history patterns include

- any first-degree relative (parents, siblings, or children) with breast or ovarian cancer
- two second-degree relatives (aunts, uncles, nieces, nephews, grand-parents, or half-siblings) on the same side of the family with breast or ovarian cancer

For non-Ashkenazi Jewish women, high-risk family patterns include

- two first-degree relatives with breast cancer, one of whom received the diagnosis before age 50
- three or more first- or second-degree relatives with breast cancer

▸ both breast and ovarian cancer among first- and second-degree relatives
▸ any first-degree relative with cancer in both breasts
▸ two or more first- or second-degree relatives with ovarian cancer
▸ one first- or second-degree relative with both breast and ovarian cancer
▸ a male relative with breast cancer

Women with any of the above family history patterns should talk to their doctor about being referred for genetic counseling and evaluation for BRCA genetic testing. Note that they should not necessarily *receive* BRCA genetic testing; rather, they should be referred to a genetic counselor to allow for informed decision making about whether BRCA genetic testing is right for them.

What about women without these family history patterns?

Most women with a family history of breast or ovarian cancer—even a strong family history—do not have mutations in the BRCA genes. Only one in every thousand women in the general population carries a mutation; in women without these family history patterns, the likelihood is even lower. Thus, the benefits of routine screening or referral for genetic counseling would be small to zero. There are also important negative ethical, legal, and social consequences that could result from routine referral and testing. Thus, the USPSTF *recommends against* routine referral for genetic counseling in women without one of the family history patterns described above.

What if I have a relative with a BRCA mutation?

These recommendations do not apply to women with a *known* BRCA mutation in their family. Women with a first- or second-degree relative with a BRCA mutation are generally referred for genetic counseling.

What happens during genetic counseling and evaluation?

During genetic counseling, you will meet with a specialist who will help you understand your risks of breast and ovarian cancer and make an informed decision about whether to undergo BRCA testing. Elements of counseling include assessing your risk of breast cancer, analyzing your family tree of breast and ovarian cancer, discussing the potential benefits and harms of BRCA testing, and outlining next steps whether you test positive or negative.

Can you tell me more about the BRCA test itself?

The primary recommendation put forth here is that women with certain family history patterns of breast and ovarian cancer should be referred for genetic counseling and evaluation for BRCA testing. It is best to discuss testing and its implications within the context of genetic counseling. A comprehensive discussion of BRCA testing is outside the scope of this book.

SECTION V: BREAST CANCER CHEMOPREVENTION

Chemoprevention is the use of medicines to reduce the risk or delay the development of cancer. In the case of breast cancer, there are two FDA-approved medicines for the prevention of breast cancer in high-risk women—tamoxifen and raloxifene.

In a recent large clinical trial, both tamoxifen and raloxifene were found to reduce the risk of developing invasive breast cancer by about 50 percent among postmenopausal women at increased risk of the disease. In addition, they promote bone health and are used for the prevention and treatment of osteoporosis. However, these drugs are not without harm. Both medications increase the risk of blood clots and uterine cancer, and tamoxifen increases the risk of cataracts. As a result, every woman considering chemoprevention must weigh the beneficial effects of these medications against the potential harms.

The USPSTF advises doctors to discuss chemoprevention with women at high risk for breast cancer and at low risk of harm from the medication. In women at low or average risk of breast cancer, the task force recommends against the routine use of tamoxifen or raloxifene to prevent breast cancer.

While these recommendations are directed toward doctors, you should talk to your doctor about chemoprevention for breast cancer to find out if it is right for you. This is particularly important in women who are postmenopausal, are over age 55, have a family history of breast cancer in one or more first-degree relatives, or have a personal history of an abnormal breast biopsy.

What is tamoxifen? What is raloxifene?

Tamoxifen is a medicine that has been used for more than thirty years to treat breast cancer. More recently, studies have shown that women who have never had breast cancer but who are at increased risk for the disease also benefit from tamoxifen. Raloxifene, a newer medicine in the same drug class as tamoxifen, was originally used for the treatment and prevention of osteoporosis. In 2007, it was also approved for use in reducing the risk of invasive breast cancer in postmenopausal women.

Tamoxifen and raloxifene belong to a family of medications called *selective estrogen receptor modulators*, or SERMs. They were given this name because they modulate the effects of the hormone estrogen in the body but do so "selectively." In some tissues, such as in the breast, SERMs block the effects of estrogen. In other tissues, such as in bone, blood vessels, and the uterus, they do the opposite and actually increase the effects of estrogen. Understanding the many effects of SERMs on the body therefore stems from understanding the effects of estrogen in different tissues. Estrogen promotes cell growth throughout the body, including in the breast, uterus, and bone, and increases blood clotting. Thus, by blocking the effects of estrogen in the breast, SERMs prevent the growth of breast cancer cells and reduce the risk of invasive cancer. In bone, blood vessels, and the uterus, by promoting the effects of estrogen, SERMs increase the risk of uterine cancer, decrease the risk of bone loss, and increase the risk of blood clots.

What are the benefits of chemoprevention?

In a recent large clinical trial involving postmenopausal women at increased risk of the disease, tamoxifen and raloxifene reduced the risk of invasive breast cancer by 50 percent over five years. The benefits are not the same for all women, however. The greater a woman's risk of breast cancer, the more likely she is to benefit from chemoprevention. This means that the older you are and the more risk factors for breast cancer you have, the more likely you are to benefit. For the purposes of the clinical trial, women were required to have at least a 1.66 percent five-year risk of breast cancer. Using the risk calculator described in section II, you can calculate your five-year risk of breast cancer to use as a starting point for discussing chemoprevention with your doctor.

What are the harms?

The major side effects of tamoxifen and raloxifene are uterine cancer and blood clots. *Uterine cancer* is cancer of the uterus, or womb, the place where a baby grows during pregnancy. The most common uterine cancer is endometrial cancer, which is cancer that starts in the inside lining of the uterus. The usual treatment is surgical removal of the uterus, called *hysterectomy*. Blood clots usually develop in the legs (called *deep vein thrombosis*) but from there may travel to the lung and cause a potentially fatal condition called *pulmonary embolism*. Less commonly, the clots may travel to the brain and cause a stroke. In addition to these serious health problems, tamoxifen and raloxifene can cause bothersome side effects, such as hot flashes and vaginal discharge.

As with its benefits, the risks of chemoprevention are not the same for all women. Women who are younger; who have no history of risk factors for blood clots or stroke; or who have no uterus are at lower risk of harm.

Which drug is better for preventing breast cancer?

Early results of a recent study show that tamoxifen and raloxifene are equally effective at reducing the risk of invasive breast cancer.[5] However, they differed significantly in their side effects. Women who took raloxifene had 36 percent fewer uterine cancers and 29 percent fewer blood clots than women who took tamoxifen. In addition, unlike tamoxifen, raloxifene did not increase the risk of cataracts. These data suggest that while tamoxifen and raloxifene are equally effective at preventing breast cancer, raloxifene is preferable in postmenopausal women because of its side effect profile. In menstruating women, only tamoxifen is available for chemoprevention. Because these data are still preliminary, however, it is best to discuss the most up-to-date information with your doctor before deciding.

How should I decide?

The higher your risk of breast cancer and the lower your risk of harm, the more likely chemoprevention is to benefit you. However, your ultimate decisions will also depend on how you as an individual weigh an increased risk of breast cancer versus an increased risk of uterine cancer and blood clots. An open discussion with your doctor is the best way to weigh these factors and arrive at a shared decision.

REFERENCES

"American Cancer Society Guidelines for Breast Screening with MRI as an Adjunct to Mammography," *CA Cancer J Clin* 57 (2007): 75-89.

National Cancer Institute (NCI). National Institutes of Health (NIH). U.S. Department of Health and Human Services. www.cancer.gov.

———. *What You Need to Know About Breast Cancer*. NIH Publication No. 05-1556. Bethesda, Md.: Department of Health and Human Services, National Institutes of Health, September 2005. Revised May 2005. www.cancer.gov/cancertopics/types/breast.

Vogel VG et al. "Effects of Tamoxifen vs. Raloxifene on the Risk of Developing Invasive Breast Cancer and Other Disease Outcomes: The NSABP Study of Tamoxifen and Raloxifene (STAR) P-2 trial," *JAMA* 295, no. 23 (June 2006): 2727-41. Epub 2006, Jun 5.

Cervical Cancer Screening and HPV

One of the most exciting developments in medicine over the past few decades has been the tremendous growth in our understanding of the molecular biology of cervical cancer and in our ability to effectively prevent it through screening. More recently, this excitement has increased with the introduction of a vaccine that prevents infection by some of the viruses that cause cervical cancer. This is the first vaccine ever developed and approved by the Food and Drug Administration (FDA) to prevent cancer.

The impact of these advances on women's health cannot be understated. Cervical cancer was once the leading cause of cancer death in women in the United States; now it is not even in the top ten. Since the introduction of the Pap smear, the death rate from cervical cancer has dropped over 70 percent.[1] And these figures have yet to reflect the impact of the cervical cancer vaccine.

However, these important developments have also brought with them increasing confusion in the general public and even among health professionals about the causes of cervical cancer and the role of preventive and screening services. Questions include the causative agent of cervical cancer, the human papillomavirus (HPV); its relationship to cervical cancer and genital warts; and its transmission. In addition, there are questions about the HPV vaccine (also known as the cervical cancer vaccine) and the role of Pap smears and other screening methods for cervical cancer.

The United States Preventive Services Task Force (USPSTF) recommends cervical cancer screening with the Pap smear in sexually active women who have a cervix.[2] The Centers for Disease Control and Prevention (CDC) recommends administering the HPV vaccine to all girls 11 or 12 years of age and women ages 13 to 26 who did not receive the vaccine earlier.[3]

The following sections provide an introduction to cervical cancer, HPV, and the relationship between HPV and cervical cancer, and detail the recommendations for cervical cancer screening and HPV vaccination.

SECTION I: CERVICAL CANCER AND HPV 101

Cervical cancer is a malignant tumor, or cancer, that starts in the cells that line the surface of the cervix. The *cervix* is the narrow lower part of the uterus.

Virtually all cases of cervical cancer are caused by HPV. However, the vast majority of HPV infections do not result in cervical cancer. The virus spreads through unprotected sexual contact with an infected individual. Thus, HPV is a sexually transmitted infection, or STI. The majority of people infected with HPV have no symptoms of infection. As a result, HPV is often passed from partner to partner unknowingly. Recently, a vaccine has become available that prevents infection with certain types of HPV.

HPV, or *human papillomavirus* (pap-ah-LO-mah-VIE-rus), is a family of over one hundred viruses, each of which is assigned a number (e.g., HPV 11). Not all types of HPV cause cervical cancer. A group of HPV viruses called the low-risk types—6, 11, 42, 43, and 44—cause ordinary genital warts and virtually never cause cancer. Most cases of cervical cancer are caused by the high-risk types—16, 18, 31, and 45. These viruses have also been linked to other, less common, skin cancers of the vulva, vagina, penis, and anus. Most HPV infections—even those with the high-risk types—go away on their own after one to two years and do not lead to cancer.

In women who do not clear the infection on their own, it takes several years from the time they are infected with a cancer-causing type of HPV for cervical cancer to develop. During this time, the cells of the cervix undergo gradual changes that give them a different appearance from normal cells. Through a routine screening test, called a *Pap test,* or *Pap smear,* a doctor can sample the cells from the cervix and have them examined under a microscope to look for any evidence of these precancerous cells. If abnormal cells are detected, they can be removed before they have a chance to progress into cancer. The several years between the time of infection and the development of cancer allows for multiple opportunities to find these precancerous cells through screening and to prevent cancer.

HPV infection, precancerous cervical changes, and even the early stages of cervical cancer are not usually associated with any symptoms. As a result, in women who do not get screened, cervical cancer is usually not diagnosed until an advanced stage of the cancer, when symptoms develop. Through regular screening with Pap smears, cervical cancer should be a completely preventable disease. However, at present, over 11,000 women are diagnosed with invasive cervical cancer each year in the United States, and nearly 4,000 die from complications of the disease. Getting informed about cervical cancer as well as making sure you are appropriately screened with regular Pap smears and immunized against HPV are the keys to staying free of cervical cancer.

How common are HPV and cervical cancer?

HPV

HPV is the most common sexually transmitted infection in the United States. Seventy-five percent of Americans—three out of every four—have been infected with HPV at some point in their lives. Because the infection does not usually cause symptoms or any long-term medical problems, most infected people clear the infection on their own without ever knowing they had it. Every year in the United States, over 6 million people are newly infected with HPV. The highest rates of infection are in women and men in their late teens and early twenties.

Cervical Cancer

Of the 11,000 women in the United States who are diagnosed with invasive cervical cancer in a typical year, more than 50 percent have never had a Pap smear, and another 10 percent have not had a Pap smear in the past five years, according to the National Cancer Institute.

Can I get reinfected with HPV?

Once you have been infected with one type of HPV virus, you usually cannot get infected with that type of HPV again. However, protection against one type of HPV does not provide protection against the others. Because there are many types, it is definitely possible to get HPV again.

How does cervical cancer develop?

If you have not read the "Special Section on Cancer" in part I, you may want to read it now to gain a better understanding of cancer in general.

A *cancer,* or a *malignant tumor,* can be understood as a mass of abnormal cells that develops from normal tissue. Cancer cells are abnormal because they do not grow and die as normal cells do but instead grow larger and more disruptive over time. In cervical cancer, the cancer develops from the cells that line the surface of the cervix.

Cervical cancer develops through gradual changes in the cervix following infection with HPV. When cells are infected by an HPV virus, they often undergo small changes over a few months to a year. Most of the time, HPV goes away on its own and the cervical cells go back to normal within one to two years. But sometimes HPV persists, and the cervical cells undergo further changes, becoming *precancers* (cells that are abnormal but are not yet cancer). If untreated, some of these precancers may develop into cervical cancer (see figure 6.1).

The time between the cervical cells first undergoing changes and the development of cervical cancer presents a window of opportunity. By periodically sampling the cells of the cervix and examining them under a microscope (i.e., a Pap smear), doctors can see if these early precancerous changes have developed, and if so, the precancers can be removed before they develop into cancer.

How do I know if I'm at risk for HPV?

HPV is an STI, so everyone who is sexually active is potentially at risk for infection. You are at higher risk of getting HPV if

- you have had more than one sex partner, or
- your sex partner has had other partners.

Just because someone has few sexual partners or does not engage in "risky behaviors" does not mean he or she cannot have HPV. Remember, most Americans are infected with HPV at some point in their lives.

How do I know if I'm at risk for cervical cancer?

As discussed above, cervical cancer is caused by infection with certain types of HPV. Most infected women, however—even those infected with the high-risk HPV types—do not develop cervical cancer. What causes some infected women to develop cervical cancer and not others is a question that scientists are still trying to answer. So far, the following risk factors have been identified.

Major Risk Factors

- irregular (or no) screening with Pap smears
- smoking
- HIV infection or other immune deficiency
- other sexually transmitted infections (STIs)

Other Risk Factors

- a family history of cervical cancer
- multiparity (giving birth to many children)
- multiple sexual partners

A
Uterus

Cervical canal

Cervix

Area
magnified in
views B – E

Vagina

Female reproductive organs

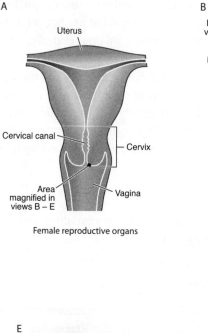

B
Blood
vessel

Basal
cell
layer

Deeper
cervical tissue

Cells lining
the surface
of the cervix

Healthy cervix
(microscopic view)

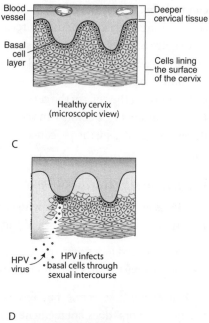

C

HPV
virus

HPV infects
basal cells through
sexual intercourse

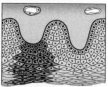

E

Infected cells become cancerous
and invade deeper cervical tissue

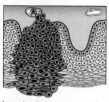

D

Infected cells become abnormal
and precancerous

Figure 6.1. (A) The cervix is the portion of the female genitourinary system that connects the vagina to the uterus. During a routine gynecologic exam, cells from the opening of the cervix can be sampled (called a *Pap smear* or *Pap test*). (B) On a microscopic level, the cervix comprises two cell layers, the surface lining of the cervix and the deeper cervical tissues. In a healthy cervix, the surface lining is maintained by the basal cells. (C) Through sexual contact, the HPV virus can enter the surface lining of the cervix and infect the basal cells. In most women, the infection is transient, and the HPV virus is successfully eradicated by the body's immune defenses. (D) In some women, however, the infection persists and disrupts the normal function of the basal cells. This causes the cells of the surface lining to undergo precancerous changes, which are evident at the microscopic level. (E) Over time, unless treated, some of these precancerous cells grow increasingly abnormal and eventually develop into cancer. Once they become cancerous, they gain the ability to invade the deeper cervical tissue and to spread through the blood vessels to other parts of the body (a process called *metastasis*).

▸ early age of first sexual intercourse
▸ oral contraceptive use (birth control pills)

Although some of these risk factors are out of your control, two of the most potent risk factors for cervical cancer—smoking and lack of screening—are not.

How can I prevent cervical cancer?

There are three ways to prevent cervical cancer: vaccination, risk reduction, and screening.

Vaccination

The cervical cancer vaccine protects against four types of HPV: two high-risk types (16 and 18) and two low-risk types (6 and 11). The vaccine *prevents* infection with these four types of HPV; it cannot cure people already infected, nor can it treat existing genital warts, precancers, or cancers. It also does not provide any protection against other types of HPV, including some that cause cervical cancer. Currently, the vaccine is recommended for all girls between ages 11 and 12 (although it can be given as early as age 9), and for girls and women up to age 26 who have not been previously vaccinated. Women who receive the vaccine still require regular cervical cancer screening. Unfortunately, only one in four teenagers receive the HPV vaccine. In women ages 18 to 26, only one in ten are vaccinated. Section III covers the vaccine in greater depth.

Risk Reduction

HPV is an STI, transmitted from one person to another through sexual contact. The only sure way to prevent HPV is to abstain from all sexual activity. In sexually active people, practicing safer sex (e.g., condom use) can significantly reduce the risk of infection.

Screening

Regular Pap smears can prevent most cases of cervical cancer. Pap smears can lead to the detection and removal of precancers before they develop into cancer. This form of screening can also detect most cervical cancers at an early, curable stage. Section II covers screening in greater depth.

What are the symptoms of HPV?

Most people who are infected with HPV—including those with precancerous changes—do not have any symptoms. Some people, however, usually those infected with the low-risk HPV types, get genital warts. Genital warts appear as soft, moist, pink, or flesh-colored swellings in the genital area. Warts usually appear within weeks or months after sexual contact with an infected person, and without treatment, they usually disappear on their own. Genital warts do not lead to cancer, nor do they predispose a person to cancer, because they are usually caused by different types of HPV than those that cause cervical cancer.

What are the symptoms of cervical cancer?

Symptoms of cervical cancer usually do not develop until the cancer is advanced. Even then, they develop gradually and often go unnoticed at first. Waiting for symptoms to develop leads to a delay in diagnosis that may limit treatment options and chances of survival. Furthermore, the goal of screening is to detect precancerous cervical changes, not cervical cancer. The fact that nearly all women with precancers have no symptoms underscores the dangers of relying on symptoms before seeking medical care. When they develop, symptoms of cervical cancer include vaginal discharge, particularly bloody, foul smelling, and thick; pelvic pain; abnormal vaginal bleeding; and pain during urination. These symptoms can also be found in many other illnesses. If you have any of them, please see a doctor.

How is an HPV infection treated?

There is no current treatment for HPV. However, genital warts, cervical precancers, and cancers of the cervix, vulva, vagina, and anus are treatable diseases that result from infection.

SECTION II: CERVICAL CANCER SCREENING

The USPSTF makes the following recommendations about cervical cancer screening:

- Screening for cervical cancer should be done in women who have been sexually active and have a cervix.
- Screening for cervical cancer is not recommended in women older than 65 if they have had adequate recent screening with normal Pap smears and are not otherwise at high risk for cervical cancer.
- Screening for cervical cancer after total hysterectomy (surgery to remove the uterus and cervix) is not recommended unless the surgery was performed to treat cervical cancer.

The USPSTF suggests that screening be performed using Pap smears. It should begin within three years of onset of sexual activity or at age 21 (whichever comes first) and occur at least every three years. Many health care providers perform more frequent screening than outlined by the USPSTF. In addition, some providers use newer screening techniques, including liquid cytology and HPV testing.

What is a Pap smear?

Most women are familiar with getting a Pap smear, although it is not uncommon to not know much about the test. A Pap smear (or Pap test) is used to find abnormal cells in the cervix. As described above, cervical cancer develops over many years from gradual changes in cells of the cervix infected by HPV. As the cells become precancerous, they begin to undergo changes in their appearance. During a Pap smear, cells are sampled from the cervix and later examined under a microscope to look for the presence of abnormal cells that *may* be the first sign of a developing cancer.

How is it done?

Pap smears are performed during a pelvic, or gynecologic, examination. The following brief overview is for women who have never had a pelvic exam or Pap smear:

1. After changing into a grown or drape, you will be asked to lie down on the examining table and place your heels in footrests called stirrups.
2. Your doctor will place a slender metal or plastic instrument called a *speculum* into your vagina. It is typically lubricated to ease insertion.
3. Once the speculum is in place, your doctor will gently open it in order to get a clear view of the cervix.
4. At this point, your doctor will collect a few cells from the cervix using a small brush. This is the sample that will be used for the Pap smear.
5. Depending on the reason for the exam, your doctor may continue with the remainder of the pelvic exam or simply remove the speculum and complete the examination.

The sample of cervical cells will be sent to a lab for analysis. The results are generally available within one week.

What does an abnormal Pap smear mean?

Interpreting a Pap smear can be complex, so *read this part carefully*.
When a Pap smear comes back as abnormal, it means just that: under the

microscope, the appearance of a few cells in the sample differed in some way from the usual appearance of healthy, intact cervical cells. An abnormal Pap smear does not suggest anything about why the cells were abnormal—only that they were. Besides HPV and early precancerous stages, abnormal cells may signify local irritation or infection, hormonal changes, or simply an error in sample collection or preparation.

Keep in mind that the purpose of the Pap smear is to screen for cervical cancer, not to diagnose it. An abnormal result is meant only to suggest the need for further testing.

If the Pap smear is abnormal, what is the next step?

An abnormal Pap smear *may* mean that you have evidence of precancerous changes or, rarely, cervical cancer. But most of the time, an abnormal Pap smear is due to reasons unrelated to HPV infection, precancerous changes, or cervical cancer. So first step, take a deep breath.

To help sort out the reason for the abnormal Pap smear, you may be asked to come back and have another Pap smear in two to three months. Most benign reasons for an abnormal result are temporary, so repeating the Pap smear after a few months usually allows doctors to differentiate these from more serious causes.

What if the repeat test is also abnormal?

A second abnormal Pap smear usually suggests that you have early precancerous cells in the cervix. Only rarely does it mean that these cells have already progressed to cancer. Again, Pap smears are screening tests, not diagnostic tests. Your doctor will likely recommend colposcopy (a special microscope that helps visualize the cervix) and biopsy (taking a tissue sample of the cervix to study under a microscope) to further evaluate the abnormality and remove potentially abnormal cells.

If the Pap smear is normal, what is the next step?

With a normal Pap smear, no further testing is required. Make sure you document the result and test date for your records. Decide with your doctor when your next screening should be. Per the guidelines, it should typically be no more than three years from now unless you undergo a hysterectomy for benign disease or turn 65.

While this result is reassuring, keep in mind that it may be a false negative. Pap smears sometimes appear normal even when a woman has abnormal cells of the cervix that warrant treatment. Don't let this possibility overly concern you, however. The guidelines for screening were developed with the expectation that sometimes Pap smears miss cervical changes. These changes occur very slowly. By getting regular Pap smears at least every three years, you ensure that most cervical abnormalities are detected before cancer develops.

What is the difference between conventional Pap smear and liquid-based testing?

Liquid-based Pap test, or *liquid-based cytology,* is a newer test for cervical cancer screening. Instead of collecting cells directly onto a glass microscope slide, in this test, the doctor places the sample into a special preservative liquid. Studies show that liquid-based testing is no better at detecting cervical cancers than are conventional Pap smears. However, liquid-based testing reduces the chance that the test will need to be repeated due to technical problems, and it offers the advantage of being able to run the HPV test on the same liquid sample.

What is an HPV test?

The Pap smear detects abnormal cells in the cervix that may be the result of infection with HPV. In contrast, the HPV test looks directly for the HPV virus. The test is done no differently than the Pap smear, and often both can be done at the same time. A few additional cells are brushed from the cervix during a pelvic exam and then sent to a lab to check for the presence of an HPV virus.

The USPSTF does not recommend routine use of the HPV test as the primary screening test for cervical cancer. However, some doctors use the HPV test in two ways:

▸ For women with indefinite Pap smear results, the HPV test is used to "break the tie," to determine whether further evaluation and testing should be done.

▸ For women over age 30 with a history of normal annual Pap smears, the HPV test is used in conjunction with the Pap smear to decrease the frequency of screening to every three years.*

SECTION III: HPV VACCINE GUIDELINES

The CDC makes the following recommendations regarding the HPV vaccine:

---

* This usage is relevant to health care settings in which cervical cancer screening is done annually. Per the USPSTF guidelines, Pap smears need not be done more frequently than every three years, regardless of HPV status.

- ▸ routine administration for girls 11 or 12 years of age
- ▸ administration in girls and women ages 13 through 26 who did not receive the vaccine when they were younger

Studies have found the vaccine to be almost 100 percent effective in preventing diseases caused by the four HPV types it protects against—including genital warts and precancers of the cervix, vulva, and vagina. So far it has been found to be safe and effective in girls and women ages 9 to 26.

Girls and women who have been vaccinated *still* need regular cervical cancer screening for two important reasons. One, the vaccine does not protect against all types of cancer-causing HPV. About 30 percent of cervical cancers will not be prevented by the vaccine. Second, sexually active women who get the vaccine may have already acquired one of the four types of HPV the vaccine protects against and therefore are still at risk of developing cervical cancer from their existing infection.[4]

Why is the HPV vaccine recommended for such young girls?

Ideally, females should get the vaccine *before* they are sexually active because the vaccine only prevents infection and cannot treat those already infected. It provides the greatest benefit to females who have not already acquired any of the four HPV types covered by the vaccine.

Do sexually active females also benefit from the vaccine?

Because HPV infection is so common, a sexually active female has likely been exposed already to one or more HPV types. For these types, the vaccine would not provide any benefit. However, she would still get protection from those types she has not been infected with. Because it is uncommon to be infected with all four HPV types covered by the vaccine, most sexually active females will get some benefit from vaccination.

Why is the HPV vaccine recommended only for females ages 9 to 26?

The vaccine has been widely studied in females ages 9 to 26, so the recommendations to date pertain only to this age group. Research on the vaccine's safety and efficacy has only recently begun in women older than 26 years. Once those studies are complete, the recommendation may be extended to a wider age group.

What about vaccinating boys and men?

Studies to evaluate the safety and effectiveness of the HPV vaccine in boys and men are ongoing. In theory, vaccinating males will prevent penile and anal cancer caused by the same high-risk HPV types that cause cervical cancer in women. It is also possible that vaccinating males will have indirect health benefits for females through the reduction of male-to-female transmission of the virus. If these studies demonstrate significant benefits of male vaccination, the vaccine will likely be recommended for boys and men as well.

How is the vaccine given?

The HPV vaccine is administered in three separate doses, much like many childhood vaccines. The second and third doses should be given two and six months after the first dose, though there is considerable flexibility in the exact timing.

Is the vaccine safe during pregnancy?

The vaccine is not recommended for pregnant women. Studies suggest that the vaccine has *not* caused health problems during pregnancy, nor has it caused health problems for the unborn child—but more research is needed before the safety of the vaccine during pregnancy is confirmed. Until then, pregnant women are being advised to complete their pregnancy before starting the vaccination series or receiving any more doses.

Is it safe? What are the side effects?

The HPV vaccine has been studied in over 11,000 females, ages 9 to 26 years, around the world. These studies have shown no serious side effects, though the medical community is continuing to monitor the safety of the vaccine now that it is in general use. The most common side effect is soreness at the injection site.

REFERENCES

Centers for Disease Control and Prevention (CDC). U.S. Department of Health and Human Services. "Human Papillomavirus (HPV) Infection." www.cdc.gov/STD/HPV.
———. "Quadrivalent Human Papillomavirus Vaccine: Recommendations of the Advisory Committee on Immunization Practices (ACIP)." *MMWR* 56, RR02 (2007).
National Cancer Institute (NCI). National Institutes of Health (NIH). U.S. Department of Health and Human Services. www.cancer.gov.

CHAPTER 7

Chlamydia Screening

C hlamydia is a common sexually transmitted infection (STI). It is often called a silent disease because the symptoms are deceptively mild. As a result, many infected people do not get tested and treated. The infection brews and over time may cause serious complications, such as pelvic inflammatory disease, ectopic pregnancy, and infertility. Untreated infection can also be passed to sexual partners and, during vaginal delivery, to the newborn baby.

Regular screening makes it possible to detect and treat infections with antibiotics before complications develop. Despite the ease of screening, however, many women are not being appropriately tested and treated for chlamydia.

The United States Preventive Services Task Force (USPSTF) recommends screening for chlamydia infection in all sexually active women age 24 or younger and in women age 25 or older with risk factors for infection.[1] The following sections provide an introduction to chlamydia and detail the guidelines for screening in nonpregnant women. Screening for chlamydia in pregnancy is discussed in chapter 19.

SECTION I: CHLAMYDIA 101

Chlamydia (kluh-MID-ee-uh) is an infectious disease named after the bacteria that causes it, *Chlamydia trachomatis.* It is an STI that can be transmitted to a partner during vaginal, anal, or oral sex, or to a baby during vaginal childbirth if the mother is infected.[2]

Chlamydia is one of the most common STIs in the United States and affects over 2 million Americans annually. Men and women in all age groups are susceptible to the disease. However, the risk of infection in teenage girls and young women is particularly high because the cervix is not mature and because the rates of infection among young people are high.

What are the symptoms of chlamydia?

Symptoms usually occur within one to three weeks of infection, if at all. About three-quarters of infected women and half of infected men have no symptoms, which is why a person can be infected with chlamydia and not even know it.

Symptoms in men:

- painful urination or burning sensation while urinating
- penile discharge
- testicular pain

Symptoms in women:

- painful urination or burning sensation while urinating
- lower abdominal pain
- vaginal discharge
- painful sexual intercourse

The presence or absence of symptoms does not correlate with disease severity. People without symptoms of infection are just as likely as people with symptoms to develop complications. In fact, because they are less likely to seek medical attention, people without symptoms may actually fare worse.

What complications can it cause?

If untreated, chlamydia can cause serious and permanent health problems:

- The infection can spread in women to the uterus or fallopian tubes, leading to *pelvic inflammatory disease* (PID). PID is a serious disease that can permanently damage the uterus, fallopian tubes, and adjacent tissues, which in turn can cause infertility, chronic pelvic pain, and *ectopic pregnancy,* a potentially fatal pregnancy outside the uterus. As many as 30 percent of women with untreated chlamydia develop PID.

- Chlamydia infection in women makes them up to five times more likely to contract an HIV infection.

- In men, chlamydia infection can cause nongonococcal urethritis (infection of the inside of the penis) and acute epididymitis (infection of the tube that carries sperm from the testis). These painful infections cause fever and can rarely lead to sterility. Long-term complications include infertility, chronic prostatitis (inflammation of the prostate), reactive arthritis (inflammation of the joints), and urethral strictures (scarring of the opening of the penis).

▸ In pregnant women, chlamydia infection is associated with preterm delivery and postpartum endometritis (infection of the uterus).

▸ Between 20 and 50 percent of babies born to women with active chlamydia infection will develop conjunctivitis, an infection of the eye that may lead to blindness. They are also at risk of infant pneumonia.

With treatment, most of these complications can be avoided. However, treatment cannot take place until the disease is diagnosed, which means that people must be made aware of the disease and the need for screening.

What can I do to prevent chlamydia?

The best ways to avoid chlamydia infection are to abstain from sexual contact or have sex only with a long-term partner who is monogamous, has been tested, and is known to be free of infection. You can practice safer sex in other ways that minimize your risk. The following practices can help prevent chlamydia and other STIs:

▸ *Use condoms correctly and consistently.* The correct use of protective barriers such as male or female condoms during every sexual encounter drastically decreases the risk of chlamydia and other STIs.

▸ *Limit your number of sexual partners.* Having multiple sexual partners increases the risk of infection.

▸ *Get regularly screened for STIs.* Become informed about how often you should get screened for STIs and make sure you are up to date.

▸ *Encourage your sexual partner(s) to be screened regularly for STIs.* When you enter into a new sexual relationship, find out if your partner has been recently tested, and if not, work with him or her to get tested before becoming sexually intimate.

SECTION II: CHLAMYDIA SCREENING

The USPSTF recommends that sexually active women age 24 or younger be routinely screened for chlamydia. In addition, the task force recommends screening women age 25 or older who have one or more risk factors, including

- multiple sexual partners in the past three months or a new sexual partner
- inconsistent condom use during sexual intercourse
- a history of chlamydia or other STIs (including gonorrhea, syphilis, hepatitis B, genital herpes, and HIV)
- a history of exchanging sex for drugs or money

These recommendations are based on evidence that screening tests for chlamydia are accurate and that screening at-risk women reduces the risk of complications.

The Centers for Disease Control and Prevention (CDC) recommends that women at increased risk be screened at least annually. For women who have tested negative for chlamydia, when to get screened next is an individual decision. If you are in the same monogamous relationship you were in during your last test, it is probably safe to wait one year. However, if you are with a new partner or have multiple sexual partners, you may want to get screened more often.

Screening for chlamydia is relatively simple. Two tests are most common:

- *Swab test:* For women, a mucous sample is taken from the cervix using a swab. In men, a sample can be taken from the penis. In addition, a culture swab of the anus can be performed.
- *Urine test:* A sample of urine is collected and then analyzed in a laboratory.

Both tests are acceptable for screening purposes. In women, obtaining a swab may require a pelvic exam; in men, the swab can be painful and is not routinely done. In comparison, a urine test is easier to perform and better tolerated. Thus, the swab test is generally used only in women already having a pelvic exam for another reason (e.g., Pap smears). In men and in women not otherwise requiring a pelvic exam, the urine test is preferred. Because the risk factors and screening tests for chlamydia and gonorrhea are similar, doctors routinely screen people for both STIs at once.

Why do only women need screening?

Chlamydia affects both men and women. It causes health problems in both men and women and can be transmitted to others by men and women. So it is a fair question to ask why screening is recommended only for women.

To date, the USPSTF has concluded that the evidence is insufficient to recommend routine screening in men. The direct benefit to men of screening is small because infection is more likely to be associated with symptoms, and the health risks of untreated chlamydia infection in men are relatively low. Although screening in men may still be beneficial if it leads to decreased chlamydia in women, there is insufficient evidence to support this reasoning.

That being said, it is not unreasonable to screen men for chlamydia. Screening for chlamydia in men is safe and may provide health benefits to the screened individual and his sexual partners. If you are a man and are at increased risk of chlamydia or have concerns about being infected, talk to your doctor about whether screening is right for you.

What does being age 24 or under have to do with anything?

Just as studies have shown that women who have multiple sexual partners or a history of STIs are at higher risk for chlamydia, they have also shown that sexually active women age 24 or under are at increased risk. Not only are the majority of chlamydia infections in women age 24 or under, but this age group also has the highest rate of complications.

What are the risks of screening?

The screening tests are safe and have no risks. However, if the test is positive and you are diagnosed with chlamydia, you will need antibiotic treatment, which can have side effects.

What happens if the screen is negative?

A negative screen means that you do not have chlamydia. Rarely, the screen will be falsely negative, but the chances of this are less than 1 percent. Be sure to document the results for your records. And be sure to talk to your doctor about when you should schedule your next screening test and about what you can do to lower your risk of infection.

What happens if the screen is positive?

A positive screening test is equivalent to a diagnosis. This means you are infected with chlamydia. Treating chlamydia effectively requires two components. First, chlamydia can be easily treated and cured with antibiotics. Depending on the antibiotic your doctor chooses, your treatment course may be a single dose or a weeklong course. The second component is to test and, if necessary, treat sexual partner(s) for chlamydia infection. Chances are high that your sexual partner also has chlamydia. Antibiotics treat the disease, but they don't prevent you from getting it again. If you are treated for chlamydia but your partner isn't, your risk of getting infected again is extremely high.

Because you have chlamydia, you are considered at high risk for having other STIs, including gonorrhea, syphilis, and HIV. Talk with your doctor about getting tested for them. And be sure to talk to your doctor about how you can lower your risk of STIs through safer sex practices. Everyone who has a history of sexually transmitted infection in the past year is advised to receive STI counseling (see chapter 20 for more details).

REFERENCES

Centers for Disease Control and Prevention (CDC). U.S. Department of Health and Human Services. "Sexually Transmitted Diseases." www.cdc.gov/std.

Cholesterol Screening

Cholesterol disorders are one of the major risk factors for cardiovascular disease. Despite its importance, cholesterol is often misunderstood. First, even though older people are at higher risk for cardiovascular disease, they are not the only people who need to pay attention to cholesterol. Knowing about cholesterol is important for *everyone:* young, middle age, and older adults; women and men; and people with cardiovascular disease as well as people without it. Cardiovascular disease is the result of decades of cholesterol buildup. Indeed, atherosclerosis and the fatty buildup of plaque begin when we are teenagers. Preventing heart attacks and strokes requires a lifetime of attention to eating right, exercising regularly, not smoking, and monitoring risk factor levels.

Second, there are generally no signs or symptoms of cholesterol disorders. Furthermore, it is difficult to predict who has a cholesterol disorder and who does not. Eating healthy helps keep cholesterol under control but by no means guarantees normal cholesterol. The same goes for being young, exercising regularly, not smoking, and maintaining a healthy weight—all of these help, but none guarantees normal cholesterol levels. *The only way to truly know your cholesterol level is to have it checked periodically.*

Finally, keeping cholesterol under control is easier today than ever before. Doctors now have a solid understanding of how diet and lifestyle affect cholesterol levels, and they have a wide array of medications to help people maintain heart-healthy cholesterol levels.

The United States Preventive Services Task Force (USPSTF) recommends cholesterol screening in all men age 35 or older and in women and younger men at increased risk for coronary heart disease.[1] The following sections provide an introduction to cholesterol and cholesterol disorders and explain how cholesterol screening can help you lead a healthier life.

SECTION I: CHOLESTEROL 101

Cholesterol is a waxy, fatlike substance that is present in all the cells in the body. Cholesterol isn't all bad! It is used to make vital hormones and vitamins and to help maintain cells. But too much cholesterol—in particular the bad kinds of cholesterol—can harm the body and lead to cardiovascular disease. *If you have not read the "Special Section on Cardiovascular Disease" in part I, you may want to read it now to gain a better understanding of that disease.*

The terms *cholesterol* and *lipids* are used interchangeably, but the term *lipid* is more general because there are other types of lipids besides cholesterol. In this book, the term *cholesterol* is used. However, if your doctor is talking about lipids, chances are he or she is talking about the same thing.

Most cholesterol is stored in the cells, but some of it can be found in the blood. Excess cholesterol in the blood can be harmful.

Cholesterol is transported in the blood on particles called *lipoproteins*. The most important lipoproteins to know about are low-density lipoproteins (LDL) and high-density lipoproteins (HDL). Medical studies have shown that elevated levels of LDL cholesterol are associated with an increased risk of coronary heart disease (CHD), whereas elevated levels of HDL cholesterol reduce that risk and protect the heart. Thus, doctors refer to LDL as "bad cholesterol" and to HDL as "good cholesterol."*

How does cholesterol cause harm?

Too much cholesterol in the blood leads to *atherosclerosis* (ath-er-o-skle-RO-sis), or the buildup of deposits of cholesterol inside the arteries. These deposits, or plaque, can narrow an artery enough to slow blood flow and over time can lead to symptoms such as chest pain (called *angina*). More seriously, a plaque can rupture and completely block an artery, leading to a heart attack, stroke, or sudden death. Fortunately, the buildup of plaque can be slowed, stopped, or even reversed through lifestyle modifications and medications.

Wait, so not all types of cholesterol are bad?

Exactly. LDL, or bad cholesterol, increases the amount of cholesterol in the blood by depositing cholesterol in the artery walls, where it can lead to plaque formation. HDL, or good cholesterol, helps eliminate cholesterol

---

* VLDL is another type of "bad cholesterol" like LDL. However, there is no simple way to measure VLDL levels, so much of the attention in cholesterol disorders is focused on HDL and LDL.

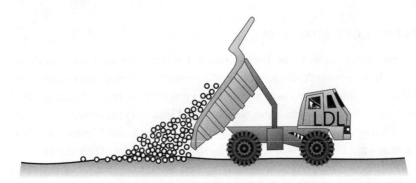

LDL deposits plaque-forming cholesterol on artery wall

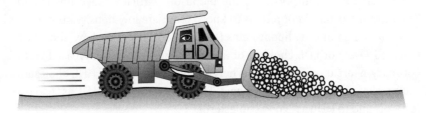

HDL clears away the cholesterol, preventing plaque formation

Figure 8.1. Not all cholesterol is bad for you. LDL is the bad cholesterol. It unloads cholesterol in the arteries, clogging them up like grease in a kitchen pipe. We want *Low* LDL. HDL is the good cholesterol. It scoops cholesterol out of the arteries. We want *High* HDL. Remember, H is great and L is lousy.

from the blood by removing cholesterol from cells and plaques and carrying it to the liver. Furthermore, studies have shown that increasing the level of HDL and lowering the level of LDL helps prevent cardiovascular disease (see figure 8.1). The big picture? The higher your LDL and the lower your HDL, the greater your risk for atherosclerosis and cardiovascular disease. We want our LDL to be *Low* and our HDL to be *High*. Or think of H as great and L as lousy. This is worth remembering; try committing it to memory.

What are triglycerides?

Triglycerides (tri-GLISS-er-ides) are another type of lipid found in the blood. They also exist in fat cells and play an important role in fat metabolism. When we eat, excess calories are converted into triglycerides and stored as fat. Between meals, triglycerides can be released back into the bloodstream to meet our energy needs. Like LDL cholesterol, excess triglycerides (called *hypertriglyceridemia*) is a risk factor for CHD. Because triglycerides are in the same family as cholesterol and are routinely measured by cholesterol tests, doctors often consider triglycerides and cholesterol together. However, because the recommendations for cholesterol screening and treatment primarily relate to LDL and HDL cholesterol, the focus of this chapter is on cholesterol.

SECTION II: CHOLESTEROL DISORDERS 101

Someone is said to have a *cholesterol disorder* when his or her LDL level is too high or HDL too low—or both.

Cholesterol disorders can be confusing because many terms describe the same disease. The following all refer to the same medical problem:

- cholesterol disorder
- lipid disorder
- dyslipidemia (diss-lip-uh-DEE-mee-uh)
- hypercholesterolemia (hi-per-kuh-less-tuh-ruh-LEE-mee-uh)
- hyperlipidemia (hi-per-lip-uh-DEE-mee-uh)
- abnormal cholesterol
- abnormal lipids

In addition, the general public often hears the phrase "high cholesterol." All of these terms and phrases are equivalent. They basically describe someone whose LDL is too high or HDL is too low. To avoid confusion, the term *cholesterol disorder* is used throughout this book.

How common are cholesterol disorders?

No matter what you call them, cholesterol disorders are common. It is estimated that among adults in the United States,

- one in every three people has too much LDL (bad) cholesterol;
- one in every four men and one in every fifteen women have too little HDL (good) cholesterol; and
- nearly one in every two people has too much total cholesterol.

What causes cholesterol disorders?

The following factors put a person at risk for developing a cholesterol disorder:

▸ *Smoking:* Smoking increases LDL (bad cholesterol) and decreases HDL (good cholesterol). The more you smoke, the more likely you are to develop a cholesterol disorder.

▸ *Family history:* Genes influence LDL cholesterol. Some people are born at high risk for having a cholesterol disorder. One specific inherited cholesterol disorder is *familial hypercholesterolemia,* a genetic disease that one in five hundred people are born with. But even if you do not have a specific genetic cause of abnormal cholesterol, your genes influence your cholesterol levels. This is why people with a family history of cholesterol disorders, especially in first-degree relatives, are at higher risk.

▸ *Diet:* What you eat affects LDL cholesterol. Recent studies show that the types of fats are more important than the amount of cholesterol you consume.

▸ *Exercise:* Regular physical activity lowers triglycerides and raises HDL cholesterol.

▸ *Age and gender:* As you age, LDL cholesterol increases. Before the age of menopause, women usually have lower total cholesterol levels than men. After menopause, women often have higher cholesterol levels than men. Cholesterol isn't just a man's problem.

▸ *Diabetes:* High sugar levels coat LDL cholesterol, causing it to stay in the blood longer. People with diabetes also tend to have low HDL and high numbers of triglycerides.

▸ *Weight:* Excess weight tends to increase LDL cholesterol. Weight loss has been shown to decrease LDL, increase HDL, and decrease triglycerides— all of which can decrease the risk of cardiovascular disease.

What diseases do cholesterol disorders cause?

Cholesterol disorders are one of the major risk factors for atherosclerosis. Through atherosclerosis, cholesterol disorders can cause the following diseases:

- coronary heart disease (including angina, heart attacks, heart failure, and sudden cardiac death)
- high blood pressure
- stroke
- carotid artery disease
- peripheral vascular disease (including claudication and gangrene)
- abdominal aortic aneurysm (AAA)
- retinopathy (eye damage)
- nephropathy (kidney damage)

Rarely, cholesterol disorders can cause symptoms or complications directly, such as pancreatitis from very elevated triglyceride levels.

How can people improve their cholesterol levels?

There are two ways to improve cholesterol: lifestyle modifications and cholesterol-modifying medications. Lifestyle modifications include healthier eating, regular aerobic exercise, weight management, and smoking cessation. Studies show that even a 10 percent decrease in total cholesterol can reduce the risk of heart attack by 20 to 30 percent. Below, healthier eating, exercise and cholesterol-modifying medications are discussed in more detail.

Healthier Eating

A common myth is that the key to improving cholesterol is reducing the amount of cholesterol you eat. While limiting dietary cholesterol is still recommended, studies show that changing the amount and types of fat that you eat is more important. Cholesterol in the blood comes from two sources: it is either absorbed from the food or made in the body. Of the two sources, more of the cholesterol in the blood comes from the body, which in turn depends largely on the amount and types of fat that you eat. *The biggest influence of the diet on blood cholesterol level is the mixture of fats in the diet, not the total amount of cholesterol.* Reducing trans fat and saturated fats and substituting monounsaturated and polyunsaturated fats can significantly shift the balance of the bad and good cholesterol in favor of reducing the risk of CHD, as illustrated in table 8.1.

Exercise

Physical inactivity is a major risk factor for CHD. Not only does regular aerobic exercise lower your risk of CHD by reducing obesity, high blood pres-

Table 8.1: The four fats

Type of fat	Main source	Effect on cholesterol
Monounsaturated	Olives; olive, canola, and peanut oils; cashews, almonds, peanuts, and most other nuts; avocados	Lowers LDL; raises HDL
Polyunsaturated	Corn, soybean, safflower, and cotton-seed oils; fish	Lowers LDL; raises HDL
Saturated	Whole milk, butter, cheese, and ice cream; beef, pork, and lamb; chocolate; coconuts	Raises both LDL and HDL
Trans	Most margarines; vegetable shortening; partially hydrogenated vegetable oil; many fast foods, processed foods, and commercial baked goods	Raises LDL

Source: Adapted from Walter C. Willett, M.D., *Eat, Drink, and Be Healthy: The Harvard Medical School Guide to Healthy Eating* (Free Press, 2001).

Note: The unsaturated fats—monounsaturated and polyunsaturated—are the good fats. Saturated and trans fat are the bad fats. An easy way to remember this is to think of the UN-saturated fats as un-fat, as in un-bad for you. All other fats are bad.

sure, and diabetes, but it also directly increases HDL cholesterol and reduces triglycerides. Studies show that at least thirty minutes of moderate exercise on most days of the week can improve your cholesterol levels and overall risk of cardiovascular disease. Keep in mind that exercise does not necessarily mean running or sweating it out in the gym. Physical activity includes a range of activities, such as hiking, biking, swimming, gardening, team sports, and dancing. The only caveat is that with lower intensity activities, it is important to strive for more minutes of activity, usually between forty-five minutes to an hour. Also, there is no need to do your entire daily workout in one setting. Breaking up your exercise regimen into two fifteen-minute blocks can make it more manageable yet provide the same benefits to cholesterol levels and cardiovascular health.

Cholesterol-Modifying Medications

There are several classes of cholesterol-modifying medications, including statins, bile acid sequestrants, nicotinic acid, fibric acids, and cholesterol absorption inhibitors. Most of these medicines have excellent side effect profiles and are effective when used to complement lifestyle modifications.

The most commonly prescribed cholesterol-modifying medications are statins (STAT-ins). They work by interfering with the activity of an enzyme in the liver responsible for producing cholesterol. On average, statins produce a 25 to 55 percent reduction in LDL levels, a 5 to 15 percent increase in HDL, and a 10 to 25 percent decrease in triglycerides. More important, they are associated with a one-quarter to one-third reduction in heart attacks and strokes in people at increased risk of CHD.

SECTION III: CHOLESTEROL SCREENING

The USPSTF recommends that all men age 35 or older receive routine screening for cholesterol disorders. In addition, the task force recommends that men between ages 20 and 35 and adult women age 20 or older receive cholesterol screening if they have one or more of the following risk factors:

- diabetes
- high blood pressure
- obesity (body mass index [BMI] ≥30 kg/m²)
- tobacco use
- a family history of early cardiovascular disease (before age 50 in first-degree male relatives or 60 in female relatives)
- a personal history of CHD or noncoronary atherosclerosis (e.g., abdominal aortic aneurysm, peripheral artery disease, carotid artery stenosis)

How does cholesterol screening work?

Cholesterol disorders are screened with a routine blood test called a *cholesterol panel*, or *lipid profile*. Sometimes your doctor may ask you not to eat or drink anything other than water for the nine to twelve hours before the blood test in order to get a fasting cholesterol level. Fasting blood tests are more accurate than nonfasting tests because they directly measure the LDL level in the blood; however, they are less convenient because you often have to schedule the test for a later date after a planned fast. For screening purposes, both fasting and nonfasting tests are acceptable.

How often should I get screened?

No study has clearly defined the best interval for cholesterol screening. Some organizations recommend screening every five years as long as cholesterol levels remain normal and every one to two years when cholesterol levels are in the borderline range. Decide with your doctor what is best for you, and regardless of the decision, be consistent and follow up on your results.

I just received my results. Can you help me understand them?

The test report will show the cholesterol levels in milligrams per deciliter of blood (mg/dL). A complete fasting lipoprotein profile will show four levels:

- *Total blood (or serum) cholesterol:* Total cholesterol is made up of LDL cholesterol, HDL cholesterol, and VLDL cholesterol. A desirable level of total cholesterol is lower than 200 mg/dL.

- *HDL (good) cholesterol:* For men, an HDL lower than 40 mg/dL is considered a risk factor for cardiovascular disease. For women, an HDL lower than 50 mg/dL is considered a risk factor.

- *Triglyceride level:* Triglycerides are the most common type of fat in the body. If they are above 150 mg/dL, the risk of heart disease or stroke may be increased.

- *LDL (bad) cholesterol:* Unlike the other three measures, LDL cholesterol is more difficult to interpret because the goal range for LDL varies from person to person. For someone with one or no risk factors for cardiovascular disease, the goal LDL is under 160 mg/dL; for someone with two or more risk factors, the goal LDL is under 130 mg/dL; for someone who has a CHD risk equivalent (e.g., diabetes) or a history of CHD, the goal LDL is under 100 mg/dL. Your doctor will determine your goal LDL based on your individual risk factors and medical history.

Table 8.2 demonstrates the range of values for each number and what they mean. Keep in mind, however, that target LDL cholesterol levels vary based on individual risk of cardiovascular disease.

Understanding the cholesterol panel is important. Often, we hear someone say, "I just got my cholesterol checked, and my doctor said my cholesterol was high." Remember that there are different types of cholesterol, both good and bad. Knowing that your cholesterol is abnormal is the first step. Strive to know which of the cholesterol numbers are abnormal and how abnormal they are.

Table 8.2: Cholesterol panel reference ranges

Total cholesterol (mg/dL)	
<200	Optimal
200–239	Borderline high
≥240	High
LDL cholesterol (mg/dL)	
<100	Optimal
100–129	Near optimal
130–159	Borderline high
160–189	High
≥190	Very high
HDL cholesterol (mg/dL)	
<40	Low
≥60	Optimal
Triglycerides (mg/dL)	
<150	Optimal
150–199	Borderline high
200–499	High
≥500	Very high

Note: Classification of cholesterol reference ranges is based on the National Cholesterol Education Program Adult Treatment Panel III guidelines.

What happens if my cholesterol is within the normal range?

This means that you do not have a cholesterol disorder. Be sure to ask your doctor for a copy of the results. Find out when your next cholesterol screening should be and note the date for your records. It should typically be no later than five years from now.

What happens if my cholesterol is abnormal?

Generally, abnormal results should be confirmed with a repeat test. The results from both tests are then averaged to assess your risk and decide what steps to take. For the repeat test, the doctor may schedule you for a fasting cholesterol test. This means that you should not eat or drink anything other than water for nine to twelve hours before the blood test.

What happens if the repeat test is also abnormal?

Having two abnormal cholesterol tests is sufficient to diagnose you with a cholesterol disorder. It is important to understand what this means and what this does not mean. It doesn't mean that something bad is necessarily going to happen to you. You are not necessarily going to need cholesterol-modifying medicines for the rest of your life. It simply means that you are at increased risk for CHD and stroke and need to take measures to improve your cholesterol.

Everyone with a cholesterol disorder should undergo lifestyle modifications as discussed in section II. This includes changing your diet to eliminate harmful fats and sources high in cholesterol, maintaining a healthy weight, exercising at least thirty minutes a day on most days of the week, and quitting smoking. However, the decision to start cholesterol-modifying medications is better made between you and your doctor. Many doctors will start with a trial of lifestyle modifications to see if you can improve your cholesterol levels without medication first.

Because having a cholesterol disorder increases your overall risk of cardiovascular disease, you may benefit from additional preventive measures such as diabetes screening (chapter 11), aspirin (chapter 3), intensive healthy eating counseling (chapter 14), and smoking cessation (chapter 22).

Unfortunately, many people do not take the critical next step of addressing their cholesterol disorder. Less than half of Americans who should be taking cholesterol-modifying treatment are actually receiving it. Furthermore, only about one-third of those receiving treatment are at their goal LDL level. Getting your cholesterol under control is possible, and thousands of Americans do it every year. The key is to partner with your doctor and take action.

REFERENCES

National Heart, Lung, and Blood Institute (NHLBI). U.S. Department of Health and Human Services. National Institutes of Health. www.nhlbi.nih.gov.

———. *Third Report of the National Cholesterol Education Program (NCEP) Expert Panel on Detection, Evaluation, and Treatment of High Blood Cholesterol in Adults (Adult Treatment Panel III)*. NIH Publication No. 02-5215. Bethesda, Md.: Department of Health and Human Services, National Institutes of Health, September 2002.

Colon Cancer Screening

Colon cancer is the third most common cancer among men and women in the United States and the second leading cause of death from cancer.* The National Cancer Institute estimates that about 150,000 Americans will have been diagnosed in 2009. This means that one in every twenty people born today will develop colon cancer in his or her lifetime.

Screening is the only proven method for preventing colon cancer, and it reduces death from colon cancer by up to 33 percent.[1] Screening can detect precancerous polyps, before cancer develops, when they can be easily removed. Even if cancer has already developed, screening offers the best hope of early detection and treatment—even cure. Despite the widespread acceptance of routine colon cancer screening by doctors, fewer than 50 percent of adults age 50 or older are up to date with screening. As a result, the majority of people who develop colon cancer are diagnosed at an advanced stage, when treatment options are limited and cure is less likely.

The United States Preventive Services Task Force (USPSTF) recommends screening for colon cancer in men and women between ages 50 and 75.[2] This chapter describes colon cancer and the importance of colon cancer screening, details the screening recommendations, and explains how screening is done.

SECTION I: COLON CANCER 101

The terms *colon cancer* and *colorectal cancer* are used interchangeably. Strictly speaking, colorectal cancer includes the colon and the rectum, whereas colon cancer refers only to the colon. In practice, however, both terms are used to refer to cancer of the colon and rectum. The term colon cancer is used in this book.

* Excluding nonmelanoma skin cancers (e.g., basal cell carcinoma and squamous cell carcinoma).

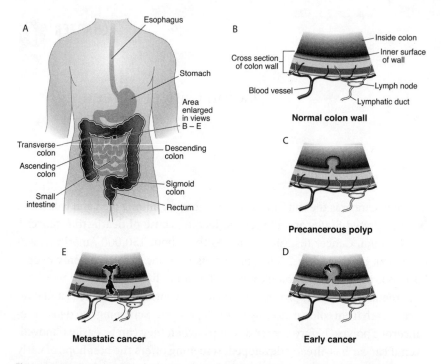

Figure 9.1. (A) The colon (also called the large intestine) is the segment of the digestive tract that connects the small intestine to the rectum. It has four parts: the ascending colon, transverse colon, descending colon, and sigmoid colon. Colon cancer can develop in any of these segments, though it most commonly forms in the descending colon and sigmoid colon. (B) Colon cancer develops on the inside wall, or lining, of the colon. (C) It starts as a precancerous polyp. (D) Unless treated, the polyp over time may develop into cancer. (E) After more time, the cancer may invade the colon wall and metastasize to other parts of the body, through the blood, or through the lymphatic system.

The digestive tract is one long tube that goes from the mouth to the anus. Different segments of the tube have different names. The colon and rectum are two segments of the tube. Together, they are called the large intestine, or large bowel. The colon is further subdivided into smaller segments, each with its own name. The last segment of the colon, which leads to the rectum, is called the sigmoid colon, or simply sigmoid. These terms are illustrated in figure 9.1.

The function of the colon is to package waste and absorb water into the body. In adults, it is about five feet long and connects the small intestine (or small bowel) to the rectum. The function of the rectum is to store waste material (feces) until it is eliminated from the body. It is about six inches long and leads from the colon to the anus.

What exactly is colon cancer?

If you have not read the "Special Section on Cancer" in part I, you may want to read it now to gain a better understanding of cancer in general.

A *cancer*, or a *malignant tumor*, can be understood as a mass of abnormal cells that developed from normal tissue. Cancer cells are abnormal because they do not grow and die as normal cells do; instead they grow larger and more disruptive. In colon cancer, the cancer develops from the lining of the colon. Through colonoscopy, which involves placing a tiny camera into the colon, doctors are able to see the cancer and sometimes cut all or part of it out.

How does colon cancer develop?

In most people, colon cancer is a slowly progressive disease that takes years to develop. The disease begins with a collection of abnormal cells so small it cannot be seen with the naked eye. Over time, the cells multiply and become more abnormal. After five years or so, the cells are numerous enough to be visible. At this phase, the collection of cells is called a *precancerous polyp*. A doctor can see the polyp and cut it out during a colonoscopy. Unless removed, the precancerous polyp may become larger and more abnormal.

Eventually, after ten to fifteen years, the precancerous polyp may develop into cancer. Once the polyp becomes cancerous, the cancer not only grows bigger but also begins to invade other parts of the colon. Eventually the cancer may spread to other parts of the body, including the liver. At this stage, it is called *metastatic cancer*. That colon cancer takes years to develop means that there are many opportunities for doctors to find and stop the disease, sometimes even before cancer develops.

How dangerous is colon cancer?

The risk of death from colon cancer varies greatly depending on the stage when cancer is found. People with early stage colon cancer have over a 90 percent chance of survival over five years. People with metastatic cancer, after the cancer has spread to other organs, have less than a 10 percent chance of survival. And people who are screened at the precancerous polyp stage have nearly a 100 percent survival rate. Colon cancer screening is designed to catch the disease before symptoms develop, at the earliest stage possible, when the chances of survival are highest.

What are the symptoms of colon cancer?

Most people with colon cancer have no symptoms. This fact often leads people to decide that they do not need to be screened for colon cancer. They may say, "I don't need testing. I can't have cancer because I feel perfectly fine." But it is common not to have any symptoms of colon cancer in its early stages. That's why screening of healthy people is recommended; screening finds disease before it causes symptoms.

Over time, symptoms develop. Changes in bowel habit, blood in the stool, and generalized symptoms such as weight loss and fatigue are symptoms of colon cancer and of other diseases too. If you have any of these symptoms, see your doctor.

Waiting to develop symptoms before getting screened for colon cancer is dangerous because symptoms usually suggest a later stage of disease. *Screening* is meant for people without any symptoms. *Diagnosis* is for people with symptoms. Clearly, screening is preferable.

What causes colon cancer? Can I do anything to prevent it?

Doctors do not fully understand why some people develop colon cancer and others do not. However, they have identified a number of risk factors:[3]

- *Age* is the most significant risk factor for developing colon cancer. Of people diagnosed with it, 90 percent are age 50 or older. The older you are, the greater your chances of developing colon cancer. The average age of diagnosis is about 70. But people in their fifties should not take this as a reason to not get screened. Half the cases of colon cancer occur in people between ages 50 and 70. And keep in mind that incurable cancer at age 70 may have been an easily removable precancerous polyp at age 50.

- As discussed earlier, some *precancerous polyps* are precursors to colon cancer. Having precancerous polyps therefore increases the risk of developing colon cancer. Finding and removing precancerous polyps reduces this risk.

- Changes or mutations in *certain genes* increase the risk of colorectal cancer. Hereditary nonpolyposis colon cancer (HNPCC) is the most common inherited disease that causes colorectal cancer. Most people with HNPCC develop colon cancer in their lifetimes and often before age 50, when screening typically begins. Familial adenomatous polyposis (FAP) is another inherited disease that causes colon cancer. It is marked by hundreds of polyps throughout the colon that predispose affected individuals to developing colon cancer by age 40, unless the colon is removed.

▸ A *family history of colon cancer* is also associated with increased risk. People with a history of colon cancer in first-degree relatives (parents, siblings, or children) are more likely to develop the disease. This is especially true if the relative had the cancer before age 60. It is important to know your family history of colon cancer because some expert organizations recommend more intensive screening for people with strong family histories—see section II for more detail.

▸ People with *a personal history of ulcerative colitis or Crohn's disease*, collectively known as inflammatory bowel disease, are at increased risk of developing colon cancer.

▸ A *low-fiber, high-fat diet* may increase your risk of colorectal cancer. Also, people with diets high in red meats and low in fruits and vegetables may be at increased risk.

▸ *Cigarette smoking* is another risk factor. People who smoke are at increased risk for colon cancer. Another reason to quit.

No diet or pill has been proven to reduce the risk of colon cancer. Smokers may decrease their risk by quitting smoking, although this has not been shown directly in medical studies. Although recent studies have suggested that low-fiber, high-fat diets are associated with colon cancer, studies have not yet conclusively shown that changing your diet can lower your risk of developing this cancer. Screening is the only proven method for preventing it. By removing precancerous polyps that may one day progress into cancer, doctors can reduce your risk of colon cancer.

SECTION II: COLON CANCER SCREENING

The USPSTF makes the following recommendations about colon cancer screening:

▸ screening in adults beginning at age 50 and continuing until age 75 using fecal occult blood testing, sigmoidoscopy, or colonoscopy
▸ against routine screening in adults age 76 to 85 years, though some considerations may support screening in an individual patient
▸ against screening in adults older than age 85

These recommendations are based on evidence that several screening methods are effective in reducing death from colon cancer and that the benefits of these methods outweigh the risks in individuals ages 50 to 75.

These recommendations do not apply to people with specific inherited syndromes, such as familial adenomatous polyposis (FAP) and hereditary nonpolyposis, or to those with inflammatory bowel disease (e.g., Crohn's disease, ulcerative colitis). For people with first-degree relatives who developed cancer before age 60, or with multiple affected first-degree relatives, an earlier start to screening may be reasonable (see below for further discussion).

The USPSTF recommends screening with one of the three following options:

- *Option 1*: high-sensitivity fecal occult blood testing (FOBT) every year. This test checks for small amounts of blood in the stool that can be a sign of colon cancer or precancerous polyps. It is a simple test that can be done at home. The primary disadvantage is that it is neither highly *sensitive* (sometimes the test does not detect colon cancer when it is present) nor highly *specific* (sometimes the test suggests that colon cancer is present when it is not).

- *Option 2*: flexible sigmoidoscopy every five years, with high-sensitivity FOBT every three years. In flexible sigmoidoscopy, doctors use a tiny camera to inspect the sigmoid colon (last segment of the colon) and rectum. If something abnormal is seen, the doctor can take a sample of the abnormal tissue to examine under a microscope. The main advantage of this test is that it has high sensitivity and specificity. The main disadvantage is that it checks only the sigmoid and rectum and may miss cancers higher up in the colon.

- *Option 3*: screening colonoscopy every ten years. As in the flexible sigmoidoscopy, in this test doctors use a tiny camera to inspect the colon. The colonoscopy, however, enables doctors to inspect the entire colon, not just the sigmoid. It is considered the gold standard test for diagnosing colon cancer (high sensitivity and specificity), and thus can be used to both screen and diagnose colon cancer at the same time. The main disadvantage is that the procedure carries greater health risks than the other screening tests.

There is no clear evidence that one of the above methods for screening is better than another. Each option has pros and cons, and the decision about which to choose is up to you and your doctor. In the following pages, each screening method is discussed in detail.

Some organizations recommend other screening tests, including *double-contrast barium enema*, *CT colonography* (also called *virtual colonoscopy*), and *fecal DNA testing*. These screening methods are discussed briefly below.

What about people at high risk for colon cancer?

The USPSTF guidelines apply to men and women at average risk for colorectal cancer. In people at higher risk (for example, those with a first-degree relative diagnosed with colorectal cancer before 60 years of age), the task force states that initiating screening at an earlier age may be advisable but makes no specific recommendations. Other respected professional organizations, however, such as the American Cancer Society (ACS) and the American Gastroenterological Association, make evidence-based recommendations on screening for colon cancer in higher risk groups. For example, in people with a history of colon cancer or precancerous polyps in a first-degree relative before age 60 or in two or more first-degree relatives with colon cancer at any age, the ACS recommends screening with colonoscopy every five years beginning at age 40 or ten years before the youngest case in the immediate family (whichever is earlier).[4]

If you are at increased risk of colon cancer because of a strong family history of colon cancer or a personal history of colon disease, talk to your doctor about whether a more intensive screening program is right for you.

Why is screening not recommended in people age 76 or older?

The primary reason for the decreased emphasis on screening older adults is that the benefits of screening are limited by competing causes of death, even though colon cancer becomes more common at older ages. It takes about seven years before the benefits of colon cancer screening can be seen; therefore, in older adults who have a limited life expectancy, the benefit of screening is diminished while the risks stay the same or increase. Because the health of older adults varies considerably, the decision about the exact age to discontinue screening is best made between you and your doctor.

Can you tell me more about option 1? High-sensitivity fecal . . . what was that again?

Option 1 is the high-sensitivity fecal occult blood test every year. First of all, *high sensitivity* distinguishes newer FOBTs from earlier ones that were less sensitive, or less likely to detect colon cancer. *Fecal* means the test is of fecal matter (or stool). *Occult* means "hidden," so *occult blood* refers to an amount of blood so small that it cannot be seen with the naked eye. So fecal occult blood testing, or FOBT, is a test done to look for the presence of small amounts of blood in the stool.

Why look for small amounts of blood in the stool?

Precancerous and cancerous polyps tend to bleed, and therefore blood in the stool can be a sign of their presence. But the bleeding, like the polyp, is very small—so small that it often cannot be detected by our eyes alone. That's where the FOBT comes in. It helps detect small amounts of blood that may be the earliest sign of precancerous polyps or colon cancer.

How does the test work?

FOBT uses a chemically treated card. To do the test, a small amount of stool is placed on the card. Then a chemical developer solution is added to see if the card changes color. It's that simple.

Normally, FOBT refers to using three of these cards to test three consecutive stool samples. Because small polyps or early cancers don't bleed all the time, doing the test three times increases the chances of detecting something abnormal. After collecting the sample at home, you take the card to the doctor's office or mail it directly to the laboratory, where the chemical developer solution is added and the card is analyzed and read by a professional.

Is any preparation required?

For seven days before and during the stool collection period, people are advised to avoid nonsteroidal anti-inflammatory drugs such as ibuprofen, naproxen, or aspirin, if possible. In addition, some doctors recommend avoiding red meat, iron supplements, and excess vitamin C for the three days prior to and during the test period.

What does it mean if one of the cards changes color?

Interpreting the result of the FOBT card is tricky, so *read this part carefully.*

First, other things besides blood may cause the card to change color. These include beets and other vegetables, red meat, vitamin and iron supplements, and certain medications. So a positive result may not mean there is blood in the stool at all. The test kits come with instructions, including information on avoiding foods that create a false positive (a result suggesting the presence of disease when it is not present). If you follow the kit's instructions, you will decrease the chances of a false positive result.

Second, there are other potential sources of blood in the stool besides colon cancer or precancerous polyps, such as hemorrhoids, stomach ulcers, anal fissures, and menstrual bleeding. For these reasons, only about 5 to 10 percent of positive FOBTs come from early stage colon cancer or precancerous polyps.

If it makes so many mistakes, what's the use of FOBT?

FOBT is not a test to *diagnose* colon cancer. It is a test to *screen* for it. It tells us, "Hey, there *may* be something going on here that needs looking into." That's why it's important not to get too concerned about a positive result.

FOBT is used because it has been proven to save lives. Studies show that people who get FOBTs every year are up to 33 percent less likely to die of colon cancer than people who don't. Imagine that! A simple one-minute test you can do in your own home could save your life.

What are the risks of taking the test?

FOBT is a simple test and has no potential for direct harm. There are indirect harms of FOBT, however, because abnormal, or positive, tests must be followed up with colonoscopy. People choose FOBT because it is simple and safe but sometimes without realizing that if the test is positive, further testing is necessary. The FOBT saves lives only because it helps doctors diagnose and treat colon cancer earlier than they would otherwise. This is a critical point—please read it again.

If the test is positive, what's the next step?

A positive result means you *may* have colon cancer or an early precancerous polyp. Remember that the test can only screen for colon cancer, not diagnose it. Most people with a positive FOBT do not have colon cancer. So first step: take a deep breath.

The next step is a colonoscopy, a procedure in which a flexible tube-shaped instrument is used to inspect the colon (more details below). Through colonoscopy, doctors may be able to determine the source of the bleeding. Keep in mind that the source of bleeding may be something other than colon cancer. After additional testing, your doctor may discover that you have anal fissures, hemorrhoids, or stomach ulcers that may require medical attention.

If the test is negative, what's the next step?

Make sure you note the result and test date for your own records. Because you have chosen to get screened with FOBT every year, your next screening will be one year from now. *Good documentation is the key to making sure you get your next FOBT no later than one year from now.*

Can you tell me more about option 2? What exactly is flexible sigmoidoscopy?

Sigmoidoscopy (sig-moi-DAHS-co-pee) is a test doctors use to scope, or visually examine, the rectum and sigmoid colon. The sigmoid is the last segment of the colon and leads to the rectum. In colon cancer screening, sigmoidoscopy is used to look for any evidence of precancerous polyps or cancer in the sigmoid or rectum.

During the exam, a sigmoidoscope—a flexible tube the thickness of a finger—is inserted into the anus. A tiny video camera at its tip allows the doctor to view the inside of the colon on a video monitor, while he or she safely guides the sigmoidoscope. The instrument also allows doctors to biopsy any suspicious masses to examine under a microscope.

With sigmoidoscopy doctors can evaluate only the rectum and the sigmoid, whereas with colonoscopy, they can evaluate the entire rectum and colon (see figure 9.2). Therefore, sigmoidoscopy may miss cancers in the other parts of the colon. This is a major drawback of the procedure. On the other hand, colon cancer most often develops in the very places sigmoidoscopy is able to check. In addition, studies have shown that it is unlikely to have cancer in the earlier parts of the colon without at least some abnormalities in the sigmoid colon. Thus, checking the sigmoid alone is a reasonable substitute for checking the entire colon.

Although sigmoidoscopy is more likely than colonoscopy to miss cancers, the risks of sigmoidoscopy are fewer than those of colonoscopy. Deciding between the two tests is a matter of personal preference; one is not clearly better or worse than the other.

How is the test done?

To provide the clearest view possible, the colon must be emptied. The day before the test, you will be asked to adhere to a clear liquid diet. This means no solid foods but includes water, juice (without pulp), tea, coffee, and soda. In some cases, a laxative or bowel prep will also be recommended.

The day of the test will be like a normal morning for you, except without any breakfast. At the doctor's office, you will change into a patient gown and lie face down on the examining table. The doctor will apply a lubricant to the entrance of your anus to ease the insertion of the sigmoidoscope. Once the instrument is inside, your doctor will inflate the colon with air to make the inside of the colon easily visible and to smooth the safe passage of the sigmoidoscope. It is normal to experience some discomfort or cramps at this point, but usually they are mild.

By guiding the sigmoidoscope, your doctor will carefully inspect the rec-

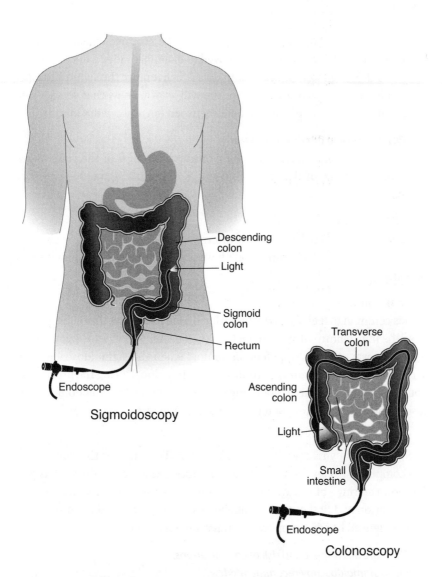

Figure 9.2. Through colonoscopy and sigmoidoscopy, doctors can directly examine the colon and look for suspicious masses. They use a flexible, lighted instrument called an endoscope to inspect the colon wall. If a suspicious mass is identified, they can pass an instrument through the endoscope to biopsy the mass and in some cases remove it entirely. The difference between the two procedures is that in sigmoidoscopy, only the sigmoid colon, the last segment of the colon, is inspected, while in colonoscopy, the entire colon is inspected.

tum and sigmoid. Any suspicious masses will be biopsied, meaning that a small sample of the tissue will be removed to examine under a microscope.

After a thorough examination, your doctor will remove the sigmoidoscope. After making sure you are okay, he or she will let you know that you are safe to go home. The entire procedure takes between ten and twenty minutes.

Will I be knocked out during the test?

Generally no anesthesia is used for this test. Because of the risks of anesthesia, this is one of the major advantages of flexible sigmoidoscopy over colonoscopy.

Will I miss work?

Most people are back to work the afternoon of the test or the next day. You will be able to drive home and won't have any restrictions on your activities or diet.

Does it hurt?

It is common to feel uncomfortable during the procedure, but a few people describe it as painful. If you are feeling anxious, let your doctor know about your concerns. Most people feel discomfort when the sigmoidoscope is inserted and again when air is introduced into the colon. During the procedure, you can expect to feel mild cramping or pressure in the lower abdomen. This discomfort may continue for a few hours after the test.

What are the risks?

Sigmoidoscopy risks are very low. The USPSTF estimates the rate of serious complications as 3.4 per 10,000 procedures. The most severe risk is perforation (tearing) of the wall of the colon. Ask about your doctor's rates of complication and find out how often he or she has performed the procedure. In experienced hands, complication rates are nearly zero.

Given the discomfort and risk of complications, why is sigmoidoscopy recommended?

Every decision in medicine is a tradeoff between risk and benefit. Here the risk is abdominal discomfort and the rare chance of perforation. The benefit is reducing the odds of death from colon cancer. Compared with patients who don't get any form of screening, patients who get regular sigmoidoscopy have a 33 percent lower chance of death from colon cancer. Sigmoidoscopy can find disease early and therefore treat it before cancer develops or, if cancer is already present, can find the cancer early and improve chances of survival.

What happens if my doctor finds something?

First of all, remember that finding "something" does not necessarily mean finding cancer. During the procedure, any suspicious masses will be biopsied and examined under the microscope to determine whether they represent a precancerous polyp, cancer, or simply normal tissue.

It may take a few days to get the results of the biopsy. Once the results come back, you and your doctor will talk about what they mean and what the next steps are. Generally an abnormal sigmoidoscopy needs to be followed up with a colonoscopy before a diagnosis can be made. However, because sigmoidoscopy involves tissue biopsies, a diagnosis of cancer can be made with this procedure alone.

What if it's cancer?

With screening, the hope is to catch the disease earlier than it would be found otherwise. Every day cancer has the potential to grow bigger and more difficult to treat. If you are diagnosed with colon cancer, you know that the road ahead will not be easy, but you can take some comfort in knowing that by catching it early, you have put yourself one step ahead.

If the doctor doesn't find anything, what is the next step?

Confirm the results of the test and be sure your doctor documents them. Note the results in your own records as well. Because you have chosen screening with sigmoidoscopy and FOBT, your next test will be an FOBT in two to three years. *Good documentation is the key to making sure your next sigmoidoscopy is no later than five years from now and that you have an FOBT no later than three years from now.*

What about option 3? How does colonoscopy work?

Colonoscopy (col-on-AHS-co-pee) is a test that allows doctors to visually inspect the entire colon and rectum. In colon cancer screening, colonoscopy is used to look for precancerous polyps or cancer.

During the exam, a colonoscope—a long, flexible tube the thickness of a finger—is inserted into the anus. A tiny video camera at its tip allows the doctor to view the inside of the colon on a video monitor while he or she guides the colonoscope through the colon. Any suspicious mass is biopsied to examine under a microscope. In addition, precancerous polyps can be removed. Because some polyps may progress into cancer, their removal can prevent colon cancer.

What is the difference between colonoscopy and sigmoidoscopy?

The key difference is that in sigmoidoscopy, doctors inspect the rectum and the sigmoid colon, whereas in colonoscopy, doctors inspect the entire colon and rectum. Colonoscopy is a lengthier procedure that is done under anesthesia and carries more risks. The benefit is that it enables doctors to catch precancerous polyps and cancer in parts of the colon where sigmoidoscopy is unable to see. In addition, colonoscopy is considered the gold standard for diagnosing colon cancer.

How is the test done?

So your doctor can get the clearest view possible, your colon must be emptied before the test. The day before, you will be asked to take a laxative or bowel prep and adhere to a clear liquid diet. A clear liquid diet means no solid foods but includes water, juice (without pulp), tea, coffee, and soda.

The day of your test will be like a normal morning for you, except that you will not eat any food. Your doctor will probably ask you not to drink anything in the six hours before the procedure.

At the doctor's office, you will change into a patient gown and lie down on the examining table. A nurse or an assistant will place an IV (intravenous line) in your arm and give you anesthesia through it. Once you are sedated, your doctor will apply a lubricant to the entrance of your anus and insert the colonoscope. Once the instrument is inside, your doctor will introduce air into the colon. This air will inflate the empty colon, which will allow your doctor to see inside and safely guide the colonoscope.

The procedure takes between twenty minutes and an hour. During that time, your doctor will carefully inspect the walls of your colon, looking for suspicious masses. If necessary, biopsies will be taken.

After the procedure is over, you will be moved to a recovery room for observation until your doctor feels comfortable sending you home. Your doctor will go over the preliminary results of the procedure with you, although the results from any biopsies taken will not be available for a few days.

Will I feel any pain?

Generally, no. Colonoscopy is almost always performed under anesthesia, so you will be sedated through most or all of the procedure. The anesthesia is a combination of a sedative (sleep-inducing agent) and a narcotic (pain-relieving medication). In the sedated state, you will not feel pain and will be breathing on your own. Even patients who do not receive anesthesia (for personal or medical reasons) usually experience only mild pain or discomfort.

Who will do the procedure?

Colonoscopy is a specialized procedure generally performed by a gastro-enterologist, though other clinical practitioners with specialized training can also do the procedure. Regardless of which type of doctor does your colonos-copy, make sure the person has done the procedure many times. Studies show that the efficacy and safety of colonscopies increase with volume performed. Some experts say that at a minimum, your doctor should be doing three to four colonoscopies a day.

How will I feel afterward? Will I be able to drive home or go to work?

Most people feel fine after colonoscopy, although they usually feel a bit woozy while the anesthesia wears off. Some people feel bloated for a few hours after the test. This feeling will gradually fade. Small amounts of blood in the first bowel movement after the procedure are not uncommon.

Because of the anesthesia, someone else should drive you home and you should take the rest of the day off work.

What are the risks of the procedure?

The major risks are bleeding, infection, and perforation (a tear) in the wall of the colon. The USPSTF estimates the rate of serious complications as 25 per 10,000 procedures and the rate of perforation to be 3.8 per 10,000. The most severe risk is perforation of the colon wall. Ask your doctor about his or her rates of complication and find out how often he or she has performed the procedure. In experienced hands, complication rates may be significantly lower.

Another risk is that your doctor may have to abort the procedure, or worse, miss a visible lesion because the colon was incompletely emptied. Taking your colonic prep as prescribed and doing your best to empty out your colon will increase the chance of detecting removable polyps and decrease the chance of having to cancel or reschedule the procedure.

Given the risks, why is colonoscopy still recommended?

Every decision in medicine is a tradeoff between risk and benefit. As doc-tors, we take the risks of colonoscopy seriously but also recognize the poten-tial health benefits. In the end, although physicians as a group believe that the benefits of colonoscopy outweigh the risks, it is up to you to weigh the risks and benefits and decide.

What happens if they find something?

Finding something doesn't necessarily mean finding cancer. The doctor will biopsy any unusual-looking tissue for further evaluation. After analyzing the sample under a microscope, the laboratory will determine whether the biopsies are precancerous polyps, cancer, or simply normal tissue.

The purpose of screening is to detect disease at its earliest stages and address it appropriately. If the abnormality turns out to be a precancerous polyp or even cancer, the screening test has just put you one step ahead of the disease and in a better position to treat and even cure it.

Colonoscopy is both a screening test and a diagnostic test. Unlike with the other two options, a positive colonoscopy does not require additional testing to make a diagnosis.

What happens if they don't find anything?

Confirm the results of the test and make sure your primary care doctor gets an official report for his or her records. Note the test date and results in your own records as well. Because you have chosen colonoscopy, your next screening will be in ten years, when you will do another colonoscopy. *Good documentation is the key to making sure you get another colonoscopy no later than ten years from now.*

Are any other screening tests available?

In addition to the screening tests supported by the USPSTF, at least three other tests are used to screen for colon cancer.

Double-contrast barium enema: In this test, a series of x-rays are taken after liquid barium and air are introduced into the colon. By looking for filling defects in the colon, doctors use this test to screen for colon cancer. Abnormal findings are followed up with colonoscopy. Compared with the other tests offered, double-contrast barium enema has medium sensitivity and medium specificity. The USPSTF did not include this test in its guidelines, noting that it has lower sensitivity than modern test strategies, has not been subjected to screening trials, and has been declining in use. Those organizations that support barium enema usually recommend screening every five years.

CT colonography: Also referred to as virtual colonoscopy, CT colonography is a newer screening test for colon cancer and one that has been receiving increasing attention. In this test, CT x-ray technology is used to take pictures of the colon, which computer software then assembles into a three-dimensional image that doctors use to look for colon cancer and precancerous polyps. This test is appealing because it provides the high sensitivity of colonoscopy without the attendant anesthesia and procedural risks. Unlike colonoscopy, however, CT colonography does not enable biopsies of suspicious polyps or masses, so abnormal findings still must be followed up with colonoscopy.

Another, perhaps unexpected, drawback of CT colonography is that about 10 percent of studies have "extracolonic findings." These findings are abnormalities picked up by the CT scan outside the colon, such as in the bladder, pancreas, or adrenal glands. The abnormalities are often harmless but once found may require additional follow-up studies and provoke anxiety. Because the harms of these findings are not well established, the USPSTF found insufficient evidence to assess the benefits and harms of CT colonography. Organizations that support CT colonography generally recommend screening every five years.

Stool DNA test: The newest screening test for colon cancer is a stool DNA test. Unlike FOBT, which tests for the presence of blood in the stool, the stool DNA test analyzes the sample for the presence of genetic alterations or mutations known to occur in colon cancer. Like FOBT, the sample can be collected at home and has no direct health risks. Early studies suggest it has a higher sensitivity than FOBT, though not as high as colonoscopy. Like FOBT, however, abnormal, or positive, tests must be followed up with colonoscopy. Because much is still unknown about the sensitivity and specificity of stool DNA tests, the USPSTF has found insufficient evidence to recommend it for routine screening. Even organizations that support stool DNA tests do not specify a screening interval.

How do I choose the option that is right for me?

Given the number of screening methods available and their relative equivalence, the most important element of colon cancer screening is to choose one method of screening that works for you and stick with it.

Choosing between the various options is a matter of personal preference and something to discuss with your family, friends, and doctor. To help frame this discussion, pros and cons of the three recommended USPSTF screening tests are presented in table 9.1.

Is screening for colon cancer really that important?

Colon cancer is a devastating disease. It is common, it is life-threatening, and it can occur in older adults with no other risk factors for the disease.

Currently, aside from removing precancerous polyps, doctors do not know how to reduce the risk of colon cancer. They don't know what causes the disease in most people, and they don't know how to prevent it from developing.

What they do know, and what you know now, is how to catch colon cancer early—sometimes so early that the disease is at the precancerous stage, and other times in an early stage of cancer that it is treatable and even curable.

Table 9.1: Pros and cons of three colon cancer screening options

Option	Pros	Cons
Fecal occult blood test (FOBT) every year	Noninvasive	Low sensitivity
	No direct risks	Low specificity
	No preparation required	If positive, diagnostic colonoscopy is required
		Annual follow-up required
Sigmoidoscopy every 5 years with FOBT every 3 years	High sensitivity for masses in the distal colon and rectum	Limited bowel preparation necessary
	Enables tissue biopsies and removal of polyps	Does not scope the entire colon
	Safer than colonoscopy (fewer complications, no sedation)	Risk of perforation and bleeding
		If positive, diagnostic colonoscopy generally required
Colonoscopy every 10 years	Scopes the entire colon and rectum, high sensitivity	Significant risk of perforation and bleeding
	Enables tissue biopsies and polyp removal	Risk of anesthesia
	If positive, no further testing required (gold standard for diagnosis)	Full bowel preparation necessary
	If negative, follow-up not required for 10 years	

Every major medical institution and expert scientific panel in the country recommends colon cancer screening for one simple reason: it saves lives. The USPSTF recommends that every American ages 50 to 75 get routinely screened for colon cancer.

The screening can be embarrassing, uncomfortable, and, frankly, scary. Some of us don't want our doctors to probe us with instruments. Some of us don't want to endure a risky procedure for a problem that we may not even have. And some of us simply don't want to know that something could be wrong. For all of us, there are at least three different options for screening.

Some are more invasive than others, and at least one can be done in the comfort of our own homes. All give us hope of a life free from colon cancer.

At present, less than half of Americans over age 50 are getting regularly screened for colon cancer. Get informed. Read this chapter carefully. And talk to your doctor.

REFERENCES

American Cancer Society (ACS). www.cancer.org.

Levin et al. "Screening and Surveillance for the Early Detection of Colorectal Cancer and Adenomatous Polyps, 2008: A Joint Guideline from the American Cancer Society, the U.S. Multi-Society Task Force on Colorectal Cancer, and the American College of Radiology." *Gastroenterology* 134, no. 5 (May 2008): 1570-95. Epub 2008, Feb 8.

National Cancer Institute (NCI). National Institutes of Health (NIH). U.S. Department of Health and Human Services. www.cancer.gov.

———. *What You Need to Know About Cancer of the Colon and Rectum*. NIH Publication No. 06-1552. Bethesda, Md.: Department of Health and Human Services, National Institutes of Health, July 2006. Revised May 2006. www.cancer.gov/cancertopics/types/colon-and-rectal.

CHAPTER 10

Depression Screening

We all experience sadness or "depression" in our lives, but these feelings are usually a normal response to a painful event—a death, a divorce, a setback at work. In a healthy situation, these feelings are fleeting and do not overwhelm one's ability to function in daily life. Depression is different. When someone has depression, the illness lingers for weeks to months and stymies the person's attempt to lead a healthy and productive life.

Each year depression affects 18 million adults in the United States. This means that one in every twelve adults in the United States has depression. Among younger people, depression is estimated to affect one in sixteen adolescents and one in thirty children. In certain groups—particularly the elderly, women after childbirth, people with recent life stressors, those with a personal or family history of depression, or those suffering from a chronic medical condition—the rates of depression are even higher.

Depression is an *illness* and a serious and potentially lethal one at that: An estimated 15 percent of people with depression commit suicide. According to the World Health Organization (WHO), depression and related disorders are the fourth leading cause of suffering worldwide and by 2020 will be the second leading cause after heart disease.[1] It leads not only to mental illness, but also to a host of physical problems. People with depression make poor choices, avoid medical care, and are less likely to follow their medication regimens, contributing to higher rates of medical diseases. Among these are substance abuse, stroke, heart disease, and diabetes. Overall, people over age 55 with depression have an estimated premature death rate four times higher than those without depression. Aside from its impact on health, depression affects many other aspects of life. It is a leading cause of job absenteeism, marital strife, and financial hardship. In adolescents, it is associated with early pregnancy and decreased school performance.

Fortunately, there is treatment. Multiple studies have demonstrated that antidepressant medication and psychotherapy reduce the symptoms of depression and improve quality of life, even in severe cases. Unfortunately, however, because the symptoms of depression are easily masked and often appear insidiously, half of adults with depression leave the doctor's office without being diagnosed. To compound matters, less than 30 percent of depressive episodes receive proper medical care despite the availability of effective treatments.

Screening is the first step to appropriate care and management of depression. By simply talking to your doctor, you can be evaluated for the illness. If depression is diagnosed, you will be offered counseling and medications that are proven to improve depressive symptoms and reduce recurrences. The United States Preventive Services Task Force (USPSTF) recommends that all adults and all adolescents ages 12 to 18 be screened for depression in clinical practices that are able to provide accurate diagnosis, treatment, and follow-up.[2] The following sections provide an introduction to depression and outline the recommendations for screening.

SECTION I: DEPRESSION 101

Depression has specific symptoms, and it is diagnosed and treated as a specific disease much in the way diabetes and other chronic diseases are. When doctors talk about depression, they are usually referring to one of several named depressive disorders. The most common of these is major depression.

In *major depression*, people experience a combination of depressive symptoms that impairs their normal functioning or causes significant distress. Episodes of major depression last weeks to months and tend to recur. Dysthymic (dis-THIGH-mik) disorder is another example of a depressive disorder. *Dysthymic disorder* (or *dysthymia,* dis-THIGH-mee-a) is less disabling than major depression but lasts longer, often two years or more. Other depressive disorders include postpartum depression (depression after childbirth), manic depression (also called bipolar disorder), psychotic depression, and seasonal affective disorder. It is essential that the correct diagnosis be made among the different kinds of depression because effective treatment depends on it. For the remaining sections, however, these disorders are referred to collectively as depression.

Is depression really a disease? Can't people just snap out of it?

Depression is a terribly misunderstood condition. People often assume that depression is "all in the head" or that people with depression are somehow at fault or responsible for their illness. This is untrue. In the popular media, depression is sometimes shown as an extreme or untreatable condition; this, too, is untrue. At the other extreme, depression is sometimes shown as an overdiagnosed and overtreated condition. These generalizations are false and dangerous because they perpetuate myths of depression and contribute to the social stigmas surrounding the disease.

Depression is best understood as a disease no different than any other physical ailment. Consider the analogy to heart disease. Heart disease develops from a combination of biological, environmental, and individual factors. Thus, not everyone who is overweight and smokes has a heart attack. Depression is similar. People often attribute the disease to the recent loss of a job or a loved one. But not everyone who loses his or her job develops depression. Although these factors may trigger the disease, the subsequent depressive symptoms appear in people already predisposed to depression. A depressed person cannot just "snap out of it," any more than someone can make chest pain go away through sheer willpower. Though sometimes people with depression get better without medical care, they usually fare better with psychotherapy and medication. The same is true for patients with heart disease, who do better through a combination of lifestyle counseling and heart medications.

By thinking of depression as a disease, we move away from the stigmas associated with mental health and instead focus on the more pressing matter—diagnosing and treating people who are afflicted.

What causes depression?

Scientists do not fully understand what causes depression, but they believe it is a combination of biological, genetic, and psychological factors. From imaging the brain, researchers have learned that the brains of people who have depression are structurally different from those of people without depression. In addition, depressed people have imbalances in the chemicals, called *neurotransmitters,* that relay messages between different parts of the brain. Because depression runs in families and is more common in identical twins, we know that depression is also related to genetics. Finally, depression can be triggered by personal events and can be remediated through psychotherapy, which suggests that the disease has an important psychological component as well.

What are the symptoms of depression?

Most people with depression exhibit two classic symptoms: low mood and anhedonia. People with low mood often appear down or depressed and hopeless or negative about the future. *Anhedonia* (pronounced an-hee-DOE-nee-a) is an inability to experience pleasure from normally pleasurable life events. People with anhedonia do not enjoy doing the things they used to enjoy, like eating good food, spending time with friends, or participating in their hobbies. Other symptoms of depression include

▸ feelings of guilt, worthlessness, or helplessness
▸ constant worrying
▸ irritability or restlessness
▸ generalized tiredness (fatigue)
▸ difficulty concentrating or poor memory
▸ overeating or loss of appetite
▸ poor sleep
▸ thoughts of suicide or suicide attempts
▸ persistent aches and pains that cannot be explained by other medical conditions

Keep in mind two caveats about the symptoms of depression. First, they vary greatly from person to person. Some people have such severe symptoms it's easy to tell something is wrong. Others feel unhappy or "not themselves" without ever thinking that they could have depression. Still others will not feel sad at all, but their friends and family notice that they are more irritable or confused than normal. Because the symptoms are so variable, it is important to keep a high index of suspicion for depression and be open with your doctor about your mood, even if you don't have the "classic" symptoms. Second, not everything that has four wheels and a roof is a car. Likewise, not everyone with two or three of the symptoms listed above has depression. But because having any of those symptoms *may* mean that you have depression, talk to your doctor if you are experiencing them.

How is depression diagnosed?

Depression is a clinical diagnosis, meaning that it is made through careful examination by a trained physician or psychologist. It is not a diagnosis made by checking off a list of symptoms or through casual dinner conversations. Although depression is related to structural and chemical changes in the brain, no existing blood tests or imaging studies can help diagnose it.

If you are having symptoms of depression, be sure to tell your doctor. Doctors have difficulty diagnosing depression unless patients are candid with them, so talk openly with your doctor about how you are feeling. Once you start the conversation, your doctor will ask you additional questions about your symptoms and take a complete medical history. He or she may also examine you and order blood work because depressive symptoms can sometimes be caused by other medical conditions, such as thyroid disease.

How is depression treated?

Depression is usually treated through a combination of psychotherapy and antidepressant medications. In severe, or refractory, cases, admission to the hospital for more intensive treatment may be recommended.

Antidepressants

Because depression is related to imbalances in neurotransmitters, chemicals in the brain that regulate mood, antidepressants are designed to act on these neurotransmitters and normalize these imbalances. For example, the SSRI (selective serotonin reuptake inhibitors) class of antidepressants increases the brain levels of serotonin, a neurotransmitter that is often decreased in people with depression. The other classes of antidepressants are SNRIs (serotonin and norepinephrine reuptake inhibitors), TCAs (tricyclic antidepressants), MAOIs (monoamine oxidase inhibitors), NRIs (norepinephrine reuptake inhibitors), and NRDIs (norepinephrine and dopamine reuptake inhibitors).

Most people have significant improvement in their symptoms within six weeks of starting antidepressant medications. Antidepressants also reduce the likelihood of recurrence in people who continue taking the medication even after their symptoms get better. It takes at least three to four weeks before antidepressants take full effect, although some improvement in symptoms may be noticed before that. If after two weeks of medication symptoms of depression persist, there is no need for concern. At two weeks, this is normal and even expected.

There are more than thirty types of antidepressants. Different kinds work for different people, and unfortunately a doctor cannot predict which antidepressant will work best for a given person. Finding the right medication may take some trial and error, so don't get discouraged if the first medication does not seem to work. Antidepressants cause side effects in some people. Most of these side effects are temporary and go away within a few weeks of starting treatment. People with persistent or unmanageable side effects should consult their doctor. Fortunately, each medication acts on the body differently, so having side effects from one medication does not necessarily mean you will have side effects from the others.

Largely because of side effects and slow response to treatment, 28 percent of patients being treated for depression stop taking their medication during the initial month of treatment, and 44 percent stop within three months. By partnering with your doctor and setting reasonable expectations beforehand, you can make sure you get the most benefit from antidepressant therapy.

Psychotherapy

Although often referred to as "talk therapy," psychotherapy involves much more than just talking. It requires specialized training in specific techniques to treat depression among other diseases and disorders. Three types of psychotherapy have been proven to be effective in depression: cognitive-behavioral therapy, interpersonal therapy, and problem-solving therapy. Each type has a different focus, although in practice many therapists use them in combination. Each offers practical approaches to overcoming the negative impact of depressive symptoms on the lives of people with depression.

Special Note on Treatment in Adolescents

Recently, news about antidepressants increasing the suicide risk in children and adolescents has caused concern. These developments have led to a new black box warning on all antidepressant medications stating that their use may increase the risk of suicide. This warning is the result of a large study of children and adolescents that reported a 4 percent suicide risk in those taking antidepressants compared with a 2 percent risk in those not taking them. This finding has prompted doctors to more closely monitor young people taking antidepressants, especially in the first weeks after initiating treatment, when the risk is highest. The consensus is that in clinical practices that can provide such intensive monitoring, antidepressants can still be used safely and effectively in adolescents.

Does depression go away?

The natural course of depression varies by type of depressive disorder and by individual. Major depression is usually episodic. Typical depressive episodes in major depression last from several months to a year. While some people experience only one episode of depression in their entire life, for most people major depression recurs if not treated. The risk of recurrence increases with the number of depressive episodes. In general, a person with a history of one major depressive episode has a 50 percent chance of recurrence. A person who has had two major depressive episodes has a 75 percent chance of recurrence. And a person who has had three episodes has a 95 percent chance of recurrence.

Understanding the course of depression is important. Even without treatment, depression can get better on its own. But with treatment, depression is more likely to get better and is less likely to recur.

SECTION II: SCREENING FOR DEPRESSION

The USPSTF recommends screening all adults and all adolescents ages 12 to 18 years for depression in clinical practices that have systems in place to ensure accurate diagnosis, effective treatment, and follow-up. This recommendation is based on evidence that screening for depression improves the accurate identification of depressed patients in primary care settings and that treatment of depression in these settings reduces illness. The task force does not specify how often screening should be done, although they recommend more frequent screening in people with a history of depression, other psychological conditions, substance abuse, chronic pain, or unexplained physical symptoms. Although this guideline is geared more toward doctors, you should talk to your doctor about your general mood, especially if you are feeling unhappy or depressed. If you are a parent of an adolescent, you should make sure your child has an opportunity to talk to a doctor about his or her mood, especially if you are concerned about depression.

How will talking to a doctor about my feelings help?

Many people see depression or low mood as a personal problem that does not require medical attention. They don't realize that depression is a disease and, like most diseases, is better managed with a doctor's help. Compared with depressed people who do not receive any medical treatment, people with depression who receive antidepressant medications and psychotherapy are 60 percent more likely to have significant improvements in their symptoms. Treatment also reduces the likelihood of getting depression again, which is important because at least half of people who experience an episode of depression will have a recurrence. In addition to providing treatment, your doctor can also help you understand your symptoms and dispel myths about depression. Finally, because mental health is an important part of a person's overall health, it is best for your doctor to know what is troubling you.

What about children age 11 or under?

Like adolescents and adults, children can also develop depression. After reviewing the latest evidence, however, the USPSTF found insufficient evidence to recommend screening in this age group. Screening is not as reliable in children as in older individuals, and the benefits of treatment are not as well understood. That being said, if you are concerned that your child may be depressed, talk to your child's doctor. Remember, screening only applies to people without symptoms—if you think your child has symptoms of depression, these guidelines do not apply.

How does screening work?

Screening for depression involves questions about your mental health. Some doctors use standardized forms or questionnaires, and others simply ask their patients about their mood and life in general. The USPSTF suggests that two screening questions are probably as effective as longer questionnaires:

1. "Over the past two weeks, have you felt down, depressed, or hopeless?"
2. "Over the past two weeks, have you felt little interest or pleasure in doing things?"

Patients who report a low mood or other depressive symptoms are often asked follow-up questions. Just like with any other symptom, your doctor will ask you about your mood symptoms, including when they started, how they affect your daily life, whether you have had similar symptoms before, and what seems to make them better or worse. He or she will also ask you whether you or anyone in your family has a history of depression or other mental illnesses and whether you have ever taken psychiatric medication. Your doctor will also ask if you have any thoughts of suicide or self-harm. After taking a complete history, he or she may examine you or order some tests.

Studies show that screening detects 90 percent of depression. However, 50 percent of people who come to their doctor's office with active depression leave without a diagnosis. What accounts for the difference? Not every doctor does a good job screening all patients for depression, and many patients are not as forthcoming about their mood as they could be. The lesson: Don't wait for your doctor to ask you about your mental health. Talk to your doctor if you are experiencing symptoms of depression.

What if I am diagnosed with depression?

Being diagnosed with depression is the first step to getting better. The two most common treatments for depression—antidepressant medications and psychotherapy—are highly effective at helping people with depression get better. Depending on the severity of your condition and your doctor's level of comfort treating depression, you may or may not be referred to a psychiatrist to help manage your depression. In people who require more intensive support and therapy, doctors may recommend admission to the hospital. Most of the time, people with depression are started on antidepressant medications and are asked to follow up frequently with their primary care doctors.

REFERENCES

National Institute of Mental Health (NIMH). National Institutes of Health (NIH). U.S. Department of Health and Human Services. www.nimh.nih.gov.

Diabetes Screening

Diabetes is the seventh leading cause of death in the United States. It is *the* leading cause of end-stage kidney disease, adult blindness, and nontraumatic amputations, and a major contributor to heart disease and stroke.

Despite these long-term complications, most people in early stage type 2 diabetes have no symptoms. The disease remains undiagnosed for five years or more, and in the meantime, the long-term effects of elevated blood glucose slowly damage the heart, kidney, and other vital organs. As a result, one-third of people with diabetes are undiagnosed, and one-third of those newly diagnosed already have one or more complications from untreated diabetes.

A routine blood test can determine whether you have diabetes. Given the availability of effective treatments—from exercise and weight control to glucose-lowering medications—screening for diabetes can help people get their blood glucose under control and prevent long-term complications. Screening also has important implications for blood pressure control. Studies show that in people with high blood pressure and diabetes, lowering blood pressure below conventional targets further reduces the risk of coronary heart disease (CHD). By finding out if someone with elevated blood pressure has diabetes, doctors can set a lower target blood pressure and further prevent heart attacks, strokes, and other forms of cardiovascular disease.

The United States Preventive Services Task Force (USPSTF) recommends screening for type 2 diabetes in adults with sustained blood pressure greater than 135/80 mmHg.[1] The following sections will provide an introduction to diabetes and detail the screening guidelines.

SECTION I: TYPE 2 DIABETES 101

Diabetes is a disease of excess *glucose*, or sugar, in the blood. Blood glucose is normally regulated by the hormone *insulin*, which acts on the body to decrease blood glucose. In diabetes, there is either insufficient insulin production or resistance to the effects of insulin on blood glucose. This causes glucose to accumulate in the blood, which over time may cause serious health complications. There are two main diabetes diseases: type 1 and type 2. In type 1 diabetes, the body does not make sufficient insulin. In type 2 diabetes, the body is insulin resistant, meaning that it does not respond appropriately to insulin.

Despite their similar consequences, type 1 and type 2 diabetes are different diseases. Type 1 develops in children and young adults when the body's immune system attacks the cells in the pancreas that make insulin. People with type 1 diabetes make no insulin at all and therefore are dependent on insulin to survive—thus, type 1 diabetes is also called *insulin-dependent diabetes.* Type 2 diabetes usually develops later in life, when the tissues in the body become resistant to the effects of insulin, usually in part due to increased weight and body fat. Although insulin can be part of the treatment for type 2 diabetes, people with this form of the disease make insulin, often more than normal, and do not need insulin to survive—thus, type 2 diabetes is also called *non–insulin-dependent diabetes.*

Young people who develop type 1 diabetes become sick and are readily diagnosed with their condition. People who develop type 2 diabetes, however, often appear to be well for years after the onset of the disease. People with type 2 diabetes are commonly not diagnosed for up to ten years after the onset of disease and all too often after the first complications of the disease develop. Because type 2 diabetes is much more common, and the risks of having undiagnosed diabetes is much greater with type 2 diabetes than with type 1, type 2 is the subject of the screening guidelines for diabetes. The remainder of the chapter focuses on type 2 diabetes and uses the terms diabetes and type 2 diabetes interchangeably.

How common is diabetes?

Over 20 million people in the United States have diabetes. About one-third of those who have diabetes have not yet been diagnosed or treated. Put another way, for every one hundred people living in the United States, seven have diabetes, of which two don't know it yet.

We are in the middle of a diabetes epidemic. Each year there are over 1.5 million new cases. In 1990, about 5 percent of the U.S. population had diabetes. Today that number is nearly 8 percent. And by the year 2025, diabetes is expected to increase to around 9 percent of the U.S. population. If we break the numbers down, they are even more alarming. In adults age 20 or older, almost 10.5 percent of men and 8.8 percent of women have diabetes.

In adults over age 60, more than 20 percent—or one in five—have diabetes. There are a number of potential reasons for this trend, but most experts agree that the increasing number of Americans who are overweight or obese is a major contributor.

How can people not know they have diabetes?

It is common to not have any symptoms of diabetes, especially in the early stages of the disease. For these people, elevated blood glucose levels are the only sign of diabetes. So unless they have their blood screened, they have no way of knowing they have diabetes.

Despite the absence of symptoms, early stage diabetes silently causes harm. Thus, people often go undiagnosed until the first complication of their uncontrolled diabetes develops—be it kidney problems, reduced vision, or a heart attack.

What are the symptoms of diabetes?

If symptoms develop, they might include one or more of the following:

- increased urination
- increased thirst
- unintentional weight loss
- increased hunger
- constant tiredness
- blurry vision
- tingling or numbness in the arms and legs
- sores that are slow to heal

Many other diseases can cause the very same symptoms. Furthermore, they tend to develop gradually and can be subtle to discern so that even people with symptoms of diabetes may go undiagnosed. Consult your doctor if you have any of these symptoms.

How do I know if I'm at risk?

Risk factors for type 2 diabetes include

- age over 45 years
- overweight or obesity (BMI $\geq$25 kg/m^2)
- abdominal obesity (waist circumference $\geq$35 inches in women or $\geq$40 inches in men)
- high blood pressure

▸ cholesterol disorder

▸ sedentary lifestyle

▸ family history of diabetes, especially in parents or siblings

What does weight have to do with diabetes?

Most people with type 2 diabetes are either overweight or obese. Studies show that while genes play a major role in diabetes, the effect of genes is also related to weight. People with strong family histories of diabetes may develop diabetes with more modest elevations in weight than those with no familial predisposition for diabetes. Scientists are still trying to understand the relationship between weight and diabetes, but many believe it is related to body fat increasing the body's resistance to insulin.

Can diabetes be prevented?

The results of a major trial—called the Diabetes Prevention Program (DPP)—showed that for certain people, moderate diet and physical activity improvements can delay, and sometimes entirely prevent, the onset of type 2 diabetes. The study showed that for people at risk for diabetes, exercising thirty minutes a day for five days a week and lowering their fat and calorie intake reduced their risk of type 2 diabetes by 58 percent. For those age 60 or older, the reduction was even greater—71 percent. These lifestyle changes equated to a 5 to 7 percent weight loss, or 10 to 14 pounds for a 200-pound person. This study, and others like it, suggest that through diet and exercise, diabetes can be prevented.

What health problems does diabetes cause?

Over time, excess glucose in the blood is deposited in the blood vessels and causes damage. Because every organ in the body depends on blood vessels for nutrients and oxygen, diabetes has the potential to harm many organs. Excess glucose also impairs the immune system, making people with diabetes more susceptible to infection, and disrupts metabolism. Below is a partial list of complications:[2]

Heart: Coronary heart disease (CHD) is the number one cause of death in people with diabetes. Diabetes is a major risk factor for CHD and is considered a CHD-risk equivalent (meaning that doctors consider it to be as serious a risk factor for future CHD as having had a heart attack!). This is based on studies that show that adults with diabetes are two to four times more likely to die of CHD than adults without it.

Brain: People with diabetes are two to four times more likely to suffer from a stroke than people without diabetes.

Blood pressure: Three-quarters of adults with diabetes have blood pressure greater than or equal to 130/80 mmHg or use prescription medications for hypertension.

Eyes: Diabetes causes changes to the blood vessels of the eye, which may lead to a disease called *diabetic retinopathy* (reh-tuh-NAH-puh-thee). Diabetic retinopathy is the leading cause of adult blindness among people ages 20 to 74.

Kidneys: Diabetes is the leading cause of kidney failure, accounting for nearly half the cases.

Nervous system: About 60 to 70 percent of people with diabetes have mild to severe forms of nervous system damage. The results of such damage include impaired sensation or pain in the feet or hands, slowed digestion of food in the stomach, and carpal tunnel syndrome.

Limbs: Over 60 percent of nontraumatic amputations occur in people with diabetes. Nerve damage makes people with diabetes more prone to having unnoticed wounds in the feet. These wounds can become infected, and the infection can spread into the deep tissues, necessitating amputation.

Pregnancy: Having poorly controlled diabetes during pregnancy causes major birth defects in 5 to 10 percent of these pregnancies and spontaneous abortions in 15 to 20 percent. In addition, poorly controlled diabetes can result in larger-than-normal babies and increase the risk for Cesarean section (C-section).

Infection: People with diabetes are more susceptible to infection and often have worse prognoses from common infections such as pneumonia.

Metabolism: Diabetes can lead to acute life-threatening metabolic disturbances, such as diabetic ketoacidosis or hyperosmolar coma.

Does everyone with diabetes develop these complications?

The risk of complications is directly related to glucose control. For example, people with poorly controlled glucose can develop end-stage kidney failure within ten years of diagnosis. On the other hand, those with well-controlled glucose can maintain healthy kidney function. Diabetes itself does not cause complications; high glucose levels cause them. By maintaining healthy glucose levels, people with diabetes can live a full life free from complications.

What is the treatment for diabetes?

Diabetes is a very treatable illness. Its treatment centers on three elements: controlling blood glucose, modifying associated risk factors, and preventing complications.

Blood glucose is controlled through a combination of lifestyle modifications and medications. Body fat is a major contributor to insulin resistance. Therefore, by losing weight, and especially abdominal fat, through dietary changes and physical activity, people with diabetes can improve their bodies' response to insulin. In addition, blood glucose levels are related to our diet. By eating foods low in carbohydrates, which the body converts into glucose, people with diabetes can lower blood glucose levels. In addition, many people with type 2 diabetes take oral glucose-lowering medications and sometimes insulin to further improve their blood glucose control. A wide variety of medications are proven to safely and effectively reduce blood glucose levels and lower the risk of complications.

It is also important for people with diabetes to modify their other cardiovascular risk factors, such as blood pressure and cholesterol. Because diabetes is a major risk factor for CHD, people with diabetes need to maintain even stricter blood pressure and cholesterol control than those without diabetes. Studies show that by lowering blood pressure below conventional target values, people with diabetes can further reduce their risk of CHD. This is a major reason why people with elevated blood pressure (over 135/80 mmHg) should be routinely screened for diabetes (see section II in this chapter).

Finally, there are additional screening and prevention measures available to directly reduce the risk of many major complications of diabetes. Secondary prevention of diabetic complications is outside the scope of this book. However, the following list briefly summarizes the available measures. According to the American Diabetes Association (ADA) guidelines, people with diabetes should routinely receive the following screening:

- ‣ blood pressure screening at every routine diabetes visit
- ‣ cholesterol screening at least annually
- ‣ retinopathy (eye disease) screening regularly
- ‣ nephropathy (kidney disease) screening at least annually
- ‣ neuropathy (nerve disease) screening at least annually
- ‣ comprehensive foot care regularly

In addition, people with diabetes are recommended to receive the pneumococcal vaccine and the annual influenza vaccine per the CDC guidelines

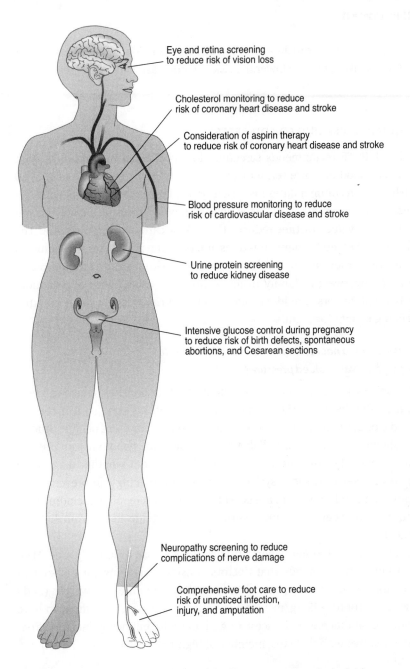

Eye and retina screening
to reduce risk of vision loss

Cholesterol monitoring to reduce
risk of coronary heart disease and stroke

Consideration of aspirin therapy
to reduce risk of coronary heart disease and stroke

Blood pressure monitoring to reduce
risk of cardiovascular disease and stroke

Urine protein screening
to reduce kidney disease

Intensive glucose control during pregnancy
to reduce risk of birth defects, spontaneous
abortions, and Cesarean sections

Neuropathy screening to reduce
complications of nerve damage

Comprehensive foot care to reduce
risk of unnoticed infection,
injury, and amputation

Figure 11.1. Diabetes is a systemic disease that affects many organs in the body.
Complications of uncontrolled diabetes include heart disease, stroke, kidney
disease, vision loss, nerve damage, and problems in pregnancy. In addition to
glucose control, many established secondary preventive services are designed to
reduce the rate of these complications.

(see chapter 23 for more details). They should also discuss with their doctors whether to take aspirin to lower the risk of cardiovascular events (see chapter 3).

SECTION II: SCREENING FOR DIABETES

The USPSTF recommends screening for type 2 diabetes in adults with sustained blood pressure (either treated or untreated) greater than 135/80 mmHg. This recommendation is based on evidence that in adults with elevated blood pressure and diabetes, lowering blood pressure below conventional target values further reduces the risk of cardiovascular disease. The USPSTF makes no recommendations for or against diabetes screening in adults with other cardiovascular or diabetes risk factors (e.g., cholesterol disorders, overweight, family history); however, adults with one or more of these risk factors should consider talking to their doctor about whether screening is right for them.

Why is screening not recommended for adults besides those with elevated blood pressure?

Effective screening tests and treatments exist for diabetes, which can help diagnose the disease early and prevent its harmful effects, so it is reasonable to wonder why screening is not recommended for more people. Studies have shown that diagnosing diabetes in people with symptoms can prevent complications, but they have been inconclusive about whether diagnosing diabetes in people without symptoms through screening can prevent complications. In addition, there are potential harms of screening, including stigmatization from being diagnosed with diabetes and side effects from diabetes medicines.

That being said, other expert organizations advise differently. The ADA, for example, recommends that doctors consider screening for diabetes in all adults age 45 or older, particularly in those who are overweight (body mass index [BMI] ≥ 25 kg/m^2), and in younger overweight adults who have an additional diabetes risk factor (e.g., habitually physically inactive, first-degree relative with diabetes, member of high-risk ethnic group, high blood pressure).

If all this is too much detail, don't worry. The main point is that not all doctors agree about who should be screened for diabetes. If you have one or more risk factors for diabetes (e.g., overweight, family history of diabetes) or for cardiovascular disease (e.g., cholesterol disorder), or if you are simply concerned about having diabetes, talk to your doctor about whether screening is right for you.

How is screening done?

There are multiple tests to screen for diabetes: fasting blood glucose, random blood glucose, hemoglobin A1c, and oral glucose tolerance test.

Fasting blood glucose: In this test, a blood sample is drawn after fasting—not having any food or drink except water—for at least eight to twelve hours. For the sake of convenience, this is often done in the morning before breakfast. Normal fasting blood glucose is between 60 and 100 mg/dl (milligrams per deciliter). The diagnosis of diabetes is usually made after two separate blood tests greater than 125 mg/dl.

Random blood glucose (or casual blood glucose): In this test, a blood sample is drawn at random, regardless of when the person last ate. This test is generally more convenient because it can be done in the same office visit. Normal random blood glucose is between 100 and 180 mg/dl. A glucose level greater than 200 mg/dl suggests diabetes.

Hemoglobin A1c: Hemoglobin A1c, or glycosylated hemoglobin, is a measure of the amount of sugar coating the surface of red blood cells. Practically speaking, it provides a running average of how much sugar has been in the blood over the past three months. It can be obtained from a routine blood draw taken any time of the day. A normal hemoglobin A1c is between 4 and 5.9 percent; greater than 6.5 percent suggests diabetes.

Oral glucose tolerance: In this test, a blood sample is drawn two hours after the ingestion of a standard amount of glucose (usually 75 grams). Generally the glucose is in a sweet-tasting liquid that you drink. This test is not used much anymore except to test for diabetes during pregnancy. Normal blood glucose two hours after glucose ingestion is between 100 and 180 mg/dl; greater than 200 mg/dl suggests diabetes.

All four screening methods are acceptable, but most doctors recommend the fasting blood glucose test because it is easy and quick to perform, convenient and acceptable to patients, and less expensive than other screening tests. The following sections are based on using the fasting blood glucose test to screen for diabetes.

What if my fasting blood glucose is greater than 125 mg/dl?

A fasting blood glucose test greater than 125 mg/dl is considered a positive screening test for diabetes but not yet diagnostic. Sometimes elevated fasting blood glucose can result from slow digestion of food, stress or pain, or a laboratory error. Diagnosing diabetes typically requires a second fasting blood glucose test on a separate visit.

What if my repeat test is also greater than 125 mg/dl?

Having two fasting blood glucoses over 125 mg/dl is diagnostic of diabetes. It is important to understand what this means and what it does not mean. It does not mean you have experienced any long-term complications from diabetes, nor does it mean you necessarily will. Being diagnosed with diabetes simply means you have persistently elevated blood glucose levels and are at risk for diabetes-related diseases. Because there are effective treatments for diabetes, getting diagnosed is often the first step to reducing this risk and staying healthy and symptom-free.

Your doctor will likely perform various tests to determine the stage of your diabetes, including tests of kidney function, cholesterol levels, blood pressure, and vision. He or she will also test your hemoglobin A1c, which is a three-month running average of your glucose control. You may be referred to other health care providers, including nurses, nutritionists, and diabetes specialists, to help you learn about the disease and take steps to keep your blood glucose levels under control. People with diabetes are encouraged to make lifestyle modifications to help them lose weight, increase physical activity, and eat a healthier diet. In addition, some will be started on one or more blood glucose–lowering medications to further improve glucose control.

Because having diabetes increases your overall risk of cardiovascular disease, you should consider additional preventive measures with your doctor. This may include daily aspirin therapy (chapter 3), intensive healthy eating counseling (chapter 14), and vaccinations (chapter 23).

If I have high blood pressure, how will finding out I have diabetes affect me?

Target blood pressure levels become stricter in people with diabetes. According to JNC VII (the Seventh Report of the Joint National Committee), which most doctors use to guide their treatment of high blood pressure, people without diabetes should aim for a blood pressure below 140/90 mmHg; those with diabetes should aim for a blood pressure below 130/80 mmHg. In addition, certain blood pressure–lowering medications are preferred over others in people with diabetes because they additionally help reduce long-term diabetes complications. Finding out you have diabetes may therefore lead to changes in your treatment regimen to meet this lower target blood pressure and to reduce your overall risk of CHD.

What if my fasting blood glucose is not greater than 125 mg/dl?

A fasting blood glucose lower than 100 mg/dl is normal. Therefore, there is no indication that you have diabetes, and no further testing is required. Because it has not been well studied, the optimal interval for screening has not been specified by the USPSTF. The ADA, on the basis of expert opinion, recommends screening at-risk individuals every three years. It is up to you and your doctor to decide when you should be rescreened for diabetes.

A fasting blood glucose between 100 and 125 mg/dl is not normal but is also not elevated enough to be considered diabetes. Some doctors call this state *prediabetes*. Studies have shown that people with prediabetes are at higher risk of developing diabetes. Although medications are generally not recommended to treat prediabetes, those with prediabetes are strongly encouraged to lose weight and make lifestyle modifications aimed at preventing the onset of diabetes. People with a fasting glucose in this range can expect to be screened for diabetes more frequently.

REFERENCES

American Diabetes Association (ADA). "Standards of Care in Diabetes 2007." *Diabetes Care* 30, supp. 1 (January 2007).
Centers for Disease Control and Prevention (CDC). "National Diabetes Fact Sheet: General Information and National Estimates on Diabetes in the United States, 2003." Rev. ed. Atlanta, GA: U.S. Department of Health and Human Services, Centers for Disease Control and Prevention, 2004.
National Diabetes Information Clearinghouse. National Institutes of Diabetes and Digestive and Kidney Disorders. National Institutes of Health. http://diabetes.niddk.nih.gov.

CHAPTER 12

Early Childhood Preventive Health

Early childhood is a wonderful time of growth, discovery, and development. By partnering with a child's health care provider, parents and other caregivers can take steps to make the most of the young child's opportunities, help him or her overcome and cope with challenges, and provide the advantages that will lead to a healthy and productive life.

Age-appropriate screenings and preventive treatments are essential to promote and protect the health of young children. The United States Preventive Services Task Force (USPSTF) makes the following recommendations:

- preventive eye drops against gonococcal ophthalmia neonatorum for all newborns at delivery
- newborn screening for phenylketonuria (PKU)
- newborn screening for congenital hypothyroidism (CH)
- newborn screening for sickle cell disease
- newborn screening for hearing loss
- routine iron supplementation for children age 6 to 12 months who are at increased risk for iron deficiency anemia (e.g., born preterm or low birthweight)
- oral fluoride supplementation for preschool children and babies older than 6 months of age whose primary water source is deficient in fluoride
- screening to detect amblyopia, strabismus, and defects in visual acuity in children younger than 5 years
- routine vaccinations as recommended by the Centers for Disease Control and Prevention (CDC)[1]

Most children who receive care from a pediatrician or family physician receive all the above preventive services. Many health care professionals go beyond these measures to provide further disease prevention, such as additional newborn screening, regular well-child visits, and anticipatory guidance.

The following sections describe the USPSTF recommended preventive measures during early childhood. Section I briefly reviews eye drops for preventing gonoccocal eye disease in newborns. Section II discusses neonatal screening for phenylketonuria, congenital hypothyroidism, and sickle cell anemia. Section III covers screening for hearing loss. Section IV describes iron supplementation. Section V provides information on preventing dental cavities. Section VI discusses routine screening for vision impairments. And section VII discusses childhood vaccines. The benefits of breastfeeding are covered in chapter 19 ("Pregnancy Preventive Health").

SECTION I: GONOCOCCAL OPHTHALMIA PREVENTION IN NEWBORNS

If gonorrhea is passed from mother to child during childbirth, one of the infections a newborn can contract is an eye infection called *gonococcal ophthalmia neonatorum* (GCON). The first symptoms of GCON usually develop between day 2 and day 5 of life. Without treatment, it can rapidly lead to blindness.

GCON can be easily and safely prevented. Instilling eye drops of silver nitrate or antibiotic immediately after birth is highly effective at preventing the infection. Since the United States mandated the use of these preventive eye drops, nearly every newborn delivered in a U.S. hospital receives them, and GCON has become rare.

The USPSTF recommends preventive eye drops against gonococcal ophthalmia neonatorum for all newborns. Acceptable regimens include a single application of silver nitrate aqueous solution, erythromycin ophthalmic ointment, or tetracycline ophthalmic ointment, all of which are effective.

When are the drops given?

The eye drops are applied to each eye immediately after birth, usually in the delivery room itself.

Are they safe?

Occasionally the eye drops (most commonly silver nitrate) can cause a mild irritation of the eyes. However, the symptoms resolve on their own and have no long-term effects on the baby.

SECTION II: NEWBORN SCREENING

Newborn screening identifies serious medical conditions that are not obviously apparent at birth. Although these diseases are rare, it is important to identify them early in order to initiate appropriate preventive measures and prevent long-term physical and mental impairments.

Newborn screening tests take place within the first few days of life. Screening identifies newborns who may have a problem and require further testing before a definitive diagnosis can be made.

A wide range of newborn screening tests can be performed. Some of these tests are mandated by state law, which differs from state to state. In addition, there are many optional tests you and your doctor can order.

The USPSTF recommends that all newborns be screened for phenylketonuria (PKU), congenital hypothyroidism (CH), and sickle cell disease. Each of these three newborn screening tests is required by law in all fifty states and in the District of Columbia. It is extremely rare for an infant born in the United States not to be screened for these disorders. The following sections briefly discuss these three diseases and the screening guidelines.

What is phenylketonuria?

Phenylketonuria (PKU; fen-uhl-kee-tuh-NURE-ee-yuh) is a hereditary disease that affects 1 in every 13,500 to 19,000 newborns. It is caused by the lack of a liver enzyme required to digest the amino acid phenylalanine. Because of this enzyme deficiency, phenylalanine accumulates in the blood and tissues and, if untreated, over time causes irreversible neurological damage, including severe mental retardation and seizures.

Newborns affected by PKU usually do not show any signs of the disease at birth. However, by 6 to 12 months of age, they begin to exhibit signs of impaired development, which is irreversible. The most effective way to diagnose PKU before this damage occurs is through neonatal screening.

The treatment for PKU is to restrict dietary sources of phenylalanine, such as milk and various meats, through special infant formulas and, later in life, a low-protein diet. Properly treated, children with PKU can expect to live normal, healthy lives.

What is congenital hypothyroidism?

Congenital hypothyroidism (CH; hi-po-THI-royd-iz-em) is caused by insufficient production of thyroid hormone. Because thyroid hormones play an important role in normal physical growth and mental development, CH may result in growth failure, deafness, and mental retardation if untreated.

CH occurs in an estimated 1 of every 3,000 to 4,000 births, and 15 to 20 percent of the cases are inherited.

Affected infants do not show any signs or symptoms of CH at birth. The first signs usually appear at 3 to 4 months of age, after some irreversible brain damage has already occurred. Newborn screening is the best way to diagnose CH early and prevent long-term complications. Screening is done with a simple blood test after birth, which must be followed by confirmatory testing if abnormal. Try not to be overly concerned about an abnormal screen. False positives are common, and only one in twenty-five positive screening tests are confirmed to be CH.

CH is treated with daily thyroid hormone supplements. Affected infants who begin treatment within the first few weeks of life typically retain full cognitive function.

What is sickle cell anemia?

Sickle cell anemia is a disease of red blood cells that causes them to have an abnormal "sickle" shape. It is an inherited disease that affects 1 in 375 African American infants born in the United States and smaller proportions of children in other ethnic groups. Because sickle-shaped cells do not move easily through the blood vessels, children with sickle cell anemia are at risk for serious complications from blockages in blood flow, the most dangerous of which are major infections.

Infants with sickle cell anemia commonly do not have any symptoms of their disease yet remain at risk for life-threatening infections. Through screening, children with sickle cell anemia can be diagnosed early and benefit from interventions that maximize protection against infection. These include the initiation of preventive antibiotics, vaccination against the pneumococcus bacteria, and parental education about signs and symptoms of early infection.

Screening is done through a simple blood test at birth. Children with two defective copies of the gene that causes sickle cell anemia are diagnosed with sickle cell disease. Those who have one defective copy of the gene and one normal copy have sickle cell trait and are generally healthy.

How is newborn screening done?

Unlike standard blood tests, newborn screening is done by pricking the baby's heel for a few drops of blood. Often the blood sample is taken while the baby is in the nursery, so it is not uncommon for parents to be unaware that the test was performed.

It is important that the sample be obtained after the first day of life because certain screening tests are not as effective if done too soon after birth. As a result, some states routinely test all infants twice to ensure proper testing, but many do not. If you are concerned that your child's screening was done improperly, talk to your child's doctor.

If your child's test shows an abnormal result, you should be notified. However, if you don't hear anything it is a good idea to follow up with your child's doctor and verify the results.

What other newborn screening tests should my child have done?

There are over fifty disorders that can be detected through newborn screening. Other organizations, including the American Academy of Pediatrics (AAP), recommend additional newborn screening tests, and almost every state mandates testing for more than these three disorders for all newborns. Although the USPSTF does not make formal recommendations for or against screening for any other disorder, you and your doctor may decide that other screening tests are right for your child, based on family history or other concerns.

What if a test has to be repeated or shows a possible health problem?

Try not to get overly anxious or concerned. There are many reasons a baby may need to be retested, including if the first test was done too early or if there was something wrong with the sample. Even if the screening test is abnormal, this does not necessarily mean that your child has a health problem. For example, as stated earlier, only one in every twenty-five abnormal screening tests for congenital hypothyroidism represents a true case.

To determine the significance of an abnormal screening result, additional testing is required, for which your child's doctor may refer you to a specialist. If further evaluation confirms a problem, your child will be started on treatment that can prevent most of the serious physical and mental problems associated with newborn diseases.

SECTION III: NEWBORN SCREENING FOR HEARING LOSS

Not all children hear and listen from birth.[2] About two or three out of every one thousand children in the United States are born deaf or hard of hearing, a condition called *congenital permanent hearing loss* (PHL). Because hearing is critical for language development, congenital PHL is associated with delayed language, learning, and speech development, which may have lifelong consequences.

Hearing loss is often difficult to detect in young infants, so diagnosis and treatment of congenital PHL is often delayed until 1 to 2 years of age. Unfortunately, this is long after what is called "the critical period"—the first 6 months of life, when development of early speech and language occurs. Through simple bedside tests, newborns can be screened for hearing loss and, if found to have PHL, can benefit from early interventions designed to improve hearing and minimize developmental delays.

The USPSTF recommends screening for hearing loss in all newborn infants by 1 month. This recommendation is based on evidence that newborn screening is highly accurate and leads to early identification and treatment of infants with hearing loss and improved language outcomes. Many hospitals routinely screen all children for hearing loss, but not all do. Make sure that your baby's hearing has been screened either before you leave the hospital or immediately afterward. If your child's hearing has not received a screening, schedule one before he or she reaches 1 month of age.

Should all infants be screened for hearing loss?

Yes! Risk factors for congenital PHL include spending two or more days in the neonatal intensive care unit, a family history of hereditary childhood hearing loss, craniofacial abnormalities, and congenital infections. However, studies show that 50 percent of newborns affected by congenital PHL have none of these risk factors. This underscores the importance of screening in all newborns, regardless of risk factors.

Aren't all newborns automatically screened?

No. Many U.S. states have enacted legislation that mandates newborn hearing screening. Even in states in which screening is not mandatory, many hospitals routinely perform it on all newborns. Unfortunately, this is not always the case. In addition, not all newborns who have abnormal hearing screens receive appropriate follow-up care. Partner with your child's doctor to find out if your child's hearing has been screened and ensure that he or she receives the right care.

How is screening done?

Two hearing tests are used to screen babies. Both tests are done painlessly while the infant is resting quietly.

- *Otoacoustic emissions* (OAE) tests show how your child's ears respond to sound. During this test, the ear is stimulated with sound through an earphone, and the presence of a normal reflection of the sound waves (or echo) is measured. The absence of an echo suggests hearing loss.

▸ *Auditory brain stem response* (ABR) checks how the brain responds to sound. During this test, electrodes are placed on the head and are used to record brain wave activity as sound is transmitted to the ears via earphones. An inadequate response to the sounds suggests hearing loss.

Often these tests are administered in a two-step screening process. All infants receive the OAE test, and those who do not pass then receive the ABR. If both tests suggest a hearing problem, the infant is referred for further testing.

What are the benefits of screening?

Evidence shows that screening leads to earlier detection and treatment of hearing loss. In addition, there is a growing body of evidence that earlier intervention results in improved language skills.

What are the risks?

The screening tests themselves are harmless. However, positive test results can provoke anxiety, and false positives (that is, the screening test suggests a problem when there isn't one) occasionally occur. In addition, certain treatments for congenital PHL can cause harm. For example, cochlear implant surgery carries the risks of surgery and an increased risk of meningitis, an infection of the covering of the brain, for several years after implantation.

What happens if my child does not pass the hearing screening?

Hearing screening tests are just that—screening tests. They are not diagnostic. The purpose of screening is to discover as many children with hearing problems as possible so that they get the appropriate treatment. If your child does not pass his or her screening, the next step is for him or her to be evaluated by an audiologist, a specialist in hearing. Through further testing, an audiologist can determine whether your child has hearing loss and, if so, can help develop a treatment plan.

Schedule the follow-up appointment immediately. Because the critical window for language development is the first 6 months of life, appropriate care for your child's hearing should not be delayed beyond 3 months of age.

What treatment options are available if my child has hearing loss?

Treatment options include interventions designed to improve hearing, such as hearing aids and cochlear implants (an electronic device that is surgically implanted in the inner ear), and those designed to improve communication, such as assistive technologies and language therapy (e.g., sign language, lip reading). Often a combination approach is used to ensure the best possible outcome.

The fact that several effective interventions are proven to improve hearing and long-term language and developmental outcomes in children with hearing loss underscores the importance of screening.

SECTION IV: IRON SUPPLEMENTATION FOR AT-RISK INFANTS

When there is not enough iron in the body, over time the deficiency can cause anemia, a condition in which the number of red blood cells is lower than normal.

Children are at increased risk of iron deficiency anemia, in part because of an increased demand for iron to support growth. While estimates vary widely, some experts report that one in ten children under age 2 have iron deficiency anemia. Symptoms of anemia depend on the severity and course of the condition. Children with mild anemia or anemia that has developed very slowly may have no symptoms at all. Still, despite the absence of symptoms, children with anemia are at risk for psychomotor and cognitive abnormalities, which may lead to poor school performance.

The USPSTF recommends iron supplementation for infants ages 6 to 12 months who are at increased risk of iron deficiency anemia. The task force recommendation is based on evidence that iron supplementation reduces the risk of iron deficiency anemia and may improve neurodevelopmental outcomes in at-risk children. The following sections provide a brief introduction to iron deficiency anemia and detail the guidelines for iron supplementation.

What is iron deficiency anemia? How do children get it?

The body needs iron to build new cells. During childhood, because of the high rate of growth, there is an increased demand for iron, which can deplete a child's iron stores. Because iron is an essential component of hemoglobin—the oxygen-carrying protein that gives blood its red color—a lack of iron can lead to anemia. *Anemia* (uh-NEE-me-uh) is a condition in which there are fewer red blood cells in the blood than normal. There are many types and causes of anemia. *Iron deficiency anemia* is one type of anemia caused by having too little iron in the body. In children, iron deficiency anemia is usually due to accelerated rates of growth, as seen in low-birthweight and preterm infants, and insufficient amounts of iron in the diet.

Can it be prevented?

The best way to prevent iron deficiency anemia is to optimize your child's nutrition. Iron in foods is variably absorbed. Although only 5 percent of iron from formula milk is absorbed, and only 10 percent from whole cow's milk, 50 percent of iron in breast milk can be absorbed by infants. Therefore, in addition to its many other health benefits, exclusively breastfeeding your baby for the first 6 months of life is the best way to prevent your child from developing iron deficiency anemia. Later, when solid foods are introduced, it is best to include iron-enriched products, such as iron-fortified cereals, in your baby's diet.

For children at risk for iron deficiency anemia, however, these measures are sometimes not enough, and iron supplementation is needed.

Should my child receive iron supplementation?

The USPSTF recommends iron supplementation for infants ages 6 to 12 months who are at risk for iron deficiency anemia. Infants who are preterm (born before 37 weeks) or low birthweight (under 5.5 pounds at birth) are considered high risk for iron deficiency anemia and should receive iron supplementation.

It has not been as well established whether children with other risk factors for iron deficiency anemia also benefit from iron supplementation. These include children living in poverty; those from families who recently emigrated from developing countries; babies fed cow's or goat's milk; and children of African American, Native American, or Native Alaskan descent. If your child has one or more of these risk factors, talk to your doctor about whether iron supplementation is right for your child.

What about at-risk children younger than 6 months?

The USPSTF does not address iron supplementation in infants younger than 6 months. However, other organizations, such as the AAP, recommend that iron supplementation begin at 2 to 3 months of age for preterm and low-birthweight infants. Your child's doctor can help you decide which guideline to follow.

What about children ages 6 to 12 months not at increased risk?

The USPSTF has not found good evidence that iron supplementation improves the health of children ages 6 to 12 months not at increased risk for iron deficiency anemia. Thus, the task force makes no recommendation for or against supplementation in this age group. It is best to discuss this with your child's doctor.

How is iron supplementation given? What are the harms?

There are many types of iron preparations available, including iron drops, syrups, elixirs (also called oral iron supplements), and iron-fortified formulas and cereals. Your child's doctor can help decide which is the best form of supplementation for your child.

The most worrisome danger of oral iron supplements is accidental overdose, so keep them out of sight of young children. Oral iron supplements can also cause gastrointestinal upset and constipation, but these go away by simply stopping the medicine. With iron-fortified foods and formula, there are no known side effects or risks of overdose, but the tradeoff is that iron-fortified foods do not provide as much iron as oral supplements do.

Shouldn't my child just get tested for iron deficiency anemia?

The USPSTF did not find sufficient evidence to make a recommendation for or against screening for iron deficiency anemia in children ages 6 to 12 months. For children at increased risk, the task force recommends initiating iron supplementation without screening. For those not at increased risk, the USPSTF does not recommend iron supplementation or screening. Other groups, including the AAP, advise screening all infants for anemia at age 9 months.

In children at increased risk, supplementation may be preferable to screening. Iron deficiency anemia is an advanced stage of iron deficiency, so a child who is iron deficient may not yet have anemia but may still be at risk of developing it. In such a child, screening would not detect the iron deficiency. Children not at increased risk of iron deficiency anemia are less likely to have the condition. Not screening spares your child from having what is likely to be an unnecessary blood test. In the end, the decision is best left up to you and your child's doctor.

SECTION V: PREVENTION OF DENTAL CAVITIES IN PRESCHOOL CHILDREN

Dental cavities are a common disease of childhood. As many as one in five children between ages 2 and 5 have them. If untreated, cavities in primary teeth may lead to cavities in permanent teeth and a possible loss of arch space. Treatment for cavities subjects young children to painful dental procedures and is costly.

One of the most effective ways to prevent dental cavities is through drinking fluoridated water. Research shows that fluoridated water reduces cavities and helps repair the early stages of tooth decay. While many communities in the United States have access to fluoridated water, some do not. Even in areas with fluoridated water, children may not be exposed to sufficient levels of fluoride if their families' primary source of water is unfluoridated (e.g., bottled water, filtered water, or well water). For these children, oral fluoride supplementation is an effective way to assure adequate fluoride intake and has been shown to prevent 32 to 81 percent of dental cavities.

The most common harm from fluoride is *dental fluorosis* (fluh-RO-sis). Dental fluorosis is not a disease or harmful condition but a cosmetic problem that may result in faint white lines or streaks on the teeth. By making sure children are getting just the right amount of fluoride, the risk of both cavities and fluorosis can be minimized.

The USPSTF recommends oral fluoride supplementation for preschool children older than 6 months whose primary water source is deficient in fluoride. This recommendation is based on evidence that in preschool children with low fluoride exposure, prescription of oral fluoride supplements leads to reduced dental cavities.

What is fluoride? What is fluoridated water?

Fluoride is an element that helps prevent cavities. It occurs naturally in varying amounts in all water sources and is commercially available in most brands of toothpaste. Fluoridated water is water that has been treated so that its fluoride content is optimal for dental health (0.7–1.2 ppm, or parts per million). Although community water fluoridation is proven to reduce tooth decay and is widely recommended by public health experts, not everyone has access to fluoridated water.

How do I find out if my water is properly fluoridated?

There are several ways in which you can find out the fluoride levels in your water:

- Contact your local water provider.
- Check your annual water quality report.
- Visit the Environmental Protection Agency (EPA) online at www.epa.gov and search for the annual water quality report for your area.[3]
- Ask your doctor.

Having access to fluoridated water in your home is only part of the equation. For example, if you live in a community with access to fluoridated water but exclusively drink bottled water, you still may not be getting enough fluoride. The key is to have sufficient amounts of fluoride in your *primary water source*. For some people, their primary water source may be at work, school, or day care rather than at home; for others, their primary water source may be filtered water, bottled water, or well water instead of tap water.

How is oral fluoride supplementation given?

Oral fluoride supplements come as tablets, drops, or lozenges that your child will take daily. They are available only by prescription. Supplements are not recommended for children under 6 months old. Fluoride varnishes, which are professionally applied topical fluorides, are also effective and can be administered by your child's dentist during routine visits or sometimes by his or her primary care doctor.

Can fluoride be dangerous?

Fluoride is safe and effective when used properly. At extremely high doses, it can be toxic, but these levels are difficult to reach when using fluoride products at home. A much more common side effect of fluoride supplementation is dental fluorosis, which results in faint white lines or streaks on the teeth and is not at all harmful or dangerous.

SECTION VI: VISION SCREENING IN CHILDREN YOUNGER THAN AGE 5

About 5 to 10 percent of preschool children have problems with their vision. The most common causes of visual impairment in this age group are amblyopia, strabismus, and defects in visual acuity (see figure 12.1). Each of these conditions can lead to poor school performance and self-image. Other vision problems, such as amblyopia, must be diagnosed and corrected as early as possible to prevent permanent vision loss and blindness in the affected eye.

About 3 percent of preschoolers have visual impairments. Unlike adults, children often do not complain about problems with vision. Furthermore, certain problems, such as strabismus, are difficult to detect without careful examination by an experienced clinician. Because visual impairment in children has an early window period when interventions lead to better outcomes, early detection, referral, and treatment are important.

The USPSTF recommends routine screening to detect amblyopia, strabismus, and defects in visual acuity in children younger than 5 years. Screening is done through simple office tests that can signal the need to refer the patient to an experienced pediatric eye care professional for proper diagnosis and treatment.

What is amblyopia?

Amblyopia (am-blee-OH-pee-uh), commonly known as lazy eye, is a serious condition marked by reduced vision that cannot be attributed to any eye disease and cannot be corrected with eyewear.[4] Rather, the disease relates to the brain ignoring the electrical signals coming from one or both eyes. Crossed or turned eye (strabismus) is often incorrectly referred to as "lazy eye." Although strabismus is a common cause of amblyopia, they are not the same condition.

Amblyopia is the most common cause of visual impairment in childhood and affects two to three out of every one hundred children. While sometimes easily spotted, amblyopia can be subtle and may go unnoticed. If not detected and treated early in life, it can cause a permanent loss of vision, including blindness.

Anything that causes large differences in vision between the two eyes in young children can result in amblyopia. This includes strabismus (deviation of one eye), *anisometropia* (different prescriptions in each eye), and obstructions in vision, such as lid droop or cataracts. This is because the brain will tend to favor the eye with clear vision and ignore the one with bad vision, which over time prevents critical connections between that eye and the brain from developing. Once this happens, even corrective surgery or glasses cannot fix the impaired vision in the affected eye.

The treatment for amblyopia involves correcting the underlying problem early and getting the child to use the weaker eye. In some cases, glasses or contact lenses are sufficient to correct the underlying problem; in other cases, surgery may be needed. In addition, the stronger eye is temporarily weakened by blurring it with eye drops or simply placing an adhesive patch on it to get the child to use the weaker eye most of the time and make it stronger.

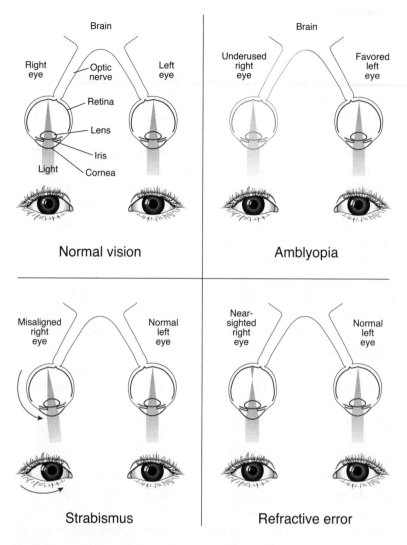

Figure 12.1. The eye is a complicated organ with many parts that work together to provide vision. In normal vision, light travels through the cornea and is focused by the lens onto the retina, a light-sensitive tissue in the back of the eye. The retina then transmits the light as electrical signals that travel to the brain through the optic nerve. In amblyopia, one of the eyes is favored by the brain so that electric signals from the unfavored eye, sometimes called the "lazy eye," are not transmitted to the brain. Over time, this lack of stimuli from the lazy eye can lead to permanent vision loss. Strabismus is a condition in which the eyes are misaligned. In some people, this turning of the eye is constant, and in others, it occurs intermittently. In young children, strabismus can lead to amblyopia. Refractive error occurs when a defect in the cornea prevents light from being perfectly focused on the retina; instead the light is focused in front of the retina (causing myopia, or nearsightedness) or behind the retina (causing hyperopia, or farsightedness).

What is strabismus?

Strabismus (struh-BIZ-muss) is an eye condition in which the eyes are misaligned and point in different directions. It is also referred to as crossed eyes, eye turns, wandering eyes, or deviating eye. Although strabismus may lead to amblyopia, they are not the same condition.

When the misalignment is present all the time, it is called *constant strabismus*. When the misalignment is observed only occasionally, such as when the child is tired or ill, it is called *intermittent strabismus*. Up to the first 6 months of age, intermittent strabismus is considered normal; thereafter, it needs to be evaluated. Constant strabismus requires medical attention at any age.

People often think of strabismus as a cosmetic problem, but it is more serious than that. Normal vision requires both eyes to look in the same direction at the same time. When a child's eyes are misaligned, he or she gets a different picture from each eye, which causes the child's brain to ignore the picture from the weaker eye. If strabismus is not detected or treated at a young age, it can result in amblyopia. As discussed above, children with amblyopia are at risk of permanent vision loss, even blindness.

Strabismus is a treatable condition. In intermittent strabismus, eye patching or eye drops can help the child to use the weaker eye more frequently and make it stronger. In constant strabismus and refractory cases of intermittent strabismus, surgery is the preferred method of correction.

What is refractive error?

A refractive error is an optical defect in the eye that prevents light from being perfectly focused onto the retina (back of the eye). It is the type of vision problem we are most familiar with and that is typically corrected by glasses or contacts. Refractive errors include myopia (nearsightedness), hyperopia (farsightedness), presbyopia (inability to focus up close that occurs with age), and astigmatism (imperfections in the surface of the eye or cornea).

An estimated 5 percent to 7 percent of preschool children have refractive errors. Unlike adults, young children do not complain about blurry vision or difficulty seeing, and therefore without proper vision testing, they remain undiagnosed and untreated. Refractive errors can lead to poor school performance and low self-esteem. Rarely, if the refractive error between the two eyes differs greatly, it can lead to amblyopia and risk of permanent vision loss.

The treatment for refractive error in this age group is usually eye glasses; in older children, contact lenses and corrective laser surgery are also options.

How is screening done?

While the USPSTF recommends routine screening for visual impairment in preschool children, they do not specify what screening tests should be performed, how often, or by what type of clinician (e.g., pediatrician, optometrist, ophthalmologist). This is in part because not many studies have been done to compare the large number of screening tests available.

The AAP recommends that children undergo vision screening at all well-child visits starting at birth. These are the particular tests they recommend:

Birth to 3 years:

1. *ocular history:* family history of eye problems or eye diseases; concerns about child's eyes, vision, or unusual behavior (e.g., tilting head to one side)
2. *vision assessment:* ability to fixate on and track a moving object
3. *external inspection of the eyes and lids:* checking for cataracts, lid droop, asymmetries; testing for alignment
4. *ocular motility assessment:* ability to fully move eyes in all directions
5. *pupil examination:* testing for symmetrical response to direct and consensual light
6. *red reflex examination:* looking for the presence of a reflection of light from the back of the eye

Three years and older:

- exams 1 through 6 plus
- *age-appropriate visual acuity measurement:* using cards, charts, or a machine to test vision; and
- *attempt at ophthalmoscopy:* using a lighted instrument to see the retina and nerve structures at the back of the eye

A similar set of tests is recommended by the American Optometric Association (AOA), although it recommends screening less frequently: 6 months, 3 years, and before entering school. Ask your child's doctor what his or her plan is for vision screening.

What happens if something abnormal is found?

The eye exam is a series of screening tests, not diagnostic tests. Usually, an abnormal finding needs to be evaluated further by a more experienced eye care professional such as a pediatric optometrist or pediatric ophthalmologist before a definitive diagnosis can be made. The reason screening for visual impairment in preschool children is so important is that effective treatments exist for most of the common pediatric eye conditions. By getting screened and referred early to an eye specialist your child has the best chance of recovery.

SECTION VII: VACCINES IN EARLY CHILDHOOD

Vaccines save millions of children from serious harm and death. Before children were routinely vaccinated in the United States, every year

- 10,000 children were paralyzed by polio. Today, none are.
- 20,000 newborns developed birth defects and cognitive impairment from rubella. This disease is practically nonexistent today.
- 4 million children were afflicted by measles. Now a couple hundred infections occur annually (largely due to outbreaks among unvaccinated children).
- 200,000 people, mostly children, were infected by diphtheria, and 15,000 would die. Since 2000, there have been fewer than 10 cases in the United States total.
- 1 in every 200 children suffered from meningitis (an infection of the covering of the brain) caused by *Haemophilus influenzae* type b (Hib), leaving many with permanent brain damage. Now fewer than 300 cases per year occur among children under 5.
- 200,000 people would develop pertussis (whooping cough). Today the incidence is 25,000.[5]

Now, thanks to universal vaccination, many of these diseases have become rare and, in some cases, been eliminated. Most children today are routinely vaccinated against these and other infectious illnesses. In recent years, however, a growing number of children are being left unvaccinated by their parents and caregivers, who question the continued need for vaccination against diseases that have now become rare and are concerned about reports that vaccines cause diseases such as autism and attention deficit hyperactivity disorder (ADHD).

The Centers for Disease Control and Prevention (CDC) recommends routine vaccination of children against common vaccine-preventable diseases. In general, your child should receive vaccinations against the following infections (displayed alphabetically):

- diphtheria, tetanus, pertussis (DTap)
- *Haemophilis influenza* (Hib)
- hepatitis A
- hepatitis B
- human papillomavirus (HPV)
- influenza (the flu)
- measles, mumps, rubella (MMR)
- meningococcus
- pneumococcus
- polio
- rotavirus
- varicella (chickenpox)

The best way to ensure your child is up to date on all vaccines is to partner with your child's doctor. The following brief introduction to vaccines addresses some of the common concerns parents and other caregivers have about vaccination. The 2009 vaccination schedule for children is provided in the appendix as are the CDC fact sheets on each vaccine. Chapter 6 discusses the human papillomavirus (HPV) vaccine in greater detail. Chapter 15 discusses the hepatitis vaccine.

What's the difference between vaccines and immunizations?

Vaccines are any substance administered to produce immunity to, or protection against, a particular disease. Immunization is the process of inducing immunity to a particular disease. Strictly speaking, vaccines are a form of immunization, but in practice, the terms are interchangeable. Here the term vaccine is used.

What exactly is a vaccine?

Let's break down the definition of a vaccine: "any substance administered to produce immunity to a particular disease."

Vaccines are commonly made of one of four *substances*: killed microorganisms (e.g., flu vaccine); live, weakened microorganisms (e.g., measles, mumps, rubella vaccine); toxoids or modified toxins rendered nontoxic (e.g., tetanus vaccine); or subunits of microorganisms (e.g., hepatitis B vaccine). Vaccines must be *administered*. People usually think of getting shots when they think of vaccines, but there are other ways to get vaccinated. For example, the flu vaccine is available in a vaporized form, which is inhaled, as well as in an injectable form, given as a shot. Other vaccines can be administered by mouth.

Vaccines produce *immunity*, or protection. The immune system is adaptable. Most adults are immune to chickenpox. However, when you were born, you didn't have natural protection against it. Usually, we develop immunity to a microorganism after the first time we are exposed to it. That's why people ordinarily get chickenpox only once in their lives. But through vaccination, immunity develops without having to get sick. Thus, today children who get the vaccine against chickenpox are immune to the disease, even though they have never had it.

Finally, they provide protection against a *particular* disease. Each vaccine provides protection against one or more microorganisms that cause disease. Getting a vaccine against one microorganism does not usually provide protection against any others. This is true even if the two microorganisms cause the same disease. That is why, for example, the pneumococcal vaccine provides protection against only some causes of pneumonia. Pneumonia is caused by over a dozen different types of bacteria, but the pneumococcal polysaccharide vaccine protects against only the pneumococcus family of bacteria, also called *Streptococcus pneumoniae,* and even then only certain members of that family. Vaccines are so specific that sometimes you need a new shot every time the microorganism mutates, or changes its genetic material. That is why, for example, people who need the flu shot are advised to get it every year. The virus that causes the flu, the influenza virus, mutates every year, so last year's flu shot often does not provide adequate protection against this year's flu.

How do vaccines prevent infection?

Vaccines themselves do not prevent infection. Instead, they rev up the body's immune system, which in turn prevents infection. Vaccines teach the immune system how to recognize a microorganism and how to defend against it. Normally, the immune system learns these skills after the first infection. Thus, the first time the immune system encounters one of these microorganisms, it is slow to respond. But if the same microorganism attacks the body a second time, the immune system is more prepared, often so much so that it prevents the second infection altogether. The trouble is that the first infection can sometimes cause serious harm to the body—even death. Vaccines work by *simulating* the first infection so that when the immune system encounters the microorganism for the first time, it will be as if it were the second time.

Vaccines do this in surprising ways; they basically have the look, smell, and taste of a microorganism without its disease-causing capabilities. Some vaccines, for example, are dead microorganisms; by being vaccinated with these dead microorganisms, the body learns how to recognize them, but because they are dead, they do not harm the body. Other vaccines are living microorganisms that have been weakened, called *attenuated vaccines*. Still others are made of one part of the microorganism, such as its outer coating. The idea behind all of these is the same—to simulate the microorganism without harming the body.

This concept helps explain why the most common side effects of any vaccine are mild flulike symptoms—a low-grade fever, a rash, or just feeling tired and worn out. The purpose of a vaccine is to simulate an actual infection by activating the immune system. When we get sick, the fevers, rashes, and tiredness we experience are not because of the infection; instead they are by-products of the immune system being activated. So the flulike symptoms we sometimes experience after a shot are actually a sign that the immune system is being activated and that the vaccine is working.

I get the flu shot every year and I still get the flu. Do vaccines really work?

No vaccine is 100 percent effective. Most childhood vaccinations prevent 85 percent or more of infections; for the 15 percent or fewer children who still get the infection, the illness is often milder and less dangerous than it would have been without the vaccine. For adult vaccinations, the result is often to prevent life-threatening illness rather than to prevent infection. This is true, for example, with pneumonia. Pneumonia, or infection of the lung, can be caused by many different types of bacteria. But the vaccine against pneumonia, called the *pneumococcal polysaccharide* (PPV23) vaccine, protects against the type of bacteria that causes the most deadly type of pneumonia, pneumococcal pneumonia. So even after receiving the PPV23, you may still get pneumonia, but it is much less likely to be fatal or disabling than it would be otherwise.

The flu shot is a special case. The flu shot protects against a specific microorganism called the influenza virus. But the "flu" as most people know it can be caused by many different viruses. That's why your doctor might say you have "flulike" symptoms without necessarily saying you have the specific "flu" virus. Part of the reason that doctors vaccinate against the influenza virus and not other viruses that cause flulike symptoms is that infection with the influenza virus is the most dangerous. The most important thing to keep in mind is that the flu shot is meant to protect you against life-threatening flu illnesses but unfortunately may not protect you against other, less dangerous but still troublesome flulike illnesses.

Why does my child need vaccines for diseases that people no longer get?

Outbreaks of measles, whooping cough, and chickenpox commonly occur when vaccination rates drop. In fact, in recent years, measles has been on the rise, an alarming trend that scientists have linked to increasing rates of vaccine refusal by parents. Unvaccinated children not only are at greater risk of infection themselves, but their communities are also at greater risk, especially those too young to be vaccinated or who cannot receive vaccines for medical reasons. This is in part because diseases that have become rare in the United States are still common in other parts of the world where access to vaccines is limited. As the world gets smaller and international travel more frequent, exposure to diseases that no longer exist here is becoming more probable. A recent outbreak of measles in Washington State that affected nineteen people (of whom eighteen were unvaccinated) was traced back to a church conference attended by people from five different countries.[6] As further evidence, one of the most recent cases of polio paralysis in the United States was an American who traveled to Costa Rica and got infected with the polio virus—this person was also unvaccinated.[7]

Do vaccines have side effects? Can they cause harm?

Vaccines are very safe. Many of the recommended vaccines have been used by doctors for decades. Newer vaccines, although they have not been around as long, are extensively studied for their safety and effectiveness.

That being said, vaccines are not harmless. Every vaccine has potential side effects. The most common side effect is pain and redness at the site of injection. In addition, it is not uncommon for vaccines to cause mild flulike symptoms, such as low-grade fevers and general tiredness. As noted earlier, these symptoms are actually a sign that the vaccine is working. They are generally mild and improve on their own or with over-the-counter remedies. Rarely, vaccines can cause more serious side effects, such as a severe allergic reaction. The specific side effects vary with each vaccine and are listed in the appendix. As with any medication, be sure to tell your child's doctor if your child has any allergies, including a history of a reaction to medications or foods.

The risks of vaccination must be weighed against the risks of not vaccinating. The Centers for Disease Control and Prevention (CDC) recommends a vaccine based on its assessment of the risks and benefits. It is up to you, however, to weigh these risks and benefits and decide what is right for your child.

I heard that some vaccines can cause autism. Is this true?

No. After extensive review, scientists have not found any relationship between vaccines and autism. While there is still considerable controversy about this in the lay press and certain advocacy groups, doctors and scientists as a group agree that vaccines do not cause autism.

How do I decide?

The risks of vaccinating must be weighed against the risks of not vaccinating. The CDC, through expert scientific consensus, recommends that the benefits of vaccination outweigh the risks. However, it is up to you to decide how you weigh these benefits and risks for your child. Be sure to weigh them one vaccine at a time. Too often parents decide against vaccinations altogether, without considering each vaccine as an independent decision.

REFERENCES

American Academy of Pediatrics (AAP). www.aap.org.

American Dental Association (ADA). www.ada.org.

American Optometric Association (AOA). www.aoa.org.

Atkinson, W., S. Wolfe, J. Hamborsky, and L. McIntyre, eds. Centers for Disease Control and Prevention (CDC). *Epidemiology and Prevention of Vaccine-Preventable Diseases*. 11th ed. Washington, D.C.: Public Health Foundation, 2009.

Centers for Disease Control and Prevention (CDC). U.S. Department of Health and Human Services. www.cdc.gov.

Cooper, J., and R. Cooper. "All About Amblyopia (lazy eye)." www.strabismus.org/amblyopia_lazy_eye.html.

National Institutes on Deafness and Other Communication Disorders. National Institutes of Health (NIH). www.nidcd.nih.gov.

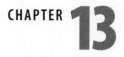

Gonorrhea Screening

Gonorrhea is a common sexually transmitted infection (STI). The symptoms of gonorrhea are usually mild, but if untreated, infection can cause serious health problems and be transmitted to sexual partners and from mother to child during childbirth.

Gonorrhea is often difficult to detect because infections are commonly asymptomatic. Even when symptoms occur, they are often mild and transient —and therefore easy to overlook. As a result, many infected people do not get tested and treated, and they remain at risk for irreversible damage, including male and female infertility, pelvic inflammatory disease, and ectopic pregnancy.

Gonorrhea is a treatable disease, and accurate diagnostic tests are available to identify asymptomatic individuals with infection. Through regular screening, gonorrhea can be detected and cured with antibiotics, before complications develop or the infection is spread to others. Despite this, only 20 to 25 percent of sexually active women are routinely screened for gonorrhea.

The United States Preventive Services Task Force (USPSTF) recommends screening for gonorrhea in all sexually active women age 24 or younger and in women age 25 or older at risk for infection.[1] The following sections provide an introduction to gonorrhea and outline the guidelines for screening in nonpregnant women. Screening in pregnancy is discussed in chapter 19.

SECTION I: GONORRHEA 101

Gonorrhea (gone-uh-REE-uh) is an infectious disease caused by the bacteria *Neisseria gonorrhoeae*. It is sometimes referred to as "the clap."[2]

How common is gonorrhea?

Gonorrhea is one of the most common STIs in the United States, affecting over 700,000 Americans each year. The disease affects both men and women and occurs in all age groups. Three out of four reported cases of gonorrhea in the United States occur in people younger than 30. The highest rates of infection are present in 15- to 19-year-old women and 20- to 24-year-old men.

How does gonorrhea spread? Who is at risk?

Gonorrhea is transmitted during unprotected vaginal, anal, or oral sex. It can also be passed from an infected mother to her baby during vaginal childbirth. It is highly contagious and spreads easily from infected people to noninfected ones.

Every sexually active person is potentially at risk for gonorrhea infection. As with all STIs, the greater the number of sexual partners, the greater the risk of infection. Gonorrhea infection is so common among young people that just having one partner can put someone at risk. In addition, because their cervix is not fully matured, sexually active adolescents and young women are at particularly high risk for infection.

What are the symptoms of gonorrhea?

Many people infected with gonorrhea have no symptoms of infection. Symptoms, when present, may include

- thick, cloudy, or bloody discharge from the penis or vagina
- pain or burning sensation when urinating
- frequent urination
- pain during sexual intercourse
- for women, lower abdominal pain, vaginal bleeding between periods, or heavier periods
- for men, painful or swollen testicles

Women get symptoms less often than men. Often, the only clue that a woman has gonorrhea is when her sexual partner becomes infected and experiences symptoms.

The severity of symptoms is not related to the risk of developing serious complications. A person with no symptoms of infection is no less likely to develop complications than someone with symptoms. In fact, because the person with symptoms is more likely to seek medical attention, the one without symptoms may actually have worse outcomes.

What kinds of complications can gonorrhea cause?

If untreated, gonorrhea can lead to major and permanent health problems in women, men, and the newborn babies of infected women.

‣ In women, gonorrhea is a common cause of *pelvic inflammatory disease* (PID), which develops when the gonorrhea bacteria spread into the uterus and fallopian tubes. PID can cause very severe, even disabling symptoms. It can also lead to internal abscesses (collections of pus) and damage the fallopian tubes, increasing the risk of infertility or a potentially fatal ectopic pregnancy (pregnancy outside the uterus).

‣ In men, gonorrhea can cause *epididymitis*—inflammation of the part of the testicles where the sperm ducts are located—a painful condition that requires antibiotics and can lead to infertility.

‣ In both men and women, gonorrhea can spread to the blood or joints and cause a life-threatening condition called *disseminated gonococcus*. It also causes skin breakdown and increases the likelihood of contracting HIV if exposed.

‣ Newborns who contract gonorrhea as they pass through the birth canal can develop *gonococcal ophthalmia* (an eye condition that can lead to blindness), joint infection, or widespread blood infection.

How do I prevent gonorrhea?

The best ways to avoid gonorrhea are to abstain from sexual contact or have sex only with a long-term partner who is monogamous, has been tested, and is known to be free of infection. If these situations are not possible, take the following steps to minimize your risk:

‣ *Use condoms correctly and consistently.* The correct use of protective barriers, such as male or female condoms, during every sexual encounter drastically decreases the risk of chlamydia and other STIs.

‣ *Limit your number of sex partners.* Having multiple sex partners puts you at a high risk of contracting gonorrhea and other STIs.

‣ *Get regularly screened for STIs.* Get informed about how often you should be screened for STIs like gonorrhea and partner with your doctor to stay up to date.

‣ *Get your partner regularly screened for STIs.* When you enter into a new sexual relationship, find out if your partner has been recently screened for sexually transmitted infections, and if not, work with him or her to get tested before becoming sexually active.

SECTION II: SCREENING FOR GONORRHEA

The USPSTF recommends that all sexually active women age 24 or younger be routinely screened for gonorrhea. In addition, the task force recommends screening women age 25 or older who have one or more risk factors, including

- multiple sexual partners in the past three months or a new sexual partner
- inconsistent condom use during sexual intercourse
- a history of gonorrhea or other STIs (including chlamydia, syphilis, hepatitis B, genital herpes, and HIV)
- a history of exchanging sex for drugs or money

These recommendations are based on evidence that screening tests for gonorrhea are accurate and that screening at-risk women reduces the risk of pelvic inflammatory disease.

The Centers for Disease Control and Prevention (CDC) recommends that women at increased risk be screened at least annually. For women who have tested negative for gonorrhea, when to get screened next is an individual decision. If you are in the same monogamous relationship you were in during your last test, it is probably safe to wait one year. However, if you are with a new partner or have multiple sexual partners, you may want to get screened more often.

Screening for gonorrhea is relatively simple. Two tests are most common:

- *Swab test:* For women, a mucous sample is taken from the cervix using a swab. In men, a sample can be taken from the penis. In addition, a culture swab of the anus can be performed.
- *Urine test:* A sample of urine is collected and then analyzed in a laboratory.

Both tests are acceptable for screening purposes. In women, obtaining a swab may require a pelvic exam; in men, the swab can be painful and is not routinely done. In comparison, a urine test is easier to perform and better tolerated. Thus, the swab test is generally used only in women already having a pelvic exam for another reason (e.g., Pap smears). In men and in women not otherwise requiring a pelvic exam, the urine test is preferred. Because the risk factors and screening tests for chlamydia and gonorrhea are similar, doctors routinely screen people for both STIs at once.

Why do only women need screening?

Gonorrhea causes symptoms and long-term complications in men and women, and both can spread the infection to others. So it is a fair question to ask why screening is only recommended for women. To date, the USPSTF has found insufficient evidence to support routine screening in men. The direct benefit to men of screening is small because infection is more likely to cause symptoms and the health risks of untreated gonorrhea infection in men are relatively low. Although screening in men may benefit women through reduced transmission of infection, there is insufficient evidence to support this reasoning.

That being said, screening men for gonorrhea infection is not unreasonable. Screening is safe and may provide health benefits to the screened person and his sexual partners. If you are a man and are at increased risk for gonorrhea infection or have concerns about being infected, talk to your doctor about whether screening is right for you.

What does being age 24 or under have to do with anything?

Just as studies have shown that women who have multiple sexual partners or who have a history of STIs are at higher risk for gonorrhea, they have also shown that sexually active women age 24 or under are at increased risk. Not only are the majority of gonorrhea cases in women age 24 or under, but this age group also has the highest rate of complications.

What are the risks?

The screening tests are safe and have no risks. However, if the screen is positive, you will be given antibiotics, which may have side effects.

What happens if the screen is negative?

A negative screen means that you do not have gonorrhea. Rarely, the screen will be falsely negative, but the chances of this are less than 1 percent. Be sure to document the results for your records. And be sure to talk to your doctor about when you should schedule your next screening test and about what you can do to lower your risk of infection.

What happens if the screen is positive?

A positive screen is equivalent to a diagnosis. This means you are infected with gonorrhea. Fortunately, gonorrheal infection can be treated and cured with antibiotics. The most common treatment is a single dose of antibiotics given orally or by injection. In most cases, the infection resolves within one or two weeks.

The CDC recommends that everyone treated for gonorrhea be treated for chlamydia as well, regardless of whether they test positive or negative for chlamydia. This is because people infected with gonorrhea are commonly co-infected with chlamydia.

Chances are high that your sexual partners also have gonorrhea. By continuing to have sexual contact with them, you risk becoming reinfected. Therefore, it is critical to inform your sexual partners of your infection and encourage them to be tested and, if necessary, treated. You should abstain from sexual contact until you and your sexual partners complete the treatment course.

Because you have gonorrhea, you are considered at high risk for having other STIs, including chlamydia, syphilis, and HIV. Talk with your doctor about getting tested for them. And be sure to talk to your doctor about how you can lower your risk of STIs through safer sex practices. Everyone who has a history of sexually transmitted infection in the past year is advised to receive STI counseling (see chapter 20 for more details).

REFERENCES

Centers for Disease Control and Prevention (CDC). U.S. Department of Health and Human Services. "Sexually Transmitted Diseases." www.cdc.gov/std.

CHAPTER 14

Healthy Eating Counseling

"You are what you eat" goes the popular saying. While this may not be entirely true, research shows that our diet is a major determinant of our health. In fact, unhealthy eating is one of the leading causes of illness and death in the United States. It is associated with a variety of diseases—coronary heart disease (CHD), stroke, certain types of cancer, osteoporosis, diverticular disease, and type 2 diabetes, to name a few.

Far from being the constant enemy, our eating habits can affect health in one of two ways. Having an unhealthy diet—that is, consuming too many calories and not enough nutrients—can lead to illness and disease. But having a healthy diet—consuming the right number of calories and the right nutrients—can stave off major illness and improve health. Indeed, studies show that people whose diets are low in fat (especially saturated fat and trans-fatty acids) and cholesterol and high in fruits, vegetables, and fiber have lower rates of cardiovascular disease and arguably several forms of cancer.

Despite the well-established benefits of healthy eating, more than 80 percent of Americans eat fewer than the recommended number of daily servings of fruit, vegetables, and grain products and more than the recommended daily calories and servings of saturated fat, total fat, and trans fats.[1] Part of the problem is that the science of healthy eating seems to change daily, and it is difficult to keep up. Even when we know what we should be eating, limited access to healthy foods, imperfect nutritional information, and our ingrained habits and lifestyles frequently get in the way of making the right choices.

One approach to overcoming these challenges that is too often neglected is partnering with our doctors. Studies show that in at-risk adults, intensive dietary counseling from doctors and other health care professionals can lead to sustained improvements in diet—increasing fruit, vegetable, and fiber intake and decreasing fat and excess calorie intake. For certain diseases, such as high blood pressure and type 2 diabetes, dietary counseling has also been shown to improve and in some cases prevent disease altogether. Despite this, less than one-third of patients report receiving advice from their physicians about healthier eating.

The United States Preventive Services Task Force (USPSTF) recommends intensive dietary counseling for adults with cholesterol disorders and other known risk factors for cardiovascular and diet-related chronic disease.[2] The following sections provide a brief introduction to healthier eating and outline the guidelines for dietary counseling.

SECTION I: HEALTHY DIETS 101

Different images come to mind when we think about dieting: failed New Year's resolutions, eating rice cakes three times a day, and feeling hungry all the time. Before reading on, put away those images and try to read the words below from a new perspective.

The concept of dieting is somewhat misguided. Most of us think of dieting as temporary changes we make to our eating habits to achieve a desired goal. Usually that goal is losing weight. But in this chapter, healthy eating means something different. Rather than "going on a diet," think about "improving eating patterns and habits." The changes to the diet advocated here are long term. The goal is not weight loss but healthier living and disease prevention.

Dieting can be an effective way to lose weight, but it is just one aspect of healthier eating. Here, the focus is on creating and maintaining a healthy diet that provides sufficient calories and nutrients (e.g., calcium, iron, fiber, vitamins). To underscore the distinction, the term *healthy eating* is used in this chapter instead of *dieting*. Healthy eating is a huge topic, too large to cover in depth in one chapter. The goal of this section is simply to provide a basic framework.

Most diets are overwhelming. Are there any basic guidelines I can follow to start eating right?

Every five years the federal government publishes dietary guidelines as a joint effort between the U.S. Department of Health and Human Services (HHS) and the U.S. Department of Agriculture (USDA). The guidelines are based on the recommendations of a committee of independent scientific experts who are responsible for reviewing and analyzing the most current dietary and nutritional information and incorporating them into a scientific evidence-based report. The most recent report published by this group is *Dietary Guidelines for Americans 2005*. The authors estimate that about 16 percent and 9 percent of deaths from any cause in men and women, respectively, could be eliminated by the adoption of the dietary habits advocated in the report. Although the *Dietary Guidelines* should not be considered the end-all and be-all of healthy eating, it provides a starting point for establishing a basic framework. Below are their key recommendations, organized by topic, some of which are taken directly from the report.[3]

Adequate Nutrients within Calorie Needs

▸ Consume a variety of nutrient-dense foods and beverages within and among the basic food groups, choosing foods that limit the intake of saturated and trans fats, cholesterol, added sugars, salt, and alcohol.

▸ Meet recommended nutritional needs by adopting a balanced eating plan according to the USDA Food Guide or the DASH Eating Plan,* for example.

Weight Management

▸ To maintain body weight in a healthy range, balance calories from foods and beverages with calories expended.

▸ To prevent gradual weight gain over time, make small decreases in food and beverage calories and increase physical activity.

Food Groups

▸ Consume a sufficient amount of fruits and vegetables while staying within energy needs. Two cups of fruit and 2 ½ cups of vegetables per day are recommended for a person who requires 2,000 calories a day, with higher or lower amounts depending on the calorie level.

▸ Choose a variety of fruits and vegetables each day. In particular, select from all five vegetable subgroups (dark green, orange, legumes, starchy vegetables, and other vegetables) several times a week.

▸ Consume three or more ounce-equivalents of whole-grain products per day, with the rest of the recommended grains coming from enriched or whole-grain products. In general, at least half the grains should come from whole grains.

▸ Consume 3 cups per day of fat-free or low-fat milk or equivalent milk products.

---

* DASH stands for Dietary Approaches to Stop Hypertension because it was initially designed as a dietary approach to preventing and treating high blood pressure.

Fats

▸ Limit intake of fats and oils high in saturated or trans fats. Consume less than 10 percent of calories from saturated fatty acids and less than 300 mg/day of cholesterol. Keep trans-fatty acid consumption as low as possible.
▸ Keep total fat intake between 20 and 35 percent of calories, with most fats coming from sources of polyunsaturated and monounsaturated fatty acids, such as fish, nuts, and vegetable oils.
▸ When selecting and preparing meat, poultry, dry beans, and milk or milk products, make choices that are lean, low fat, or fat free.

Carbohydrates

▸ Choose fiber-rich fruits, vegetables, and whole grains often.
▸ Choose and prepare foods and beverages with few added sugars or caloric sweeteners.

Sodium and Potassium

▸ Consume less than 2,300 mg (approximately 1 tsp of salt) of sodium per day.
▸ Choose and prepare foods with little salt.
▸ Consume potassium-rich foods, such as fruits and vegetables.

Alcoholic Beverages

▸ People who choose to drink alcoholic beverages should do so in moderation—defined as the consumption of up to one standard drink* per day for women and men over age 65, and up to two drinks per day for younger men.
▸ Some people should not drink alcohol, including those who cannot restrict their alcohol intake, women of childbearing age who may become pregnant, pregnant and lactating women, children and adolescents, people taking medications that can interact with alcohol, and those with specific medical conditions.

Keep in mind that these recommendations will need to be tailored in a few ways. One, daily serving sizes are estimated for a 2,000-calorie diet. Calorie

---

* The definition of "standard drink" is discussed in chapter 2.

requirements per day vary with age, activity level, and gender, and therefore the recommended servings should also vary with these factors. Furthermore, if you are trying to lose weight, your daily calorie requirements will be lower. Two, serving sizes are based on recommendations for the average American adult. If you have lactose intolerance, for example, you may choose to consume fewer than the recommended milk and dairy servings and substitute them with other calcium-rich foods. Likewise, if you have high blood pressure, a cholesterol disorder, or diabetes, you may be advised to observe stricter sodium, fat, and carbohydrate servings, respectively.

Three, while not typically considered part of the diet, alcohol is included in the basic framework. Alcoholic beverages are important contributors to calorie consumption yet contain few essential nutrients; thus, alcoholic beverages are "empty calories." Four, the above guidelines reference two specific diet plans: the USDA Food Guide and the DASH eating plan. Both eating plans follow the recommendations outlined above yet are flexible enough to accommodate a range of food preferences and cuisines. They are helpful to review because they translate the above recommendations into actual meal plans (see table 14.1). It is more important to follow the general principles of the diets than the exact diets.

What can I do to stick to a healthy eating plan?

The hardest part about healthy eating is getting the information outlined above onto your kitchen table, so to speak. Even with the exact number of servings of each type of food outlined for us, it is difficult to figure out how to actually make a meal plan that works, let alone find the motivation to follow it through. For people with certain medical problems (e.g., diabetes), with dietary restrictions (e.g., vegetarians), or with weight-loss goals, this problem is further compounded by the need to adjust and tailor the recommendations to their specific health needs.

Achieving a healthy diet is not easy by any measure, and there is no magic bullet that can help you get there. But one thing is nearly for certain: it is much harder to get there alone. Studies show that by partnering with your doctor and other health professionals, you are much more likely to make sustained improvements to your diet; this is especially true for people at risk for cardiovascular and diet-related health problems, the exact group of people that needs dietary improvements the most. Partnering with your doctor can help you create a diet regimen tailored to you and your health needs as well as troubleshoot and deal with issues as they arise. Like many areas of health, there is a science to changing habits and making lifestyle improvements. By

Table 14.1: USDA Food Guide and DASH Eating Plan (2,000 calorie diet)

Food groups and subgroups	USDA Food Guide amount*	DASH Eating Plan amount	Equivalent amounts
Fruit group	2 cups (4 servings)	2 to 2½ cups (4 to 5 servings)	½ cup equivalent is: • ½ cup fresh, frozen, or canned fruit • 1 medium fruit • ¼ cup dried fruit • USDA: ½ cup fruit juice • DASH: ¾ cup fruit juice
Vegetable group • Dark green vegetables • Orange vegetables • Legumes (dry beans) • Starchy vegetables • Other vegetables	2½ cups (5 servings) 3 cups/week 2 cups/week 3 cups/week 6½ cups/week	2 to 2½ cups (4 to 5 servings)	½ cup equivalent is: • ½ cup of cut-up raw or cooked vegetable • 1 cup raw leafy vegetable • USDA: ½ cup vegetable juice • DASH: ¾ cup vegetable juice
Grain group • Whole grains • Other grains	6 ounce-equivalents 3 ounce-equivalents 3 ounce-equivalents	7 to 8 ounce-equivalents (7 to 8 servings)	1 ounce-equivalent is • 1 slice bread • 1 cup dry cereal • ½ cup cooked rice, pasta, cereal • DASH: 1 ounce dry cereal (½–1¼ cup depending on cereal type—check label)
Meat and beans group	5½ ounce-equivalents	6 ounces or less meat, poultry, fish 4 to 5 servings per week nuts, seeds, and dry beans	1 ounce-equivalent is: • 1 ounce of cooked lean meats, poultry, fish • 1 egg • USDA: ¼ cup cooked dry beans or tofu, 1 tbsp peanut butter, ½ ounce nuts or seeds • DASH: 1½ ounces nuts, ½ ounce seeds, ½ cup cooked dry beans
Milk group	3 cups	2 to 3 cups	1 cup equivalent is: • 1 cup low-fat/fat-free milk, yogurt • 1½ ounces low-fat or fat-free natural cheese • 2 ounces low-fat or fat-free processed cheese

(continues)

Table 14.1 *(continued)*

Food groups and subgroups	USDA Food Guide amount*	DASH Eating Plan amount	Equivalent amounts
Oils	4 grams (6 tsp)	8 to 12 grams (2 to 3 tsp)	1 tsp equivalent is: • DASH: 1 tsp soft margarine • 1 tbsp low-fat mayo • 2 tbsp light salad dressing • 1 tsp vegetable oil
Discretionary calorie allowance •Example of distribution:	267 calories	18 grams	1 tbsp added sugar equivalent is: • DASH: 1 tbsp jelly or jam • ½ ounce jelly beans • 8 ounces lemonade
Solid fat†	18 grams		
Added sugars	8 tsp	~2 tsp (5 tbsp per week)	

Source: HHS/USDA Dietary Guidelines, 2005.

Note: Amounts of various food groups that are recommended each day or each week in the USDA Food Guide and in the DASH Eating Plan (amounts are daily unless otherwise specified) at the 2,000-calorie level. Also identified are equivalent amounts for different food choices in each group. To follow either eating pattern, food choices over time should provide these amounts of food from each group on average.

*The 2,000-calorie USDA Food Guide is appropriate for many sedentary males 51 to 70 years of age, sedentary females 19 to 30 years of age, and for some other gender/age groups who are more physically active. The calorie requirements of children ages 8 to 13 range from 1,200 to 2,600 depending on their activity level.

†The oils listed in this table are not considered to be part of discretionary calories because they are a major source of the vitamin E and polyunsaturated fatty acids, including the essential fatty acids, in the food pattern. In contrast, solid fats (i.e., saturated and trans fats) are listed separately as a source of discretionary calories.

working with your doctor and other health professionals, you can benefit from this science and be on your way to a healthier diet.

SECTION II: HEALTHY EATING COUNSELING

The USPSTF recommendation for adults with cholesterol disorders and other known risk factors for cardiovascular and diet-related chronic disease is intensive behavioral dietary counseling. The task force recommendation is based on evidence that counseling interventions can produce improvements in average daily intake of core components of a healthy diet (including saturated fat, fiber, fruit, and vegetables) among adult patients at increased risk for cardiovascular and diet-related chronic disease.

Although the recommendation is addressed to doctors, you should talk to your doctor about dietary counseling, especially if you are at risk for cardiovascular or diet-related diseases. Don't wait for your doctor to initiate the conversation. Studies show that only about 23 to 42 percent of physicians counsel their patients about diet.

Who is at risk for cardiovascular or diet-related chronic disease?

People with one or more of the following conditions are considered at increased risk for cardiovascular or diet-related chronic disease:

- cholesterol disorder
- high blood pressure
- diabetes
- obesity (body mass index [BMI] ≥30 kg/m^2)
- overweight (BMI of 25 to 29.9 kg/m^2)
- abdominal obesity (weight circumference ≥40 inches in men and ≥35 inches in women)

What if I don't have any of these conditions?

The USPSTF did not find sufficient evidence to support dietary counseling in people without any known risk factors for cardiovascular or diet-related chronic disease. Therefore, the task force makes no recommendation for or against counseling in these people. Those without any of the above conditions may also benefit from intensive behavioral dietary counseling; however, insufficient evidence supports this approach. The decision about whether to undergo intensive behavioral dietary counseling is best left between you and your doctor.

How is talking to my doctor going to help?

Many people see their diet as a personal problem. But considering that an unhealthy diet can lead to an increased risk of cardiovascular disease, stroke, cancer, and other serious medical conditions, your eating habits can also be a medical problem. While many people successfully maintain healthy diets without any help from their doctors, studies show that at-risk individuals are more likely to make improvements to their diet with counseling from a health professional.

What happens during counseling?

Healthy eating counseling typically begins with your doctor assessing your current diet and eating habits. Based on this assessment, he or she will give you specific advice about eating habits to change. Usually this is a two-way process, in which you both agree on a set of reasonable goals to meet and a reasonable time frame for meeting them. To help you reach these goals, your doctor may offer behavioral counseling to assist you in developing the skills needed to make sustained improvements in your diet. Examples include teaching self-monitoring (e.g., tracking calories, counting servings, reading nutrition labels), training to overcome barriers, goal setting, and guidance in shopping and food preparation. The text above uses the term "doctor" loosely. In practice, many clinics use a team of health care professionals, including nutritionists, dietitians, and trained health educators. In addition, some clinics offer group counseling sessions, which provide additional peer support.

Research from the USPSTF showed that the most effective counseling interventions involved more than six sessions, lasting longer than thirty minutes each, with a specialized health care professional. Talk to your doctor about how to best receive the healthy eating counseling you need within the norms of his or her practice.

REFERENCES

U.S. Department of Agriculture. MyPyramid.gov. www.mypyramid.gov.

U.S. Department of Health and Human Services. *Healthy People 2010: Understanding and Improving Health*. 2nd ed. Washington, D.C.: U.S. Government Printing Office, 2000.

U.S. Department of Health and Human Services and U.S. Department of Agriculture. *Dietary Guidelines for Americans, 2005*. 6th ed. Washington, D.C.: U.S. Government Printing Office, January 2005.

CHAPTER 15

Hepatitis B Vaccination and Screening

Hepatitis B is a serious liver infection caused by the hepatitis B virus (HBV). Chronic infection with HBV can lead to cirrhosis or scarring of the liver, liver failure, and liver cancer. Most individuals infected as adults recover fully and develop protective immunity against the virus. Those infected as infants and children are more likely to develop chronic infection.

The hepatitis B virus is transmitted through contact with infected bodily fluid and during childbirth. Risk factors include unprotected sex, needle sharing, living with someone infected with HBV, and travel to parts of the world where hepatitis B is common. However, because HBV is so contagious, many people infected with the virus have none of these risk factors.

The best way to prevent infection is to get vaccinated. The Centers for Disease Control and Prevention (CDC) recommends the hepatitis B vaccine be given to all babies beginning at birth. They also recommend the vaccine for children and adolescents not previously vaccinated and for unvaccinated adults who have risk factors for infection or who simply want to be vaccinated.

Because the infection often has no symptoms, screening is the best way to find out if you have hepatitis B. Screening is especially important for pregnant women because additional medications can be given at the time of birth to prevent mother-to-child transmission. Both the United States Preventive Services Task Force (USPSTF) and the CDC recommend screening all pregnant women for hepatitis B.[1] Outside of pregnancy, screening has uncertain benefits. The USPSTF recommends against routinely screening the general population for hepatitis B, while the CDC recommends screening people at high risk.

Section I provides an introduction to hepatitis B. Section II details the guidelines for HBV vaccination. Section III outlines the guidelines for screening in pregnant women. Screening for HBV in the nonpregnant population is not discussed in detail. However, the CDC guidelines are presented at the end of this chapter.

SECTION I: HEPATITIS B 101

Hepatitis B (HEP-ah-TY-tis B) is a serious disease caused by the hepatitis B virus (HBV). HBV infects the liver and can lead to liver cancer, liver failure, and cirrhosis in people chronically infected with the virus.

Hepatitis B is surprisingly common. One in every twenty Americans will get infected with HBV in his or her lifetime. Although most of these infections will resolve on their own, over 1.25 million Americans are currently living with chronic HBV.

How often does HBV resolve on its own?

The chances of clearing the infection vary with age. In 95 percent of adults, HBV resolves on its own. However, only 50 to 75 percent of children between ages 1 and 5 clear the infection. Among infected newborns, the chances are even lower—a dreaded 10 percent if additional measures are not taken.

People who clear the infection develop immunity to HBV—meaning they cannot get infected with that virus again—and are no longer at risk for passing HBV to others.

What happens to those who don't clear the infection?

People who do not recover are said to have chronic HBV infection. Some people with chronic infection later clear the infection, but most will not.

Many people with chronic hepatitis B have no serious problems from their infection and lead normal, healthy lives. However, people with chronic infection remain capable of passing HBV on to others. In addition, some will develop liver problems. An estimated 15 to 25 percent of chronically infected people will die from HBV-related liver disease, such as liver failure, cirrhosis, or liver cancer.

How is HBV spread?

Hepatitis B virus is found in blood and certain other bodily fluids—saliva, semen, vaginal fluid—of people infected with HBV. The virus is *not* found in sweat, tears, urine, breast milk, or respiratory secretions. The primary means of transmission are unprotected sexual intercourse, injection drug use, and mother-to-baby transmission. However, because HBV is highly contagious, contact with even one or two droplets of infected material can transmit infection. Furthermore, HBV can live outside the body for up to one week and still be able to cause infection.

You can only contract the hepatitis B virus from an HBV-infected person.

However, because one-third of people infected with HBV have no symptoms of their illness, many people with HBV do not know they are infected. As a result, engaging in any behaviors that expose you to another person's saliva, blood, semen, or vaginal fluid puts you at risk. Thus, according to the CDC, you may be at risk if you

- have sex with a person infected with HBV
- have sex with more than one partner during a six-month period
- are a man and have sex with a man
- share a household with someone who has chronic HBV infection
- use injection drugs
- have a job that involves contact with human blood
- were born in or have traveled to areas where hepatitis B is common (Alaska, Asia, Africa, the Amazon Basin, the Pacific Islands, Eastern Europe, or the Middle East)
- received blood transfusion before 1975, when effective blood testing became available
- have hemophilia
- are a patient or worker in an institution for the developmentally disabled
- require hemodialysis

Many people who contract HBV don't know when or how they acquired the infection. Studies show that up to 40 percent of people who acquire hepatitis B are unable to identify any of the risk factors above to explain why they got the infection.

What are the symptoms of hepatitis B?

Most people with HBV have no signs or symptoms of their disease. When present, symptoms include

- poor appetite
- nausea and vomiting
- yellowing of the skin and eyes (jaundice)
- constant tiredness (fatigue)
- abdominal pain
- dark urine, light-colored stool

These symptoms can be caused by many other diseases and conditions besides hepatitis B. If you have any of these symptoms, please see your doctor.

The general absence of symptoms of HBV is important for two reasons: one, it means that just because someone does not appear ill does not mean they could not have HBV. Two, it means that you could have HBV and not even know it.

How can I protect myself?

The best way to protect yourself from HBV is to get vaccinated. The hepatitis B vaccine is 90 to 95 percent effective and can be given safely to infants, children, and adults (see section II below).

You can also reduce your risk of contracting hepatitis B by minimizing your exposure to other people's bodily fluids. This includes practicing safer sex, making sure clean instruments are used for any haircuts or body piercing, and not sharing materials that may be contaminated with blood (e.g., razors, injection needles).

Is there a cure for HBV?

No existing medications cure hepatitis B. For chronic HBV infection, doctors can use antiviral medications to control the infection and decrease the risk of disease progression.

SECTION II: HEPATITIS B VACCINE

The hepatitis B vaccine has been in widespread clinical use for over twenty years. It has been shown to prevent HBV infection in up to 95 percent of people who receive it.* Like most vaccines, the vaccine against HBV can only prevent infection with the hepatitis B virus; it cannot treat existing infections or the complications of infection.

The CDC makes the following recommendations regarding the hepatitis B vaccine:

- universal vaccination for all babies beginning at birth
- routine vaccination of unvaccinated children and adolescents
- vaccination of unvaccinated adults who are at risk for HBV infection or who wish to be protected from HBV infection

The CDC considers adults with one or more of the following risk factors to be at risk for HBV.

---

* The phrase "up to" was added because a lower rate of immunization has been reported in immunocompromised adults and older adults.

People at Risk for Infection by Sexual Exposure

- sexual partners of people who are positive for HBsAg (hepatitis B surface antigen)
- sexually active people who are not in long-term mutually monogamous relationships (e.g., people who've had more than one sex partner during the previous six months)
- people seeking evaluation or treatment for an STI
- men who have sex with men

People at Risk for Infection by Percutaneous or Mucosal Exposure to Blood

- current or recent injection drug users
- household contacts of HBsAg-positive people
- residents and staff of facilities for developmentally disabled people
- health care and public safety workers with reasonably anticipated risk for exposure to blood or blood-contaminated bodily fluids
- people with end-stage renal disease receiving any form of dialysis

Others

- people who travel to countries with high rates of hepatitis B infection
- people with chronic liver disease
- people with HIV infection

In addition the CDC recommends giving the vaccine to anyone who wants protection against HBV, even if they have no known risk factors.[2]

These recommendations are based on evidence that hepatitis B vaccination is the most effective measure to prevent HBV infection and its consequences—including cirrhosis of the liver, liver cancer, liver failure, and death. Talk to your doctor about getting vaccinated against hepatitis B if you have not previously received the vaccine.

What if I don't know if I have been vaccinated before?

Although testing for the presence of hepatitis B antibodies in your blood can demonstrate protection from either vaccination or previous exposure, the best way to figure out your vaccination status is to locate your immunization records. Often these can be found by contacting your previous doctors, employers, or schools. Even if you have been vaccinated before, you can safely receive the hepatitis B vaccine again. Therefore, if you are still unsure, it is best to get vaccinated again.

How is the vaccine given?

The hepatitis B vaccine is given in three doses. Infants get the first dose within twelve hours after birth. They get the second dose at 1 to 2 months and the third between 6 and 18 months. Older children and adults get three doses over six months; the shots are usually given on a schedule of zero, one, and six months, but there is flexibility in the timing of these injections. You need *all three* shots to be protected.

Is the hepatitis B vaccine safe?

The hepatitis B vaccine has been shown to be very safe for people of all ages. Pain at the injection site and low-grade fever are the most frequently reported side effects, but they are mild and usually go away on their own.

Can the vaccine be given during pregnancy or breastfeeding?

Yes.

Is there anyone who should not receive the vaccine?

Anyone who had a serious allergic reaction to a prior dose of hepatitis B vaccine or a vaccine component should not receive further doses of hepatitis B vaccine. In addition, anyone allergic to yeast should not receive the vaccine because it is prepared using yeast.

SECTION III: SCREENING FOR HEPATITIS B IN PREGNANCY

Pregnant women who are infected with HBV can transmit the virus to their babies. Without appropriate treatment, up to 90 percent of these babies develop chronic (lifelong) HBV infections, placing them at increased risk of developing liver failure or liver cancer later in life. Most women of childbearing age infected with HBV have no symptoms of their disease. Thus, without testing, pregnant women with HBV may not know they carry the virus. By screening mothers early in pregnancy, doctors can diagnose HBV and take steps to prevent it from being transmitted.

The USPSTF recommends screening for HBV in all pregnant women during the first trimester. This recommendation is based on evidence that universal prenatal screening for HBV infection substantially reduces mother-to-baby transmission of the virus and the subsequent development of chronic HBV infection in the newborn.

Screening is done with a routine blood test for hepatitis B surface antigen (HBsAg).

What if the test is negative?

A negative HBsAg test means that you do not have hepatitis B. Your baby should receive only the standard hepatitis B vaccine series starting at birth. Usually, women who are negative for HBsAg do not undergo further testing. However, there is a small chance that the test is falsely negative, because in some stages of infection, HBsAg levels are too low to detect. While not routinely recommended, some doctors rescreen high-risk women near or at the time of delivery.

What if the test is positive?

A positive, or reactive, blood test means you have hepatitis B. However, from an HBsAg test alone, doctors cannot distinguish between acute or chronic infection and cannot determine your prognosis. Further blood work and testing will help your doctor determine the stage of your infection and what treatments are most appropriate.

To protect your baby from getting HBV, your doctor will give him or her a medication at birth called the *hepatitis B immune globulin* (HBIG). This medication is a direct antibody to the hepatitis B virus and is given as an injection. In addition, your baby will be vaccinated against HBV as is recommended for all babies.

If I have hepatitis B, is it okay to breastfeed?

Because hepatitis B is not present in breast milk, it is safe to breastfeed your baby. In fact, breastfeeding is encouraged because it is the optimal infant nutrition.

What are the CDC guidelines for hepatitis B screening?

The CDC recommends screening for hepatitis B in all pregnant women and in people at risk for infection:

- infants born to infected mothers
- anyone in the same household as an infected person
- sexual partners of infected people

- people with HIV
- people born in Asia, Africa, or other geographic regions with 2 percent or higher rates of chronic HBV infection
- U.S.-born people not vaccinated as infants whose parents were born in regions with HBV rates > 8 percent
- men who have sex with men
- injection drug users
- people with abnormal liver function tests not explained by other conditions
- people who require immunosuppressive therapy (e.g., chemotherapy)
- people on hemodialysis[3]

REFERENCES

Centers for Disease Control and Prevention (CDC). U.S. Department of Health and Human Services. "Hepatitis B." www.cdc.gov/hepatitis/hbv.
———. "Hepatitis B Vaccination Recommendations for Adults," *MMWR* 55, RR-16 (2006). www.cdc.gov/hepatitis/HBV/VaccAdults.htm.
———. "Hepatitis B Vaccination Recommendations for Infants, Children, and Adolescents," *MMWR* 54, RR-16 (2005). www.cdc.gov/hepatitis/HBV/VaccChildren.htm.
———. "Recommendations for Identification and Public Health Management of Persons with Chronic Hepatitis B Virus Infection," *MMWR* 57, RR-8 (2008). www.cdc.gov/hepatitis/HBV/TestingChronic.htm.

CHAPTER 16

HIV Screening

HIV/AIDS is a highly stigmatized and misunderstood disease. Let's begin by clarifying some general misconceptions. First, HIV/AIDS is a common condition. Over 1 million people are infected with HIV in the United States, and each year over 50,000 people are newly infected. Second, HIV/AIDS is not limited to certain populations but is prevalent across socioeconomic groups, geographic areas, and sexual preferences. Everyone who is sexually active is potentially at risk for infection and should at least consider being screened for the disease. Third, not everyone with HIV/AIDS is "sick." It often takes several years after infection before the first signs and symptoms of the disease become evident. As a result, one in four Americans living with HIV is unaware of being infected. Fourth, HIV/AIDS is treatable. Being diagnosed with the disease is not a death sentence. To the contrary, with proper treatment, people with HIV/AIDS can expect to live well into their 60s and beyond. And finally, HIV/AIDS is largely preventable. By engaging in lower risk sexual behaviors such as condom use, the risk of HIV transmission can be substantially reduced.

The United States Preventive Services Task Force (USPSTF) recommends screening for HIV in all adolescents and adults at increased risk for infection.[1] Other organizations, most notably the Centers for Disease Control and Prevention (CDC), recommend screening all Americans ages 18 to 64. Currently, less than half of Americans in this age group have ever been tested for HIV. Among at-risk groups, less than two-thirds have ever been tested. The following sections provide an introduction to HIV/AIDS and detail the guidelines for screening. Screening in pregnancy, which is recommended for all pregnant women regardless of risk factors, is discussed in chapter 19.

SECTION I: HIV 101

HIV is the virus that causes AIDS, and AIDS is the disease that can develop after several years of untreated HIV.

▸ HIV stands for human immunodeficiency virus. It infects humans. It is a virus. Over time it can cause immunodeficiency, or weakness of the immune system, leading to infections a healthy person would ordinarily not get.

▸ AIDS stands for acquired immune deficiency syndrome. It is acquired because a person is not born with the deficiency. It is an immune deficiency. It is a syndrome, or a group of symptoms that stem from a common medical problem.

Because of the causal link between HIV and AIDS, the spectrum of disease associated with HIV is called HIV/AIDS. To help keep things clear, in this chapter, HIV refers to the virus and HIV/AIDS refers to the clinical disease caused by HIV.

How do people get HIV/AIDS?

People get HIV/AIDS after infection with HIV, which is present in blood, semen, vaginal fluid, and breast milk of infected people. As a result, HIV can be transmitted through sexual intercourse, blood contact—through needle sharing, accidental medical exposure, or unsafe blood transfusion—and from mother to baby during pregnancy and breastfeeding.

Not every exposure to HIV-infected fluid leads to a new infection. Instead, the risk of transmission depends on various factors, including the kind and degree of exposure (e.g., condom use compared to unprotected sex).

Can you get HIV from oral sex?

Numerous studies have shown that oral sex can result in the transmission of HIV and other sexually transmitted infections (STIs). Although the risk of HIV transmission through oral sex is smaller than the risk from anal or vaginal sex, it is not zero, and it can be further lowered through the use of condoms and other protective barriers.

How can people not know they have HIV/AIDS?

Most of us probably think of people with HIV/AIDS as "being sick." However, the reality is that for the first five to ten years after infection, most people are asymptomatic. This is because HIV/AIDS is a slowly progressive disease. Although at its later stages, the disease's effects on health can be dramatic, at its earliest stages, HIV/AIDS is almost impossible to detect without screening tests.

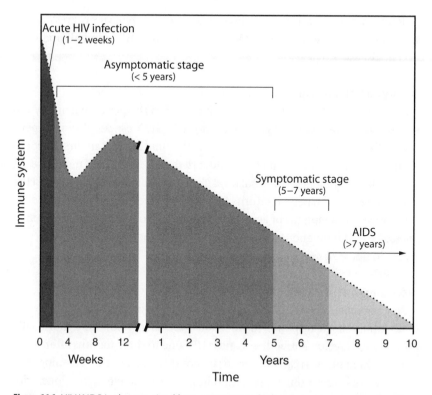

Figure 16.1. HIV/AIDS is characterized by a progressive decline in immune system function as a result of the human immunodeficiency virus. The effects of the disease on health are directly related to the extent of immune system compromise. The first stage of HIV/AIDS is called acute HIV. Seventy percent of people with acute HIV have flulike symptoms, while the remaining 30 percent have no symptoms at all. Over the next several years, although the immune system function continues to gradually decline, the body has sufficient immunity to resist infection (asymptomatic stage). After five to seven years, the decline in immune function is sufficient to make the body susceptible to nonopportunistic infections and to generalized symptoms such as night sweats, rashes, and fatigue (symptomatic stage). Eventually, the immune system deteriorates so much that the person develops opportunistic infections. This final stage of the disease is called AIDS.

How does HIV/AIDS progress?

The typical progression of HIV/AIDS is described below. The time it takes a person to go through each stage of HIV/AIDS varies, but for most people, the progression is fairly slow, taking several years from infection to the development of AIDS (see figure 16.1).

As you read the subsections below, keep in mind the following: one, regardless of the stage of infection, people with HIV/AIDS can transmit the infection to others; and two, the description is of the typical progression for people *not* receiving treatment. Medications to treat HIV can halt and even reverse disease progression.

Primary Infection (Acute HIV)

Primary HIV infection (or acute HIV) describes the period when HIV enters the bloodstream and begins to infect the body. Most people will experience flulike symptoms during this stage as the immune system first encounters the virus. Symptoms, which include sore throat, fevers, and night sweats, typically last no more than several days until the virus establishes itself in the body. Thereafter the person returns to looking and feeling completely well.

Because the symptoms of acute HIV are similar to those of more common illnesses like the flu and can be mild or absent, people with acute HIV commonly do not seek medical attention and remain undiagnosed.

Seroconversion

Seroconversion is the phase when antibodies—or proteins made by the immune system in response to infection—are first produced against HIV. Most people develop antibodies against HIV one to three months after infection, although rarely it can take up to six months. Because the screening tests for HIV work by detecting these antibodies, an HIV screening test done prior to seroconversion may give a false negative result. To be certain of your HIV status, an HIV antibody test must be done three months or longer after exposure to the virus.

Asymptomatic Stage

After the acute HIV stage, people with HIV/AIDS will typically look and feel completely healthy for several years. Beneath the surface, however, the virus is active and is slowly killing the cells of the immune system. But because the immune system has reserve, or excess capacity, people generally do not experience any ill effects from the gradual weakening in immune function. In this stage, the only reliable means of diagnosing HIV is through a positive antibody screening test. As a result, without screening, people in the asymptomatic stage remain unaware of their infection.

Early and Mid-Stage HIV Symptomatic Disease

After five to seven years of infection, some people begin to experience generalized symptoms of their illness, including chronic fungal rashes, recurrent herpes blisters, persistent night sweats and fevers, and diarrhea. In addition, they may become ill with serious, life-threatening infections that people with normal immune systems can also get but that are more severe in people with HIV/AIDS. Because these symptoms and infections are not necessarily specific to HIV/AIDS, some people even at this stage of the disease are undiagnosed.

AIDS (Late-Stage HIV Disease)

Once the immune system function drops below a critical threshold, people with HIV/AIDS become susceptible to infections that non–HIV-infected people do not ordinarily get. These *opportunistic infections* are caused by microorganisms that normally do not cause disease in humans but that take advantage of the "opportunity" created by the weakened immune system to cause disease in people with advanced HIV/AIDS. The onset of these opportunistic infections marks the beginning of AIDS, the last stage of HIV/AIDS.

How I can protect myself from HIV?

With the advent of effective HIV medications, HIV/AIDS is a treatable disease, but it is not curable. Prevention is therefore the best means of protection. The three most common modes of HIV transmission are sexual contact, needle sharing, and pregnancy.

Sexual Contact

Anytime you are exposed to another individual's semen, blood, or vaginal fluid, you put yourself at risk for HIV. The best way to protect yourself is to abstain from sexual intercourse (including vaginal, anal, and oral sex), or to be in a long-term mutually monogamous relationship with a partner who has been tested for HIV and who you know is not infected. Short of this, many other practices can help prevent HIV transmission.

Use latex condoms. For condoms to provide maximum protection, they must be used *correctly* and *consistently.* Correct and consistent condom usage can dramatically and effectively reduce the risk of HIV transmission, although not to zero. Incorrect use of condoms can lead to slippage or breakage, which reduces or even nullifies their protective effect. Inconsistent use, such as failure to use condoms with every act of intercourse, can also lead to HIV transmission.

Limit your number of sexual partners. Having multiple sexual partners, especially partners whose HIV status is unknown, increases the risk of HIV and other STIs.

Get routinely screened for HIV and other STIs. Certain STIs can increase the risk of HIV transmission if exposed. For example, being infected with chlamydia increases the risk of getting HIV five-fold if exposed.

Encourage your partner to get regularly screened for HIV. When you enter into a new sexual relationship, find out if your partner has been recently tested, and if not, insist that he or she get screened.

Needle Sharing

People who *share* syringes and other paraphernalia for injection drug use are at extremely high risk of HIV infection. The best way to protect yourself against HIV transmission through needle sharing is to stop using and injecting drugs. Injection drug users who cannot stop can reduce their risk of transmission by never reusing or sharing needles and other drug paraphernalia.

Pregnancy

To learn about preventing mother-to-baby transmission, see chapter 19.

Are there any treatments available for HIV/AIDS?

Twenty years ago, no drugs were available to treat HIV/AIDS. Today there are over thirty. Twenty years ago, HIV/AIDS was almost a uniformly fatal disease. Today it is a chronic, manageable disease, and people who are tested early, seek treatment, and take their medications regularly can expect to live long, healthy lives. Although there is no cure for HIV/AIDS and no vaccine against HIV, many effective treatments exist that improve the quantity and quality of life for those living with the disease. The availability of effective treatment is why getting screened for HIV and finding out if you are infected early is more important than ever.

SECTION II: HIV SCREENING

The USPSTF recommends routine screening for HIV in all adolescents and adults at increased risk for infection. This recommendation is based on evidence that screening tests for HIV are highly accurate and that appropriately timed treatment for infection improves the health of people diagnosed with HIV through screening. Individuals at increased risk for HIV infection include

- men and women who have unprotected sex with multiple partners
- men who have sex with men
- people with a history of an STI in the past year (e.g., syphilis, gonorrhea, chlamydia)
- injection drug users
- people who exchange sex for money or drugs
- sexual partners of people with any of the above risk factors

People who do not fit into any of these risk categories may also benefit from routine screening. The USPSTF guidelines state that simply requesting an HIV test may be sufficient grounds for doctors to offer screening.

The Centers for Disease Control and Prevention (CDC) recently published guidelines recommending that *all individuals* between 13 and 64 years of age be screened for HIV regardless of recognized risk factors. Although the USPSTF recommendations are not consistent with this approach, either guideline is reasonable to follow. In the end, the decision about screening for HIV is best left between you and your doctor.

Why get tested?

The main reason to get tested is to know your HIV status. If you are HIV-negative, you can take steps to keep yourself protected. If you are HIV-positive, you can partner with your doctor to make sure you stay healthy and take care not to spread HIV to others. You need not have symptoms or look sick to have HIV/AIDS. People with HIV/AIDS often look healthy for many years after infection. Getting tested is the only way to know with certainty that you do not have the disease.

How is screening done?

Screening is commonly performed using a routine blood sample but can also be done using saliva or urine. Results usually take between two to three days, though rapid HIV tests using saliva can give results in less than thirty minutes so that you know the outcome before you leave the office. In general, HIV screening tests are equally accurate, and which type of test you take largely depends on the testing center.

HIV screening tests work by checking for the presence of antibodies against the virus. Because it takes one to three months (and rarely up to six months) after infection with HIV to begin making antibodies, people who were infected with HIV in the past three months may not test positive. This means that even with a negative HIV test, it is still possible to have HIV.

What if the HIV screening test is negative?

A negative HIV screening test means that you do not have HIV. No further testing is needed.

Rarely, an HIV screening test is falsely negative, meaning the test suggests you do not have HIV when you are in fact infected. Because HIV screening tests look for the presence of anti-HIV antibodies, it is possible that you contracted the virus in the past one to three months but that your immune system has not had sufficient time to produce detectable antibodies. As a result, in some instances your health care provider may wish to screen you for HIV again in three months or directly test you for the presence of the HIV virus. This is not routinely recommended, however, and is typically limited to circumstances in which a known exposure occurred or in which acute HIV is suspected.

Before leaving the testing center or clinic, you should discuss two things. The first is safer sex and lifestyle choices. You were most likely tested for HIV because you have one or more risk factors for infection. The best treatment for HIV is prevention. Talk to someone at the testing center about your risk factors for HIV (e.g., unprotected sex, multiple partners, needle sharing) and find out ways you can better protect yourself.

The second is the date of your next HIV screening. The USPSTF makes no specific recommendation about the optimal interval for screening, so the decision about when to screen next is up to you and your health care provider. Depending on your risk factors, the next screening test may be as soon as one month from now or as late as one year. Make sure you document the date for your records and make an effort to get retested no later than that date.

What if the HIV screening test is positive?

A positive (or preliminary reactive) HIV screening test means that you *may* be infected. HIV screening tests sometimes produce false positives (that is, a test suggests someone has HIV when he or she does not), so to diagnose HIV/AIDS, your health care provider must perform a confirmatory test called a *Western blot*. Western blots require a routine blood sample. The results are usually available in few days to a week.

What if the Western blot is also positive?

This means you are HIV positive and are infected with the virus that causes HIV/AIDS. HIV/AIDS is a treatable condition. By getting tested for HIV early, before symptoms develop, you have given yourself the best chance of continuing to stay healthy. Clearly, from here, many additional steps will need to be taken. But you will not be alone—much support is available for people with HIV, starting with the place where you got tested.

REFERENCES

Centers for Disease Control and Prevention (CDC). U.S. Department of Health and Human Services. "HIV/AIDS." www.cdc.gov/hiv.

National HIV and STD Testing Resources. Centers for Disease Control and Prevention. U.S. Department of Health and Human Services. www.hivtest.org.

CHAPTER **17**

Obesity Screening and Counseling

The United States is currently facing an obesity crisis. One in three adults is obese today, compared with 1 in 8 adults in 1960. An additional one in three adults is overweight. All told, over 130 million adults in the United States are overweight or obese. While the reasons for this trend are many, increasing portion sizes and decreasing levels of physical activity are thought to be major contributors.

Many people consider weight to be an appearance issue. It isn't. Weight is a health issue. Obesity is a serious medical condition that accounts for 300,000 deaths each year in the United States. It puts people at risk for major illnesses ranging from cardiovascular disease and diabetes to cancers of the breast, colon, and uterus. Thus, like any other medical condition, obesity must be recognized and treated.

There are dangers to thinking of weight as a cosmetic problem. Such thinking motivates people to "cut the fat" or start dieting, instead of cultivating healthier eating and exercise habits. It also steers them to get weight-loss advice from celebrity programs and fad diets, which sometimes work at the expense of their health, instead of partnering with their doctors to develop long-term strategies that promote overall health.

The United States Preventive Services Task Force (USPSTF) recommends that doctors screen all adults for obesity and offer intensive counseling and behavioral interventions to promote sustained weight loss for obese adults.[1] The following sections provide a brief overview of obesity and explain the guidelines for screening and counseling.

SECTION I: OBESITY 101

Obesity is a condition of excess fat accumulation in the body. Although a certain amount of fat in the body is normal, in obesity, body fat is increased to unhealthy levels. Doctors define obesity as having a body mass index (BMI) above 30 kg/m². This is equivalent to 221 pounds or greater in a person who stands 6'0" tall and to 186 pounds or greater in a person 5'6" tall (male or female).

How is body fat measured?

Figuring out the amount of body fat in a person is not easy. While accurate methods for measuring body fat exist—like weighing people under water—they are not practical for the average person. Simpler methods of estimating body fat, such as skinfold thickness and bioelectrical impedance, while useful in some settings, often provide inconsistent measurements.

Doctors generally rely on BMI and waist circumference for measuring obesity. These tests do not measure fat directly, but they offer important advantages. Both measurements are simple, inexpensive, and highly consistent. In addition, they are related to important health measures, such as risk of cardiovascular disease and type 2 diabetes.

Body Mass Index

BMI is based on a person's height and weight. Doctors consider BMI to be a better measure of health risk than actual weight in pounds. The medical terms "overweight" and "obesity" are based on BMI values.

To calculate your BMI, use one of the two following equations:

1. weight in kilograms / (height in meters)²
2. 703 × weight in pounds / (height in inches)²

Using the second equation, you can calculate your BMI by dividing your weight in pounds (lb) by height in inches (in) squared, and then multiplying by a conversion factor of 703.

Example: Weight = 150 lb, Height = 5'5" (65")
Calculation: [150 ÷ (65)²] × 703 = 25 kg/m²

BMI can also be determined using a BMI table (see table 17.1) or a BMI calculator, which can be easily found on the Internet. The calculation is the same for men and women. Once you know your BMI, use the definitions below to find out its significance:

Underweight = BMI of <18.5 kg/m²
Normal weight = BMI of 18.5–24.9 kg/m²
Overweight = BMI of 25–29.9 kg/m²
Obesity = BMI of ≥30 kg/m²

Obesity is classified into mild, moderate, and extreme obesity—otherwise known as class I, class II, and class III obesity, respectively. People with class I obesity have a BMI between 30.0 and 34.9 kg/m²; class II BMI is between 35.0 and 39.9 kg/m²; and class III BMI is 40 kg/m² or greater.

While it has definite advantages, BMI is not perfect. It considers all types of weight equally, including weight from muscle and from fat. As a result, it tends to *overestimate* body fat in athletes and others who have a muscular build and *underestimate* body fat in older people and others who have lost muscle mass. It also does not account for body fat distribution, which is an independent risk factor for cardiovascular disease, as discussed below.

Table 17.1: Body mass index (BMI) chart

BMI	19	20	21	22	23	24	25	26	27	28	29	30	31	32	33	34	35
Height (inches)	Body weight (pounds)																
58	91	96	100	105	110	115	119	124	129	134	138	143	148	153	158	162	167
59	94	99	104	109	114	119	124	128	133	138	143	148	153	158	163	168	173
60	97	102	107	112	118	123	128	133	138	143	148	153	158	163	168	174	179
61	100	106	111	116	122	127	132	137	143	148	153	158	164	169	174	180	185
62	104	109	115	120	126	131	136	142	147	153	158	164	169	175	180	186	191
63	107	113	118	124	130	135	141	146	152	158	163	169	175	180	186	191	197
64	110	116	122	128	134	140	145	151	157	163	169	174	180	186	192	197	204
65	114	120	126	132	138	144	150	156	162	168	174	180	186	192	198	204	210
66	118	124	130	136	142	148	155	161	167	173	179	186	192	198	204	210	216
67	121	127	134	140	146	153	159	166	172	178	185	191	198	204	211	217	223
68	125	131	138	144	151	158	164	171	177	184	190	197	203	210	216	223	230
69	128	135	142	149	155	162	169	176	182	189	196	203	209	216	223	230	236
70	132	139	146	153	160	167	174	181	188	195	202	209	216	222	229	236	243
71	136	143	150	157	165	172	179	186	193	200	208	215	222	229	236	243	250
72	140	147	154	162	169	177	184	191	199	206	213	221	228	235	242	250	258
73	144	151	159	166	174	182	189	197	204	212	219	227	235	242	250	257	265
74	148	155	163	171	179	186	194	202	210	218	225	233	241	249	256	264	272
75	152	160	168	176	184	192	200	208	216	224	232	240	248	256	264	272	279
76	156	164	172	180	189	197	205	213	221	230	238	246	254	263	271	279	287

Source: Adapted from www.nhlbi.nih.gov/guidelines/obesity/bmi_tbl.htm. *The Clinical Guidelines on the Identification, Evaluation, and Treatment of Overweight and Obesity in Adults: Evidence Report.* Bethesda, Md.: National Heart, Lung, and Blood Institute Obesity Education Initiative, 1998. NIH Publication No. 98-4083.

Waist Circumference

The *total* amount of fat in the body is one important risk factor for obesity-associated diseases. Another important risk factor is the *distribution* of the fat in the body (where the fat is located). Body fat that accumulates in the stomach area (called abdominal obesity) poses a greater health risk than body fat that builds up in the buttocks and thigh areas. In fact, abdominal obesity is considered an independent risk factor for cardiovascular disease just like high blood pressure and smoking.

Waist circumference is a good measure of abdominal obesity. Studies show that having an increased waist circumference increases your risk of cardiovascular disease, high blood pressure, abnormal cholesterol, and type 2 diabetes. An "increased" weight circumference is defined as 40 inches or more in men (102 cm) and 35 inches or more in women (88 cm).

What is my ideal weight?

Ideal weight is a myth. There is no way to know what the "ideal" weight is for a person or even whether such a weight exists. However, what we do know is that being obese, overweight, or even underweight increases your risk of important diseases compared with having normal weight. Normal weight is defined as having a BMI between 18.5 and 24.9 kg/m². By multiplying this range by your height squared, you can determine what the equivalent normal weight range is for you.

Let's take as an example someone who is 5'10" (1.8 m). By squaring the height in meters and multiplying by the normal BMI range, we get a weight range of 59–79 kilograms. Multiply this by 2.2 to get 130–174 pounds. Therefore, as a general rule, a healthy weight for this 5'10" person is any weight between 130 and 174 pounds.

I'm confused about the best way to lose weight. Can you tell me what actually works?

The popular media bombard people with messages about weight loss and obesity. There are a seemingly endless number of "perfect" diets and "perfect" workouts out there. The often conflicting messages (carbohydrates are bad/carbohydrates are good, or total fat intake matters/does not matter) leave people who are genuinely interested in healthy weight loss confused. How do we make sense of all of this? The following is a simple model for thinking about weight and weight loss.

Picture a reservoir of water. Each day a certain amount of water pours into the reservoir, and each day a certain amount of water drains out. If the amount of water pouring in and the amount of water draining out is the same on a given day, the water level does not change. But if more water pours in than drains out, the water level rises. It doesn't matter whether the water that pours in is rain water or river water. It also doesn't matter whether the water pours in today or yesterday. The effect on the water level tomorrow is the same.

The reservoir is you, and the water level is your weight. The water pouring in is the number of calories you eat each day. The water draining out is the number of calories you burn up each day. The difference in calories—calories in minus calories out—represents the change in your weight every day.

This model of weight keeps things simple. Every dessert or every apple you eat is water pouring into the reservoir. All that matters are the total number of calories you eat. It doesn't matter if the calories come from fat, protein, or carbohydrates (although for health reasons other than weight loss, clearly this does matter). Every time you take the stairs instead of the elevator or every time you go for a swim, water drains out. All that matters are the total number of calories you burn up. You can do it running a marathon or ballroom dancing.

The model makes losing weight all about accounting. If you want to lose weight, you can decrease the number of calories you eat or increase the number of calories you burn up—or both. To decrease calories in, you can do Atkins, Weight Watchers, or a diet you make up on your own. To increase calories out, you can run, bike, or garden, for example. The key is simply to be consistently burning up more calories per day than you are eating. And to do that, you have to find a plan that works for you and keeps you motivated.

Why is my extra weight a health problem?

Make no mistake about it—being overweight or obese is a serious health issue. Obese and overweight people have more heart attacks; more strokes; more high blood pressure; more cholesterol problems; more depression; more liver problems; more diabetes; more arthritis; more respiratory problems; and more cancers of the colon, prostate, uterus, and breast than normal weight people. Obese people die younger and have a lower quality of life than normal weight people. To bring home this message, here are some compelling facts and figures from the surgeon general.[2]

Overall
- Obesity accounts for 300,000 deaths a year in the United States.
- Obese people have a 50 to 100 percent greater likelihood of premature death than people of normal weight.
- The health risks of obesity increase as the degree of obesity increases.

The more obese a person is, the more likely he or she will develop obesity-related health problems.

▸ While the health risks of being overweight are smaller than the health risks of obesity, they do exist. In addition, being overweight is considered a major risk factor for obesity.

Cardiovascular Disease

▸ A weight gain of 10 to 20 pounds increases the risk of coronary heart disease (nonfatal heart attack and death) by 25 percent in women and by 60 percent in men.

▸ High blood pressure is twice as common in adults who are obese than in those who are at a healthy weight.

▸ Obesity is associated with elevated triglycerides and LDL cholesterol ("bad cholesterol") and decreased HDL cholesterol ("good cholesterol").

Diabetes

▸ A weight gain of 11 to 18 pounds doubles the risk of type 2 diabetes.

Cancer

▸ Overweight and obesity are associated with an increased risk for some types of cancer, including endometrial, colon, gallbladder, prostate, kidney, and postmenopausal breast cancer.

▸ Women who gain more than 20 pounds from age 18 to midlife double their risk of postmenopausal breast cancer compared with women whose weight remains stable.

Arthritis

▸ For every 2-pound increase in weight, the risk of developing arthritis increases by 10 percent.

Reproductive Complications

▸ Obesity during pregnancy is associated with an increased risk of death in both the baby and the mother.

▸ Women who are obese during pregnancy are at increased risk for gestational diabetes, elevated blood pressures during pregnancy, and obstetric complications requiring a Cesarean section (C-section).

▸ Infants born to obese mothers are at increased risk for birth defects, particularly neural tube defects, such as spina bifida.

▸ Obesity is associated with irregular menstrual cycles and infertility.

Additional Health Consequences

Obesity is associated with increased risks of

▸ sleep apnea (interrupted breathing while sleeping)
▸ gallbladder disease
▸ fatty liver disease
▸ gastroesphogeal reflux disease (GERD)
▸ gout (a disease of the joint)
▸ incontinence (inability to control bladder or bowel)
▸ depression

Obesity can also affect quality of life through limited mobility and decreased physical endurance as well as through social, academic, and job discrimination.

Children and Adolescents

▸ Risk factors for cardiovascular disease—such as abnormal cholesterol, high blood pressure, type 2 diabetes—are more common in overweight children and adolescents.
▸ Overweight adolescents have a 70 to 80 percent chance of being overweight or obese in adulthood.
▸ The most immediate consequence is psychosocial—specifically discrimination from peers.

If I lose weight, will my risk of these diseases go down?

Yes! Studies show that diet and exercise leading to even a modest weight loss (5 kg, or 11 lb) improve blood sugar levels, blood pressure, and cholesterol. In addition, long-term sustained weight loss is likely to reduce the risk of obesity-associated diseases. For example, weight loss has been shown to reduce the risk of type 2 diabetes by 60 percent.

What can I do about my weight?

The treatment for obesity and being overweight is obvious—losing weight. To achieve significant weight loss, a calorie deficit must be created and maintained. For example, to lose 1 to 2 pounds a week, a daily calorie deficit of 500 to 1,000 calories is necessary. But of course, knowing that the treatment is weight loss doesn't make it any easier. The struggle to lose weight is faced by millions of Americans. Despite dieting books and exercise programs galore, shedding pounds is a daily battle. What's more, many who manage to lose weight through Herculean efforts often find themselves back to where they started only a few months later.

What is the solution? Like most hard things in life, there is no single solution, no quick-fix plan you can follow or pill you can take to lose weight or motivate yourself to diet and exercise more. But there is hope, and it comes from recognizing that it is often more difficult to try to lose weight alone. Studies show that by partnering with your doctor, you are much more likely to lose weight than if you don't. Yet most of us, despite the fact that we go to our doctors for most of our other health problems, don't talk to our doctors about our weight. And doctors, despite studies showing that they can effectively help people achieve sustained weight loss, often do not advise their patients about losing weight. It makes no sense, right?

Partnering with your doctor can help you initiate a dieting and exercise regimen tailored to you and your health needs and help you troubleshoot and deal with issues as they come up. Like most things, there is a science to changing habits and making lifestyle changes. By working with your doctor and other health professionals—dietitians, nutritionists, nurses, and therapists —you can benefit from this science. In certain people, doctors can also prescribe weight-loss medications or, in more severe, refractory cases, recommend weight-loss surgery (bariatric surgery). Not all doctors are comfortable helping people lose weight, so find a doctor or other health professional who has experience in weight-loss management and is willing to work with you in making weight loss a priority.

A recent report by the National Institutes of Health (NIH) reviewed dozens of clinical trials that studied the effects of dietary therapy, physical activity counseling, behavioral therapy, medications, and surgery on weight loss. The report concluded that medical therapy helps the average overweight or obese individual lose 8 percent of his or her baseline weight within six months and sustain that weight loss for at least one year. This means that the *average* 200-pound person will lose 16 pounds and keep it off. They further conclude that the most effective medical therapy uses a combination of dietary counseling, physical activity counseling, and behavioral therapy. In certain people, weight-loss medications and surgery can supplement this basic treatment regimen. The following subsections summarize the NIH findings.[3]

Dietary Counseling

What the data show. A decrease in calorie intake is the most important dietary component of weight loss. Low-calorie diets have been shown to reduce total body weight by an average of 8 percent over six months. Excluding those who did not lose any weight, people who initiated low-calorie diets dropped 10 percent of their baseline weight. A low-calorie diet typically has between 1,000 and 1,200 calories per day for women and between 1,200 and 1,500 calories per day for men. While total calories is most important for weight loss, for other health reasons, take care to eat servings of all the daily foods recommended by the U.S. Department of Agriculture. It is the *size* of the serving that matters.

How health care can help. Finding a way to reduce calories while maintaining a well-balanced, nutritious diet is not easy. Sitting down with a health care professional (e.g., dietitian, nutritionist) at the start of your diet program can help you create an individualized diet that meets your weight-loss goals, nutritional needs, and food preferences. In addition, regular follow-up visits geared toward reinforcement, encouragement, and monitoring can help you lose weight and stay healthy.

Physical Activity Counseling

What the data show. Studies show that physical activity contributes to weight loss and offers the additional benefit of increased cardio-respiratory fitness independent of weight loss. Initially, moderate levels of physical activity for thirty to forty-five minutes, three to five days per week, should be encouraged. All adults should set a long-term goal to accumulate thirty minutes or more of moderate-intensity physical activity on most, and preferably all, days of the week. Moderate-intensity activities include washing and waxing a car for an hour, playing touch football for forty-five minutes, gardening for forty-five minutes, social dancing for thirty minutes, walking for thirty to forty minutes, stair walking for fifteen minutes, or jogging for fifteen minutes.

How health care can help. Finding the time and motivation for physical activity can be hard. In addition, people starting a physical activity program need to avoid injury, overexertion, and long-term orthopedic problems. Your doctor and other health care professionals can help you develop a plan tailored to your weight-loss goals, fitness level, and lifestyle. In addition, frequent clinical encounters can help you troubleshoot health concerns as they arise, accelerate the intensity of your program safely, and monitor your progress.

Behavioral Therapy

Behavioral therapy is predicated on the assumption that sustained weight loss is about changing habits. The goal of behavioral therapy is to alter dietary and physical activity habits to enable sustained weight loss.

What the data show. Studies show that *beyond* dietary counseling and physical activity counseling, behavioral therapy helps people lose weight.

How health care can help. Through behavioral therapy with a health care professional, you can learn specific techniques such as self-monitoring, stress management, urge control, and problem-solving that can help you develop habits that support weight loss.

Medications

There are three FDA-approved medications for weight loss: orlistat (marketed as Xenical or Alli), sibutramine (Meridia), and phentermine (available as a generic). Orlistat blocks absorption of fat in the gut, thereby reducing caloric intake. Sibutramine and phentermine act on neurotransmitters in the brain to suppress appetite. They are all intended for use in conjunction with a physician-directed low-calorie diet.

What the data show. These drugs are effective but modest in their ability to produce sustained weight loss: typically 2.5 to 4.8 kg (5.7 to 10.6 lb). Like all medications, they have side effects. Orlistat may decrease absorption of important vitamins and cause diarrhea or loose stools. Sibutramine and phentermine can increase heart rate and exacerbate high blood pressure. Few trials have studied these medications longer than six months, and therefore the long-term health benefits and risks are not well known.

How health care can help. These medications should be taken under a doctor's direction.

Surgery

The aim of bariatric surgery—including gastric bypass surgery and other weight-loss surgeries—is to modify the digestive tract to reduce food intake. Because of the risks, surgery is generally reserved for people with class III obesity or class II obesity and additional risk factors for obesity-associated disease in whom other treatment options have been unsuccessful.

What the data show. Surgery can produce substantial weight loss—28 kg to over 40 kg (62 to 88 lb)—but poses substantial risks, from the surgery itself and postoperative complications. Despite its potential, surgery is far from a cure-all, and many people do not lose any more weight than they could through dieting and exercise.

How health care can help. Bariatric surgery can only be done under the direction of a surgeon. The decision to perform the surgery often involves multiple providers—including a family doctor or internist, a surgeon, an anesthesiologist, and often a psychologist or psychiatrist.

SECTION II: OBESITY SCREENING AND COUNSELING

The USPSTF recommends that doctors screen all adults for obesity and offer intensive counseling and behavioral interventions to promote sustained weight loss for obese adults. This recommendation is based on evidence that body mass index (BMI) is a good screening tool for obesity and that high-intensity dietary and exercise counseling along with behavioral interventions produces sustained weight loss and health benefits in obese adults.

The USPSTF recommendations are geared toward doctors, who are advised to counsel their patients about weight loss. Whether or not your doctor brings up the subject, however, you should talk to him or her about your weight, and if you are obese, find out how your doctor can help you lose weight. Don't wait for your doctor to initiate the conversation. In a large national study of adults with obesity, only 42 percent reported that their doctor advised them to lose weight.

How will talking to my doctor help?

Many people see weight as a personal problem. But as this chapter has stressed, it is also a medical problem. Although many people lose weight without any help from their doctors, people are much more likely to succeed if they partner with health care providers. Studies show that people who receive health care–based counseling and behavioral therapy lose 8 to 10 percent of their weight within six months.

How is screening done?

Body mass index (BMI) is used to screen for obesity. It is calculated using weight and height. (See section I for the formula and example calculations.) People with a BMI greater than 30 kg/m^2 are obese. People with a BMI between 25 and 30 kg/m^2 are overweight.

What if I'm obese?

The guidelines recommend that doctors offer intensive counseling and behavioral interventions to help people with obesity lose weight. In practice, not all doctors offer such treatments. Therefore, you should take the initiative to talk to your doctor about how he or she can help you lose weight. A weight-loss program might be available through your regular clinic, or your doctor might refer you to a comprehensive weight-loss center. Before selecting a program, find out what it offers. Studies show that the best results come from programs that offer both diet and exercise counseling and behavioral interventions; utilize a variety of health care professionals, including nutritionists, exercise therapists, psychologists, and nurses; and have at least one or more sessions per month for at least the first three months of treatment. Depending on your BMI and other risk factors for obesity-associated disease, you might also be offered weight-loss medications or bariatric surgery.

What if I'm overweight?

Although the health risks are smaller, overweight people are still at increased risk for obesity-related diseases and for developing obesity in the future. Not many studies have been done on the effectiveness of counseling and behavioral therapy on weight loss in overweight adults. As a result, the USPSTF has found insufficient evidence to recommend for or against offering such interventions to overweight people. Deciding how best to address your weight is between you and your doctor. The decision should take into account your risk factors for obesity-related diseases and your weight-loss history.

What if I am normal weight?

People with BMIs between 18.5 and 24.9 kg/m^2 are considered normal weight. For such individuals, no further testing or counseling is required. Keep in mind, however, that even in normal weight people, physical activity and diet are important determinants of health. Talk to your doctor about your eating and exercise habits and find out how he or she can help you reduce your health risks.

REFERENCES

National Heart, Lung, and Blood Institute (NHLBI). *Clinical Guidelines on the Identification, Evaluation, and Treatment of Overweight and Obesity in Adults.* NIH Publication No. 98-4083. Bethesda, Md.: Department of Health and Human Services, National Institutes of Health, September 1998.

National Institutes of Health (NIH). U.S. Department of Health and Human Services. "Obesity." http://health.nih.gov/topic/Obesity.

U.S. Department of Health and Human Services. *The Surgeon General's Call to Action to Prevent and Decrease Overweight and Obesity.* Rockville, Md.: U.S. Department of Health and Human Services, Public Health Service, Office of the Surgeon General, 2001. www.surgeongeneral.gov/topics/obesity.

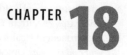
Osteoporosis Screening

O steoporosis is a common disease that weakens bone and increases the risk of fracture. Over 10 million adults in the United States have osteoporosis, and an additional 34 million have a condition called *osteopenia,* which places them at increased risk for developing osteoporosis. Each year, osteoporosis is responsible for over 1.5 million fractures, including 300,000 hip fractures, 700,000 vertebral fractures, and 250,000 wrist fractures. Women are at particularly high risk: it is estimated that half of women over age 50 will have an osteoporosis-related fracture in their lifetime.

Osteoporosis is considered a silent disease. Because the bone loss that leads to osteoporosis does not cause symptoms, without screening, the disease often goes undiagnosed until fractures develop. Unlike most fractures in younger people, osteoporosis-related fractures can lead to chronic pain, disability, and, in the case of hip fractures, death.

Fortunately, osteoporosis is preventable and treatable. Through adequate calcium and vitamin D intake, physical activity, weight control, smoking cessation, and limited consumption of alcohol and phosphate-containing sodas, osteoporosis can be prevented. In addition, through routine screening, people with osteoporosis can be diagnosed before fractures develop and benefit from treatments proven to slow the progression of disease and prevent fractures.

The United States Preventive Services Task Force (USPSTF) recommends that women age 65 or older be routinely screened for osteoporosis and that screening begin at age 60 in women at increased risk.[1] The following sections provide an introduction to bone health and osteoporosis, and detail the guidelines for screening.

SECTION I: OSTEOPOROSIS 101

Osteoporosis is a disease marked by reduced bone strength leading to an increased risk of fractures, or broken bones. Bone strength is determined by its density and structure. Bones that are more dense, or heavy, are stronger and harder to break: think of a hollow baseball bat versus a solid one. In addition, bones with a higher quality structure are less likely to break: wooden baseball bat versus a metallic one. In osteoporosis, both bone mass and bone quality are reduced. As a result, people with osteoporosis have fragile bones that are more easily broken. Compared with fractures in young people that occur from major accidents or traumatic sporting injuries, osteoporosis-related fractures occur much more easily—from falling, lifting, or even coughing.

Many people think of osteoporosis as a natural and unavoidable part of aging. Doctors used to believe this as well. But now we know that osteoporosis is a disease and one that is largely preventable and treatable.

How do I actually "lose" bone? Can I regain what I've lost?

We usually think of our bones as static, but throughout our lifetimes, old bone is constantly being broken down and new bone is constantly being formed. This process is regulated by hormones in our body, our intake of nutrients such as vitamin D and calcium, and our physical activity. The National Institute of Arthritis and Musculoskeletal and Skin Diseases has created a powerful analogy for understanding bone: "Think of bone as a bank account where you 'deposit' and 'withdraw' bone tissue."[2] When we make more deposits than withdrawals, our bone bank account increases; when we make more withdrawals than deposits, our bank account decreases.

During childhood and adolescence, more deposits of bone are made than withdrawals, and our bones grow in size, weight, and density. This pattern continues, but with deposits gradually decreasing compared with withdrawals, until we reach our *peak bone mass* (maximum bone density and strength) at around age 30, and our bone bank account starts to decrease. Thus, after early adulthood, bone mass may gradually decrease with age. If there are too many withdrawals and not enough deposits, the bone bank balance gets too low and osteoporosis develops.

To maximize deposits, we need to get enough calcium, vitamin D, and exercise—important factors in building bone. Likewise, we can minimize bone withdrawals by avoiding tobacco and excessive alcohol use, in addition to getting the nutrients and exercise we need for deposits.

Two important lessons come from understanding the life cycle of bone. One, osteoporosis is not a condition that *develops* in older age; it is only a condition that *occurs* in older age. Low bone mass at age 60 is usually a result of less-than-optimal peak bone mass at age 30 and greater-than-optimal bone loss after age 30. Therefore, preventing osteoporosis requires a lifetime of good bone health. Two, it is never too late to improve bone health. Deposits and withdrawals of bone are constantly being made; by tipping the balance more in favor of deposits, bone mass can be increased, even after osteoporosis already develops.

Am I at risk for osteoporosis?

Osteoporosis is very common: one in two women over age 50 and one in eight men over age 50 will have an osteoporosis-related fracture in their lifetime. However, which half of women and which eighth of men develop osteoporosis and to what degree is determined by their risk factors.[3]

Risk factors that cannot be changed:

- *Female sex*: Women are much more likely to develop osteoporosis than men for two reasons. One, women generally have smaller, thinner bones than men. Two, women lose bone mass more rapidly in the first several years after menopause because of decreased estrogen production.

- *Older age*: Because bone loss accumulates over time, the risk of osteoporosis increases with age.

- *Small body size or low weight*: Slender, thin-boned people are at higher risk.

- *Family history of osteoporosis*: The disease runs in families. People whose parents have a history of osteoporosis or fractures are at increased risk.

- *At-risk ethnicity*: Caucasians and Asians are at higher risk than Hispanics or African Americans.

Risk factors that can be changed or controlled:

- *Low calcium intake:* Calcium is an integral component of bone. Many people consume less than half the amount of calcium needed to build and maintain healthy bones. The recommended daily intake of calcium in adults between ages 18 and 50 is 1,000 mg; in adults over age 50, the recommended daily intake increases to 1,200 mg. To put this in perspective, consider that a cup of milk or fortified orange juice has about 300 mg of calcium.

- *Low vitamin D intake:* Vitamin D is important for calcium absorption and bone health. Although many people naturally get sufficient levels of vitamin D through exposure to sunlight and eating certain foods, studies show that the elderly, particularly those who are housebound, and people of all ages during the winter are at risk for suboptimal vitamin D intake. The recommended daily intake of vitamin D is between 400 and 800 international units (IU).

▸ *Not enough exercise*: With bone, the saying goes, "you don't use it, you lose it." Weight-bearing exercise is the best way to keep bones strong because it forces the bones to work against gravity. Examples of weight-bearing exercise include walking, hiking, tennis, weight training, and dancing.

▸ *Smoking*: Smoking is bad for your bones. Yet another reason to quit.

▸ *Alcohol*: Even in young people, daily consumption of 2 to 3 ounces of alcohol increases bone loss. Heavier drinkers are at even greater risk because they are more likely to have poor nutrition.

▸ *Low sex hormone levels*: Low estrogen levels due to menopause or missing menstrual periods increase the incidence of osteoporosis in women. Low testosterone levels likewise promote bone loss in men.

▸ *Medications*: Some medicines are associated with increased bone loss (e.g., steroids, antiseizure medications).

▸ *Phosphate beverages*: The phosphate in soda binds calcium and prevents adequate digestion and intake of calcium from the small intestine.

Can I do anything to prevent it?

Osteoporosis is largely preventable. Given the controllable risk factors outlined above, there are many steps you can take to prevent bone loss:

▸ a diet rich in calcium and vitamin D
▸ regular weight-bearing exercise
▸ abstinence from smoking
▸ limited alcohol consumption
▸ limited consumption of phosphate-containing sodas
▸ consideration of hormonal/estrogen-replacement therapy in postmenopausal women

As mentioned above, osteoporosis develops from a lifetime of poor bone health. Therefore, preventing it requires a lifetime of attention to the many important healthy choices listed above.

What are the health effects of osteoporosis?

Fractures and their complications are the major consequences of osteoporosis. The most common fractures are those of the vertebrae (spine), proximal femur (hip), and distal forearm (wrist). The health effects of fractures vary considerably, ranging from full recovery to serious complications and death.

- Hip fractures are deadly and disabling. Older people who have a hip fracture face up to a 20 percent greater likelihood of death over the following year. In addition, up to 25 percent of hip fracture patients may require long-term nursing home care, and only 40 percent ever fully regain their prefracture level of independence.

- Vertebral fractures cause significant complications, including back pain, height loss, and kyphosis (stooped posture), which in turn may limit daily activities.

- Wrist fractures cause considerable pain and are often slow to heal. While nonfatal, wrist fractures can severely limit quality of life for older adults.

In addition, fractures commonly result in loss of self-esteem and even depression because of pain, changes in appearance, and reduced independence.

How is osteoporosis diagnosed?

The diagnosis of osteoporosis is based on accurate and precise measurements of bone mass, called *bone mineral density,* or BMD.

People with severely below average BMDs are diagnosed with osteoporosis. Those with moderately below average BMDs are diagnosed with osteopenia.* Osteopenia is a less severe bone condition than osteoporosis that places people at increased risk of developing osteoporosis.

In the past, because of the absence of symptoms and the lack of screening tests, most people were diagnosed with osteoporosis only after they had already sustained an osteoporosis-related fracture. Fortunately now, thanks to screening, people are increasingly being diagnosed with osteoporosis at an earlier stage of the disease and before the onset of any complications.

---

* In statistical terms, the cutoff for severely below average is 2.5 standard deviations (SD) below the average. For moderately below average, the cutoff is between 1 and 2.5 SDs below the average. (If this doesn't make sense, don't worry about it.)

What is the treatment for osteoporosis?

Treating osteoporosis requires a comprehensive program that includes proper nutrition (e.g., vitamin D and calcium), exercise, fall prevention, and for some, medication. The importance of regular screening for osteoporosis is underscored by the effectiveness of these treatments in preventing fractures and slowing the progression of the disease.

Calcium and Vitamin D

People with osteoporosis should receive 1,000 to 1,500 mg of elemental calcium per day. They should also receive a minimum of 800 IU daily of vitamin D. If these recommendations cannot be met through sunlight exposure and diet, oral supplements may be taken. Supplements vary widely in their calcium and vitamin D content, so it is best to choose supplements with your doctor's guidance.

Fall Prevention and Exercise

Older adults often have poorer balance, muscle weakness, and diminished eyesight that put them at increased risk of falls. Because osteoporosis-related fractures often result from falls, taking measures to prevent them is essential to improving the long-term health of people with osteoporosis. Fall prevention encompasses various interventions, including regular eye exams, walking aids, rubber-soled shoes, physical therapy, and fall-proofing the home environment (e.g., improving lighting at night, removing carpets, installing grab bars in the bathroom).

Medications

Several classes of medications are available to treat osteoporosis, including bisphosphonates, selective estrogen receptor modulators (SERMs), calcitonin, and hormonal/estrogen-replacement therapy. Each of these medications is FDA approved for the treatment of osteoporosis based on its proven effectiveness in rebuilding bone and reducing fractures. The effectiveness of these medications is remarkable: as an example, in people with osteoporosis, bisphosphonates reduce the risk of fracture by 25 to 50 percent. Because these medications are usually taken chronically, it is important to discuss the risks and side effects with your doctor.

SECTION II: OSTEOPOROSIS SCREENING

The USPSTF recommends that women age 65 or older be screened routinely for osteoporosis. In addition, the task force recommends that screening begin at age 60 for women at increased risk. These recommendations are based on evidence that screening can accurately predict the short-term risk of fracture and that treating asymptomatic women reduces their risk of fracture.

- ▸ If you are a woman over age 65, regardless of the presence or absence of other risk factors, you should be screened for osteoporosis.

- ▸ If you are a woman between ages 60 and 65, talk to your doctor about whether osteoporosis screening is right for you. In general, women who are low weight (under 154 lb) or do not currently use hormone (estrogen) replacement therapy are the best candidates for earlier screening.

The USPSTF does not specify the optimal interval for screening. A reasonable approach is to screen younger women with normal bone scans every five years and older women more frequently. How often you should be screened is up to you and your doctor.

What about women under 60 years old?

The USPSTF found insufficient evidence to recommend screening in women under 60. Although screening women under age 60 may detect additional cases of osteoporosis, the task force concluded that the number of fractures that might be prevented was too small to make a general recommendation. If you are a woman under age 60 and have risk factors for osteoporosis or concerns about your bone health, talk to your doctor.

What about screening men?

Although far more common in women, osteoporosis in older men is still a considerable problem. An estimated one in eight men over age 50 will have an osteoporosis-related fracture in his lifetime. To date, most studies of osteoporosis screening have been done in women, so not much is known about the potential benefits and harms of screening in men. If you are an older man and have concerns about your bone health, talk to your doctor about whether screening is right for you.

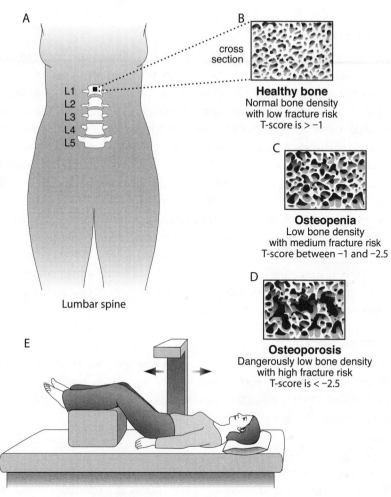

A

cross section

L1
L2
L3
L4
L5

Lumbar spine

B

Healthy bone
Normal bone density
with low fracture risk
T-score is > −1

C

Osteopenia
Low bone density
with medium fracture risk
T-score between −1 and −2.5

D

Osteoporosis
Dangerously low bone density
with high fracture risk
T-score is < −2.5

E

DXA bone densitometry scan of lumbar spine

Figure 18.1. (A) Osteoporosis commonly develops in the bones of the spine (also known as vertebrae), and in particular in the bones that support the lower back (the lumbar spine). (B) On a microscopic level, bone comprises a matrix of protein and calcium. Healthy bone is characterized by high bone density, or bone mass. (C) Osteopenic bone has reduced bone density. The "holes" in the bone matrix make it susceptible to fractures. (D) Osteoporotic bone has severely reduced bone density that may lead to fractures even with minor stresses, such as falling, lifting, or coughing. (E) DXA bone densitometry is a simple test doctors use to measure bone density and to diagnose osteoporosis. In the test, the patient lies on an examining table while the DXA machine takes x-rays of the spine. The information from the x-rays is then computed into a single number called the T-score. Having a T-score greater than -1 means that the bones are healthy. Osteoporosis is diagnosed when the T-score is less than -2.5. Between -1 and -2.5 the bone is osteopenic, meaning the person is at risk for developing osteoporosis.

How is screening done?

Screening is done through one of several tests that measure bone mineral density (BMD). The most widely used test to measure BMD is called a *dual-energy x-ray absorptiometry,* or DXA test (pronounced "dex-a"; see figure 18.1). It is similar to an x-ray, but with less exposure to radiation. The advantages of DXA over other tests of BMD are that it is easy to perform, carries low risks, and reliably predicts the near-term chances of fracture.

A DXA test is similar to an x-ray. During the test, you will be asked to lie on a table while a machine above you measures the bone density in your hip and spine. The test takes about fifteen minutes and is painless. The primary risk of the test is from exposure to radiation. However, this risk is considered low, and the total exposure is about one-tenth that of a standard chest x-ray.

The test reports your BMD and compares it to that of the average healthy young adult. If your bone density is below a certain cutoff, you are diagnosed with osteoporosis. If your bone density is decreased but not below the cutoff, you may be diagnosed with osteopenia.

What are the harms?

As mentioned above, the risks of the DXA scan itself are small. However, there are other potential harms from screening, such as side effects from medications used to treat people diagnosed with osteoporosis. It is important to discuss these risks with your doctor.

What if my test results are normal?

You do not have osteopenia or osteoporosis and no further testing is required at this time. The USPSTF does not specify the optimal interval for screening, so it is up to you and your doctor to decide when your next screening test for osteoporosis should be. Every three to five years is typical. Even though you don't have any signs of osteoporosis, you can still take steps to improve your bone health. By staying physically active, ensuring adequate intake of vitamin D and calcium, staying away from cigarettes, consuming alcohol in moderation, and avoiding phosphate-containing sodas, you can keep your bones healthy and strong.

What happens if I'm diagnosed with osteopenia?

Osteopenia is a less severe bone condition than osteoporosis, but it places you at increased risk of developing osteoporosis. Doctors generally do not prescribe medications for people with osteopenia and instead focus on aggressive preventive measures, such as vitamin D and calcium supplementation as well as weight-bearing exercise. The USPSTF does not make any specific recommendations about how often people with osteopenia should be rescreened. Therefore, it is up to you and your doctor to decide when you should be screened next. The usual interval is two to three years.

What happens if I'm diagnosed with osteoporosis?

Osteoporosis is a serious, chronic medical condition. Fortunately, there are effective treatments that can slow, or even reverse, the progression of disease and prevent fractures. In addition to aggressive preventive measures, people with osteoporosis are usually started on one or more medications, including bisphosphonates, hormone replacement therapy, selective estrogen replacement modulators (SERMs), and calcitonin. Your doctor will help you pick the medication that is right for you.

REFERENCES

National Institute of Arthritis and Musculoskeletal and Skin Diseases. "Bone Health Overview." National Institutes of Health. U.S. Department of Health and Human Services. www.niams.nih.gov/Health_Info/Bone/Bone_Health/default.asp.

National Institutes of Health (NIH). U.S. Department of Health and Human Services. "Osteoporosis." www.health.nih.gov/topics/Osteoporosis.

National Institutes of Health Osteoporosis and Related Diseases National Resource Center. "Osteoporosis Overview." www.niams.nih.gov/Health_Info/Bone/Osteoporosis/overview.pdf.

U.S. Department of Health and Human Services. *Bone Health and Osteoporosis: A Report of the Surgeon General.* Issued October 14, 2004. www.surgeongeneral.gov/library/bonehealth.

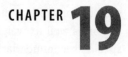

Pregnancy Preventive Health

Pregnancy is a vital time in the development of the child and in the health of the mother. By partnering with her health care provider, a pregnant woman can optimize her chances of staying healthy during pregnancy and having a healthy baby.

The United States Preventive Services Task Force (USPSTF) recommends the following pregnancy-related preventive health measures:

- folic acid supplements for all women planning or capable of pregnancy
- asymptomatic bacteriuria screening at the end of the first trimester
- Rh(D) blood typing at the first prenatal visit
- iron deficiency anemia screening
- breastfeeding education and counseling[1]
- chlamydia screening in women at increased risk
- gonorrhea screening in women at increased risk
- HIV screening at the first prenatal visit*
- hepatitis B screening at the first prenatal visit
- syphilis screening at the first prenatal visit
- tobacco use counseling
- alcohol misuse counseling

In addition, the Centers for Disease Control and Prevention (CDC) recommends immunization with seasonal influenza vaccine for women who are or will be pregnant during the flu season.

The majority of women who receive prenatal care in the United States receive at least these preventive services. Often additional services, such as screening for gestational diabetes or group B streptococcus, are offered to

---

* The USPSTF does not specify when to screen for HIV but the first prenatal visit is a reasonable time.

pregnant women based on recommendations from professional organizations, such as the American College of Obstetricians and Gynecologists and the American Academy of Pediatrics (AAP).

The following sections describe the USPSTF-recommended preventive measures related to pregnancy. Section I describes folic acid supplementation, which is recommended to start before pregnancy. Sections II to V discuss the four recommendations specific to pregnancy—asymptomatic bacteriuria, Rh(D) blood typing, iron deficiency anemia, and breastfeeding—in depth. Section VI briefly covers screening for five sexually transmitted infections (STIs), which are discussed in detail elsewhere in the book (gonorrhea, chlamydia, hepatitis B, HIV, and syphilis). Sections VII and VIII close the chapter with brief discussions of tobacco and alcohol use, respectively, during pregnancy. Influenza vaccination is covered in its entirety in chapter 23.

SECTION I: FOLIC ACID SUPPLEMENTATION

The concept of prenatal vitamins is familiar to most women. By supplementing her diet with vitamins, a woman can best prepare herself for pregnancy and ensure the health of her unborn child. However, many women do not know which vitamins to take or which ones have proven health benefits. And because half of pregnancies in the United States are unplanned, many women miss the opportunity to supplement their diet during the critical phase of their child's development.

The USPSTF recommends that all women planning or capable of pregnancy take a daily supplement containing between 400 to 800 micrograms of folic acid. To be most effective, supplementation should start at least one month before conception and continue through the first two to three months of pregnancy. Because many pregnancies are unplanned, it is important that all women of reproductive age take folic acid routinely. This recommendation does not apply to women who have had a previous pregnancy affected by neural tube defects or women taking antiseizure medications, who typically require higher doses of folic acid.

What is folic acid? What is folate?

Folate, or vitamin B9, is a water-soluble vitamin that occurs naturally in foods, particularly leafy green vegetables like spinach and turnip greens, citrus fruits and bananas, avocados, and dried beans and peas. It helps produce and maintain new cells, which is especially important during periods of rapid growth such as pregnancy and fetal development. Folic acid is the synthetic form of folate that is found in supplements and added to fortified foods such as breads, cereals, and other grain products.

What are the benefits of taking folic acid?

When started at least one month before conception, folic acid supplementation has been shown to prevent up to 40 percent of neural tube defects. *Neural tube defects* are a type of birth defect that result from a malformation of the unborn baby's central nervous system. They are among the most common birth defects in the United States, affecting one in every one thousand pregnancies. Despite this, only a third or so of reproductive age women are receiving sufficient amounts of folic acid either through supplementation or fortified foods.

What are the harms of folic acid?

Folic acid supplementation is safe to take at the usual doses.

How should it to be taken?

Folic acid can be taken as an individual supplement or as part of a prenatal vitamin. While most of the other nutritional supplements found in prenatal vitamins have no proven benefit to mother or baby, they are generally considered safe when taken in the appropriate doses. Regardless of which formulation you choose, make sure it includes between 400 to 800 micrograms of folic acid and that you take it regularly. Although you do not need a prescription for folic acid, talk to your doctor about folic acid and whether it is right for you. Women with a history of a previous pregnancy affected by a neural tube defect or who take antiseizure medications are generally advised to take higher doses of folic acid and should consult their doctor for specific recommendations.

What other supplements should pregnant women take?

Folic acid is the only nutritional supplement that the USPSTF routinely recommends in women who are pregnant or who become pregnant. However, the USPSTF also recommends screening all pregnant women for iron deficiency anemia. Women diagnosed with iron deficiency anemia through screening are advised to take iron supplements. This is discussed in greater detail in Section IV.

SECTION II: SCREENING FOR ASYMPTOMATIC BACTERIURIA

Asymptomatic bacteriuria is a condition in which a significant number of bacteria are present in the urine without any of the usual symptoms of a urinary tract infection, such as pain or burning when urinating and a frequent urge to urinate. Asymptomatic bacteriuria occurs in up to 6 percent of healthy women and usually does not cause any serious health problems. As many as 10 percent of pregnant women have asymptomatic bacteriuria, however, and without treatment, they are at risk of kidney infection (pyelonephritis), preterm labor, and delivering a low-birthweight baby.

Because asymptomatic bacteriuria has no symptoms, the only way to detect it is through screening. The USPSTF recommends screening for asymptomatic bacteriuria at 12 to 16 weeks' gestation or at the first prenatal visit, if later, in all pregnant women.

How is screening done?

Screening is done through a urine culture test. In this test, a routine urine sample is sent to a lab, where it is kept under conditions that allow bacteria to grow. If few organisms grow, the test is negative. If the urine culture is positive, other tests may be done to determine the species of bacteria causing the infection and to help choose the best antibiotic to treat the infection. Results are typically available in one to three days.

What are the benefits of screening?

Pregnant women with asymptomatic bacteriuria have a twenty- to thirtyfold increased risk of pyelonephritis compared with pregnant women without bacteriuria. Studies have shown that screening for asymptomatic bacteriuria in pregnancy decreases the risk of developing pyelonephritis from 20 to 35 percent to 1 to 4 percent. It also reduces the risk of low-birthweight and preterm delivery.

What are the risks?

Urine sample collection has no health risks of any kind. However, there is a risk associated with a positive screening test. While generally safe, antibiotics can be potentially harmful to the mother and baby and carry a small risk of anaphylaxis (major allergic reaction). Be sure to tell your doctor if you have allergies to any antibiotics or other medications.

What happens if I test positive?

A positive urine culture suggests that you have asymptomatic bacteriuria. Because of the risks described above, antibiotics are recommended. The normal treatment course is three to fourteen days of oral antibiotics.

What happens if I test negative?

A negative urine culture suggests that you do not have asymptomatic bacteriuria. No antibiotic treatment or further testing is recommended.

How often should I get screened during pregnancy?

The guidelines recommend a one-time screening for asymptomatic bacteriuria at the end of the first trimester (12 to 16 weeks of pregnancy) or at the first prenatal visit, if later. No further recommendations are made about rescreening later in the pregnancy. However, if you develop symptoms consistent with a urinary tract infection, you should consult your doctor immediately. The symptoms of a urinary tract infection are burning or pain with urination, frequent urge to urinate, and difficulty starting or stopping urination.

SECTION III: SCREENING FOR RH(D) INCOMPATIBILITY

Rh(D) refers to a person's minor blood type. Most people know of the major blood types: A, B, AB, and O. But in addition, there are minor blood types: Rh(D)-positive and Rh(D)-negative. When someone is said to be A-positive, it means he or she is major blood type A and minor blood type Rh(D)-positive.

Because blood type is inherited from both parents, it is possible for a mother and her baby to have different Rh(D) blood types. *Rh(D) incompatibility* is a condition in which the pregnant woman is Rh(D)-negative and her unborn baby is Rh(D)-positive. About 85 percent of adults are Rh(D) positive. Therefore, in most couples, both parents are Rh(D)-positive and their children are Rh(D)-positive. However, if a woman who is Rh(D)-negative and a man who is Rh(D)-positive have a child, there is a 50 percent chance their baby will be Rh(D)-positive, which means that the mother and baby will be Rh(D) incompatible.

While Rh(D) incompatibility does not usually pose a health risk to the baby during the mother's first pregnancy, it can cause a life-threatening condition known as *hemolytic disease of the newborn,* or HDN, in subsequent pregnancies. HDN is a life-threatening condition characterized by anemia (low red blood cell count), jaundice (yellowing of the skin), and in severe cases, heart failure. A woman's Rh(D) status can be determined with routine blood tests. Furthermore, women who test Rh(D)-negative and are at risk of Rh(D) incompatibility can receive treatment that virtually eliminates the risk of having a child with HDN.

The USPSTF recommends that Rh(D) blood typing and antibody testing be performed in all pregnant women during their first prenatal visit. In addition, the task force recommends further testing for unsensitized Rh(D)-negative women (those who have not developed antibodies) at 24 to 28 weeks of pregnancy, unless the biological father is known to be Rh(D)-negative.

How does HDN develop?

The immune system is designed to distinguish between self and nonself (also called foreign) and to make antibodies against anything nonself. As a result, if someone with type A blood receives a type B blood transfusion, the type B blood cells are seen as foreign, and antibodies are made to defend against them. The resulting destruction of type B blood cells can cause a life-threatening condition called a *transfusion reaction.*

If the mother is Rh(D)-negative and her baby is Rh(D)-positive, the mother's immune system may interpret the baby's Rh(D)-positive blood as foreign and produce antibodies against the baby. Fortunately, in order to make these antibodies, the mother has to first be exposed to the baby's blood. During pregnancy, this exposure does not typically occur until delivery. Thus, Rh(D) incompatibility does not usually pose a health risk to the baby during the mother's first pregnancy. However, if the mother carries a second Rh(D)-positive child, her antibodies will recognize the baby's blood cells as foreign and will attack them, causing HDN.

How is testing done?

Rh(D) blood typing and antibody testing are done through routine blood tests. Often this test is done during the first prenatal visit along with several other prenatal blood tests.

What if I am Rh(D)-positive?

Women who are Rh(D)-positive are at no risk of Rh(D)-incompatibility. No further testing or treatment is required.

What if I am Rh(D)-negative?

There is a chance that your baby is Rh(D)-positive and therefore that you and your baby are Rh(D) incompatible. Testing your baby's blood type while the baby is still in the uterus can be dangerous and is generally not done. Instead, for all practical purposes, it is assumed that your baby is Rh(D)-positive so that the full preventive measures can be taken. In addition to the standard prenatal care, you will be given two doses of Rh(D) immunoglobulin (also known by its trade name RhoGAM), once at 24 to 28 weeks of pregnancy and once around the time of delivery. RhoGAM is given as an injection, similar to other vaccine shots. You will also get a repeat blood test at 24 to 28 weeks to look for the presence of antibodies to Rh(D).

Is RhoGAM safe?

RhoGAM can cause swelling, redness, irritation at the injection site, and a mild fever. Because RhoGAM is made from human plasma, there is a risk of certain viral infections, such as hepatitis C. This risk has been virtually eliminated, however, through pretesting of donors and advancements in the manufacturing process. In addition, RhoGAM no longer contains thimerosal, which has been associated with brain toxicity when taken in high doses.

SECTION IV: SCREENING FOR IRON DEFICIENCY ANEMIA

Iron deficiency anemia is a common condition in pregnancy. While estimates vary widely, some experts believe that up to half of pregnant women have this condition. Iron deficiency anemia during pregnancy has been associated with increased health risks for the baby. Because pregnant women often experience no symptoms of this anemia, without screening, their condition goes undiagnosed and untreated.

The USPSTF recommends screening for iron deficiency anemia in all pregnant women. The following subsections provide a brief introduction to this condition and explain the screening guidelines in pregnancy.

What exactly is iron deficiency anemia?

Anemia (uh-NEE-me-uh) is a condition in which there are fewer red blood cells in the blood than normal. There are many types and causes of anemia. Because iron is an essential component of hemoglobin—the oxygen-carrying protein that gives blood its red color—a lack of iron can lead to anemia. *Iron deficiency anemia* is caused by having too little iron in the body. It is a common and easily treated condition.

What causes it?

The body needs iron to build new cells. It gets iron from recycling old red blood cells and from food. There are four causes of iron deficiency:

- blood loss, either from disease or injury
- insufficient iron in the diet
- impaired absorption of iron in the gut
- increased demand for iron due to growth or pregnancy

Iron deficiency anemia in pregnancy is often due to multiple causes. Young women sometimes have low levels of iron from menstrual blood losses. With pregnancy, iron stores are further depleted because of the increased demand for iron to support the growing baby. In many women, this is further compounded by low dietary intake of iron and vitamin C, which helps absorb iron from the gut into the body.

What foods are rich in iron?

Iron is present in a variety of foods. In general, iron in meats is more easily absorbed by the body than iron in vegetables and other foods. The best source of iron is red meat, especially beef and liver, which have high iron content and are most readily absorbed by the body. Chicken, turkey, pork, fish, and shellfish also are good sources. Other foods high in iron include dark green, leafy vegetables such as spinach; beans and nuts; dried fruits; and cereals, breads, and pastas fortified with iron.

Because iron deficiency is sometimes caused not by a lack of iron but by a lack of vitamin C, increasing intake of that vitamin may help. Good sources of vitamin C in foods include fruits, especially citrus, and a variety of vegetables.

What are the symptoms of iron deficiency anemia?

Because red blood cells transport oxygen to the tissues, anemia can cause various symptoms related to the lack of oxygen in the body. The most common symptom is fatigue (constant tiredness). Other common symptoms include

- generalized weakness
- fainting or lightheadedness
- shortness of breath or chest pain with activity
- pale skin, gums, or nail beds
- cravings for ice, dirt, or paint

The severity of symptoms is related to the degree of anemia. The lower the number of red blood cells, the more severe the symptoms. Having no symptoms of anemia is common, especially in cases of mild anemia or when the disease develops gradually over months. In addition, those who have symptoms often overlook them or attribute them to pregnancy itself and therefore do not seek medical attention. For these reasons, screening for anemia in at-risk populations is essential.

What problems does it cause?

Iron deficiency anemia can range from mild to severe. In addition to causing disabling symptoms such as fatigue and shortness of breath, iron deficiency anemia can lead to serious health complications, particularly in pregnant women.

Iron deficiency anemia in pregnancy has been associated with an increased risk of low-birthweight, preterm delivery, and perinatal mortality, as well as decreased parent-child interaction and poorer developmental outcomes in infants. Recent studies suggest that it may also be associated with postpartum depression in the mother and poor performance on mental and psychomotor tests in the child.

Although the complications of iron deficiency anemia generally increase with the severity of symptoms, it is possible to have some of these complications without any symptoms of anemia.

How is it treated?

The goals of treatment are to restore normal levels of red blood cells and iron. In addition, for people whose iron-deficiency is a result of a secondary problem such as chronic bleeding, another important goal is to correct the underlying condition.

The mainstay of treatment is iron supplements. Usually oral iron tablets are taken daily for two to three months to correct low iron levels. Often vitamin C supplements are also given to help the body absorb the iron. Rarely, severe anemia may need to be treated with hospitalization, iron injections, or blood transfusions.

The primary risk of iron supplements is overdosing, so keep iron pills away from children. In addition, iron and vitamin C supplements can cause side effects, such as stomach irritation and heartburn. Iron also commonly causes constipation.

How is screening done?

The USPSTF does not specify how often and when screening should occur during pregnancy, and therefore this decision is up to you and your doctor. However, it is reasonable to get screened during the first prenatal visit.

Screening is done with a routine blood test that measures blood count levels. If you are found to be anemic, your doctor may order additional blood work to determine if iron deficiency is the cause of the anemia.

What are the benefits of screening?

Screening for iron deficiency anemia has been shown to increase red blood cell levels and, in many people, cure the anemia. Less clear is whether testing for iron deficiency anemia in pregnancy reduces complications from anemia such as the risk of preterm delivery. However, because there is a clear link between anemia and these complications, it is generally assumed that screening also reduces the risk of these complications.

What are the harms?

The screening test for iron deficiency anemia itself does not carry any risks. However, there are risks of oral iron supplementation, such as stomach irritation and constipation. Most concerning, supplements can cause serious harm or death in young children who accidentally overdose on them.

What if my test is negative?

A negative test means that you are not anemic and have normal blood levels of iron. However, it is possible that you will develop anemia later in pregnancy. It is up to you and your doctor to decide whether to screen again for anemia.

What if my test is positive?

A positive blood test for anemia will typically be followed up with further blood work. Most but not all cases of anemia in pregnancy are related to iron deficiency. If this blood work is consistent with low iron levels, you will be diagnosed with iron deficiency anemia. However, further testing may also suggest other causes of anemia, such as folate deficiency or chronic disease.

The usual treatment of iron deficiency anemia is oral iron tablets for one to two months. Some doctors recommend taking additional vitamin C supplements to improve iron absorption, and stool softeners as needed for constipation, a common side effect of iron supplements.

Pregnant women with iron deficiency have a good prognosis. Often the condition resolves within weeks, and the pregnancy is carried to term without any complications from the anemia.

SECTION V: BREASTFEEDING COUNSELING AND EDUCATION

Breast milk is the optimal infant food and provides a host of benefits to the infant and mother. In addition to providing nutrition to support infant growth and development, breast milk contains maternal antibodies that protect the newborn from infection and disease. Less well known are the benefits to maternal health. Breastfeeding helps women lose weight after pregnancy, provides partial contraception, and decreases the long-term risk of breast, ovarian, and endometrial cancer. In addition, breastfeeding is less expensive than other forms of infant nutrition, improves maternal-child bonding, and is better for the environment. As a result, many expert organizations, including the AAP, recommend breastfeeding for at least the first twelve months of the baby's life, including exclusively for the first six months, and thereafter for as long as mother and baby desire.

Despite this, less than three-quarters of mothers initiate breastfeeding. Less than one-half breastfeed past six months, and less than one-quarter for twelve months. While the reasons for this are many, studies show that physician-based programs that provide mothers with breastfeeding education and counseling can successfully increase rates of breastfeeding.

The USPSTF recommends counseling during pregnancy and after birth to promote and support breastfeeding. This recommendation is based on evidence that counseling increases rates of initiation, duration, and exclusivity of breastfeeding. Although the wording is geared more toward doctors, you should talk with your doctor about your plans for breastfeeding to learn about ways he or she may be able to help you start and continue breastfeeding your child. The following subsections describe the benefits of breastfeeding and detail the counseling guidelines.

Should all women breastfeed?

All new mothers are encouraged to breastfeed with few exceptions. Mothers with human immunodeficiency virus (HIV) should not breastfeed because there is a risk of HIV transmission through breast milk. Mothers with ongoing alcohol and drug use or dependence are also advised not to breastfeed. Finally, some medications—including prescription, nonprescription, and herbal—should be avoided in breastfeeding women. Be sure to tell your doctor about all the medications and alternative or complementary remedies you are taking so he or she can best advise you.

Smoking is not a contraindication to breastfeeding, although quitting is strongly encouraged.

What are the benefits of breastfeeding?

The benefits of breastfeeding have been well studied and include health benefits to both newborn and mother and nonhealth benefits.[2]

Infants who are breastfed have over a 20 percent lower chance of death than those who are not breastfed and a lower rate of hospitalization. Antibodies, or infection-fighting proteins, in breast milk reduce the risk of a wide range of infections including pneumonia and other lower respiratory tract infections (1.7 to 5 times lower risk), gastrointestinal tract infections (3 times lower risk), bacterial meningitis (3.8 times lower risk), and ear infections (2.4 times lower risk). For less clear reasons, studies have also shown that breast milk–fed infants have a lower risk of sudden infant death syndrome or SIDS. Later in life, breastfed infants have lower rates of many chronic diseases from diabetes, obesity, and allergies to certain cancers such as leukemia.

Equally remarkable are the benefits to maternal health, which result in part from the hormonal effects of breastfeeding. Breastfeeding mothers have less postpartum bleeding and more rapid uterine involution (return of the uterus to normal position) than mothers who do not breastfeed. They also benefit from an earlier return to prepregnancy weight than nonbreastfeeding mothers. Finally, women who breastfeed have a lifetime lower risk of premenopausal breast cancer and premenopausal ovarian cancer and a lower risk of osteoporosis.

Breastfeeding has nonhealth benefits as well. Breast milk reduces the costs of child rearing because it is less expensive than other forms of nutrition and reduces health care expenses. Because breastfed children get sick less often than children who are not breastfed, breastfeeding also decreases visits to the doctor's office and missed days of work. Finally, it also improves mother-child bonding and has been associated with better cognitive development.

Why should I try breastfeeding education and counseling?

Breastfeeding education, counseling, and support programs have been shown to improve rates of breastfeeding. Studies show that for every ten women who enroll in breastfeeding programs, two will initiate breastfeeding and four will continue to breastfeed for one to three months.

What can I expect from my doctor?

Your doctor will likely begin by assessing your willingness and comfort level with breastfeeding. Women who have experience with breastfeeding and who are committed to breastfeed through the first year of life may not require any further interventions or support. In contrast, women who are first-time mothers or have doubts or concerns about breastfeeding may benefit from a formal breastfeeding program.

Breastfeeding programs generally begin during the prenatal period (before delivery) and cover core topics: benefits of breastfeeding for infant and mother (health and other), basic physiology and anatomy, equipment (including clothing, pumps, and storage), technical training in positioning and latch-on techniques, and behavioral training. The USPSTF found that educational sessions that review the benefits of breastfeeding, principles of lactation, myths, common problems, solutions, and skills training appear to have the largest impact on breastfeeding. They often involve individual or group sessions led by specially trained nurses or lactation specialists.

Breastfeeding support should not end with the birth of the child or discharge from the hospital, and as always, you should feel comfortable bringing your ongoing concerns to the attention of your or your child's doctor.

SECTION VI: SCREENING FOR STIs IN PREGNANCY

Women who are pregnant can become infected with the same STIs as women who are not pregnant.[3] As with nonpregnant women, many of these infections are silent, with symptoms that are either absent or mild, and as a result they often go undiagnosed. Over time, these STIs can cause a range of health problems and be transmitted to sexual partners.

Of importance in the context of pregnancy is the fact that STIs can also be transmitted from mother to baby. Some STIs, like syphilis, can cross the placental barrier and infect the baby in the uterus. Others (e.g., gonorrhea, chlamydia, hepatitis B) may infect the baby during delivery as the baby passes through the birth canal. And still others, like HIV, can infect the baby at multiple points, including in the uterus, during delivery, and even later through breastfeeding. In addition, STIs can lead to complications of pregnancy, such as preterm labor and postpartum endometritis.

Most of these complications can be prevented through routine prenatal care, which includes screening tests for STIs starting early in pregnancy.

Screening can lead to effective interventions aimed at curing the underlying infection with antibiotics, as with gonorrhea, chlamydia, and syphilis, for example, or reducing the likelihood of passing the infection to the newborn, as with hepatitis B and HIV.

The USPSTF recommends the following screening measures for STIs during pregnancy:

- chlamydia screening in pregnant women at increased risk
- gonorrhea screening in pregnant women at increased risk
- hepatitis B screening
- HIV screening
- syphilis screening

All five of these STIs are discussed in greater depth elsewhere. If you have not already read these sections, read them now to gain a better understanding of these STIs. This chapter includes only the information most relevant to pregnancy.

GONORRHEA AND CHLAMYDIA

Each year 100,000 pregnant women are infected with chlamydia, and another 13,000 are infected with gonorrhea. Because both of these infections commonly cause no symptoms in women, without screening, these infections may remain undiagnosed and untreated.

Both gonorrhea and chlamydia are associated with poorer pregnancy outcomes. Gonorrhea infection in a pregnant woman increases the risk of preterm rupture of membranes, preterm labor, and chorioamnionitis (infection of the membranes that surround the fetus). Chlamydia increases the risk of miscarriage, premature rupture of membranes, preterm labor, low birthweight, infant mortality, and postpartum endometritis (infection of the uterus).

Both infections can be transmitted from mother to baby during labor and delivery. In newborn infants, gonorrhea infection can cause blindness, joint infection, or a life-threatening widespread infection of the blood. Chlamydia can cause infant pneumonia and conjunctivitis (pink eye) in newborns.

Should I be screened for gonorrhea and chlamydia?

The USPSTF recommends screening for gonorrhea and chlamydia infection in pregnant women at increased risk for infection. Pregnant women at risk for infection include those under 25 years old and those of any age with risk factors for infection, including a history of chlamydia, gonorrhea, or other STIs; new or multiple sexual partners; or a history of exchanging sex for drugs or money. Pregnant women at increased risk for either infection should be screened at the first prenatal care visit. For pregnant women who remain at increased risk or who acquire a new risk factor, such as a new sexual partner, screening should be repeated in the third trimester.

Screening for chlamydia and gonorrhea in pregnant women is done the same way it is done in nonpregnant women (see chapters 6 and 13). Pregnant women who test positive should receive antibiotic treatment to cure the infection, though the choice of antibiotics may differ from those prescribed in nonpregnant women. These antibiotics carry additional risks in pregnancy but are generally regarded as safe for mother and baby.

HEPATITIS B

Pregnant women who are infected with HBV can transmit the virus to their babies. Without appropriate treatment, up to 90 percent of these babies develop chronic (lifelong) HBV infections, placing them at increased risk of developing liver failure or liver cancer later in life. Most women of childbearing age infected with HBV have no symptoms of their disease. Thus, without testing, pregnant women with HBV may not know they carry the virus. By screening mothers early in pregnancy, doctors can diagnose HBV and take steps to prevent it from being transmitted.

The USPSTF recommends screening for HBV in all pregnant women during the first trimester. This recommendation is based on evidence that universal prenatal screening for HBV infection substantially reduces mother-to-baby transmission of the virus and the subsequent development of chronic HBV infection in the newborn. Screening is done with a routine blood test for hepatitis B surface antigen (HBsAg).

What if the test is negative?

A negative HBsAg test means that you do not have hepatitis B. Your baby should receive only the standard hepatitis B vaccine series starting at birth. Usually, women who are negative for HBsAg do not undergo further testing. However, there is a small chance that the test is falsely negative because in some stages of infection, HBsAg levels are too low to detect. While not routinely recommended, some doctors rescreen women at high risk of HBV near or at the time of delivery.

What if the test is positive?

A positive, or reactive, blood test means you have hepatitis B. However, from an HBsAg test alone, doctors cannot distinguish between acute or chronic infection and cannot determine your prognosis. Further blood work and testing will help your doctor determine the stage of your infection and what treatments are most appropriate.

To protect your baby from getting HBV, your doctor will give him or her a medication at birth called the *hepatitis B immune globulin* (HBIG). This medication is a direct antibody to the hepatitis B virus and will reduce the risk of your baby getting HBV. In addition, your baby will get vaccinated against HBV as recommended for all babies.

If I have hepatitis B, is it okay to breastfeed?

Because hepatitis B is not present in breast milk, it is safe to breastfeed your baby. In fact, breastfeeding is encouraged because it is the optimal infant nutrition (as discussed in section V above).

HIV

HIV can be transmitted from mother to baby during pregnancy, during labor and delivery, and after delivery through breastfeeding. Each year in the United States, an estimated 6,000 HIV-positive women give birth, and 300 to 400 HIV-positive infants are born. Because there are often no symptoms of HIV in the early stages of the disease, many women who become pregnant do not know that they have HIV. In 2000, 40 percent of the infants who were born with HIV were born to mothers who did not know they were infected.

Screening for HIV in pregnancy is especially important because there are effective interventions for reducing mother-to-baby transmission. Through a combination of highly active antiretroviral therapy (HAART), elective Cesarean sections, and avoidance of breastfeeding, rates of HIV transmission in pregnancy can be reduced from 25 percent to less than 2 percent.

Screening tests for HIV in pregnancy are no different from those in the general population (see chapter 16). The USPSTF recommends screening for HIV in all pregnant women, regardless of whether they have any risk factors. The USPSTF makes no specific recommendations about when or how often screening should occur. General practice is to screen once during the first trimester; however, for women at high risk for infection, it is reasonable to rescreen later in the pregnancy.

Does HIV screening during pregnancy carry any special risks?

HIV screening itself poses no additional risks during pregnancy. However, pregnant women diagnosed with HIV are typically given HAART and elective Cesarean sections, both of which carry certain risks to mother and baby. It is important to discuss these risks with your doctor.

What if I test negative for HIV?

Testing negative for HIV generally means you are not infected. However, screening tests for HIV measure antibodies to HIV, not the virus itself, which take one to three months (and, rarely, up to six months) to become detectable. So even with a negative HIV test, a woman could be infected with the virus if the infection occurred recently. In addition, it is possible to become newly infected during pregnancy. For these reasons, women at increased risk for HIV should consider getting rescreened later in their pregnancy.

What if I test HIV positive?

A positive HIV screening test must be followed up with a confirmatory test (called a *Western blot*). If the Western blot is also positive, a diagnosis of HIV / AIDS is made.

From here, additional measures will be taken to ensure your health and the health of your baby. These will include additional blood work and tests to better understand the stage of your disease and determine what treatments are appropriate at this time. HAART—a combination of medications that work together to combat the virus—will most likely be started. Your doctor may also recommend scheduling an elective Cesarean section (C-section). C-sections reduce the chance of mother-to-baby transmission tenfold, and when done electively (meaning planned well in advance) are relatively safe. Finally, because HIV can be transmitted through breast milk, you will be advised not to breastfeed.

SYPHILIS

Syphilis can cross the placenta and be passed from mother to baby during pregnancy. Untreated syphilis results in stillbirth in up to 40 percent of pregnancies. Syphilis also can put a woman at risk of giving birth to a baby who dies shortly after birth. Babies who survive the infection may develop *congenital syphilis,* which can lead to central nervous system abnormalities; deafness; multiple skin, bone, and joint deformities; and blood disorders.

Because the symptoms of syphilis are often mild and fleeting, women can develop syphilis during pregnancy yet remain undiagnosed. Screening is the only way to diagnose the infection in asymptomatic women. Antibiotic therapy is highly effective in curing syphilis and preventing the transmission of infection during pregnancy. The usual choice of antibiotic, penicillin, is considered safe to use during pregnancy for both mother and baby.

The USPSTF recommends screening for syphilis in all pregnant women. This is based on evidence that universal screening of pregnant women reduces the incidence of congenital syphilis. Screening for syphilis in pregnancy is no different than screening in the general population (see chapter 21). All pregnant women should be tested at their first prenatal visit. In high-risk women, repeat blood testing in the third trimester and at delivery should be considered.

SECTION VII: TOBACCO USE IN PREGNANCY

In addition to the long-term risks it poses to the mother, tobacco use is a serious health risk during pregnancy. Smoking during pregnancy can lead to premature births, spontaneous abortions, stillbirths, and intrauterine growth retardation (diminished growth of the fetus). Pregnant women who smoke have more obstetric complications, including placenta previa and placental abruption, and are more likely to require a Cesarean section than are pregnant women who don't smoke. In addition, smoking decreases your chances of becoming pregnant and increases the risk of infertility. Finally, infants of mothers who smoke have an increased risk of mortality and a three to four times greater risk of sudden infant death syndrome (SIDS).

Tobacco cessation should be a major component of health promotion at every health visit, but during pregnancy it takes on even greater importance. Talking to your doctor about smoking can help you better understand the risks, especially during pregnancy; learn effective behavioral and motivational techniques for quitting; and use tobacco-cessation medications that are safe to take during pregnancy. Studies have shown that intensive smoking-cessation counseling, compared with brief, generic counseling sessions, substantially increases quit rates during pregnancy.

The USPSTF recommends that doctors ask all pregnant women about tobacco use and provide augmented pregnancy-tailored counseling to those who use tobacco products. Tobacco cessation at any point during pregnancy can yield important health benefits for the mother and the baby. Although this recommendation is directed at doctors, you should talk to your doctor about your smoking habits and about ways you can successfully quit.

SECTION VIII: ALCOHOL USE IN PREGNANCY

When a pregnant woman drinks alcohol, so does her unborn baby. Each year in the United States, an estimated 2,000 to 8,000 infants are born with fetal alcohol syndrome, and many thousands more suffer from milder cognitive and physical impairments related to their mothers' alcohol use. In addition, women who drink alcohol during pregnancy are at greater risk of miscarriage and stillbirth.

A recent survey estimates that one in ten pregnant women in the United States drinks alcohol. In addition, among sexually active women who are not using birth control, over half drink, and over one in ten report binge drinking, which places them at particularly high risk of an alcohol-exposed pregnancy. Because it isn't known whether any amount of alcohol is safe during pregnancy, all women who are or may become pregnant are recommended to completely abstain from drinking alcohol. While alcohol use is largely not seen as a medical problem, counseling about alcohol misuse has been shown to be an effective way to reduce unsafe levels of alcohol consumption in women of childbearing age.

The USPSTF recommends screening and behavioral counseling to reduce alcohol misuse by pregnant women. Although this recommendation is geared more toward doctors, you should talk to your doctor about your alcohol use if you are pregnant, planning to be pregnant, or at risk for unplanned pregnancy.

REFERENCES

American Academy of Pediatrics (AAP). www.aap.org.
American College of Obstetricians and Gynecologists (ACOG). www.acog.org.
Centers for Disease Control and Prevention (CDC). "Recommendations for Identification and Public Health Management of Persons with Chronic Hepatitis B Virus Infection," *MMWR* 57, RR-8 (2008). www.cdc.gov/hepatitis/HBV/TestingChronic.htm.
———. Sexually Transmitted Diseases. www.cdc.gov/std.

CHAPTER 20

Sexually Transmitted Infection Counseling

S ex is considered a very personal matter, and rightfully so. But sex is also a health matter. Every time you engage in sexual intercourse, you expose yourself to another person's bodily fluid and in doing so put yourself at risk for sexually transmitted infections, or STIs. While the degree of risk varies with different sexual habits and practices, the risk is always there.

STIs can have a substantial effect on health. Even commonly joked about infections such as gonorrhea and chlamydia can lead to chronic pain syndromes, ectopic pregnancies, and sterility. And then there are life-threatening diseases such as hepatitis B and HIV/AIDS, which are also transmitted through sexual intercourse.

Perhaps most important, studies have shown that through counseling, individuals at higher risk for STIs can reduce their risk of infection. By teaching important STI-prevention techniques such as condom usage, role playing, and risk assessment, your doctor can help you reduce your risk of sexually transmitted infections and improve your health.

The U.S. Preventive Services Task Force (USPSTF) recommends counseling to prevent STIs for all sexually active adolescents and for adults at risk for STIs.[1] The following sections provide a brief introduction to STIs and the guidelines for counseling. For a more detailed discussion of particular STIs, review the relevant chapter in this book or consult the references provided at the end of this chapter.

SECTION I: STIs 101

Sexually transmitted infections, also known as sexually transmitted diseases (STDs) are infections transmitted through sexual contact with an infected individual. *Sexually transmitted infections* is a broad term that includes over twenty different infections, such as chlamydia and gonorrhea, syphilis, HIV, hepatitis B and C, and human papillomavirus (HPV).

Nineteen million new STIs occur each year. Nearly half of all STIs occur in persons 15 to 24 years of age. The health effects vary by STI and range from minor annoyances, such as pain on urination, to life-threatening conditions, such as liver cancer and HIV / AIDS.

Although early screening and detection can prevent many of the long-term complications of STIs, not all of these infections are curable. At the same time, because STIs do not always cause symptoms in the early stages, people with STIs often go undiagnosed and put themselves, their partners, and, in the case of pregnancy, their unborn babies at risk for serious illness. The best strategy, therefore, is prevention, which is the focus of this chapter.

How common are STIs?

Here are the number of new cases of common STIs based on data from the CDC for 2006:

Chlamydia	1,030,911
Gonorrhea	358,366
Syphilis	36,606
Genital herpes	371,000
Genital warts	422,000
Vaginal trichomoniasis	200,000
HIV	56,300
Hepatitis B	46,000[2]

How do STIs spread?

All STIs spread by sexual contact, but the way they do this differs from one infectious organism to the next. Some STIs are spread through direct contact with a sore on the genitals or mouth of an infected individual. Other STIs are spread by bodily fluids. As a result, even without signs of infection, the infectious organisms can be transmitted during oral, vaginal, or anal intercourse. These latter STIs can usually also be transmitted through blood by nonsexual contact, such as sharing needles or, during pregnancy, through the placenta from mother to baby. In the case of HIV, the virus can also be spread through breast milk.

What symptoms do STIs cause?

STIs usually do not cause any symptoms. Let me repeat that: *STIs usually do not cause any symptoms.* This is true across the board, from gonorrhea and chlamydia to hepatitis B and HIV. And in general this holds more true for women, who are less likely to experience symptoms than men.

Even if symptoms develop, they are often vague and may be confused with other common illnesses. The specific symptoms vary by infection. Most people associate genital sores, vaginal or penile discharge, or pelvic discomfort with STIs. However, these symptoms are found in only a subset of STIs (e.g., chlamydia and gonorrhea), and even then are often unreliable indicators of infection.

Because STIs often do not cause symptoms, they can be spread by people who don't know they are infected. Being asymptomatic from an STI does not make someone any less likely to transmit the infection to others. This underscores the importance of practicing safer sex (see below), regardless of how you or your sexual partner may feel or appear.

What are the risk factors for STIs?

Anyone who is sexually active is at risk for contracting an STI, but the degree of risk varies with your sexual behavior and that of your sexual partners. Your risk is higher if you have had many sex partners, have had sex with someone who has had many partners, or do not use condoms correctly or consistently. In addition, your risk is higher if you or your partner has ever had any STI, does not get regularly tested for STIs, uses drugs or alcohol in situations when sex may occur, uses injection drugs, or has anal intercourse.

How can STIs be prevented?

The only certain way to prevent STIs is to abstain from sexual contact and intercourse, which is often not desirable or practical.

Short of abstinence, you can reduce the risk of STIs by practicing safer sex. Safer sex is a relative term; there is no such thing as safe sex and not safe sex. Rather, there is a spectrum of sexual behaviors and practices that place people at varying degrees of risk. The least risky approach is to have sex only with a long-term partner who is monogamous, has been tested, and is known to be free of any STI. The following are other approaches to reducing your risk of STIs:

Use condoms. For maximum protection, condoms must be used *correctly* and *consistently*. This means knowing how to properly use a condom to avoid slippage or breakage, which can reduce or nullify its protective effects. It also means using a condom every time you have a sexual encounter, be it vaginal, anal, or even oral. Failing to use a condom one time is all it takes to become infected with an STI.

Limit sexual partners. The greater the number of sexual partners, the greater the risk of getting an STI. Remember, most people with STIs appear healthy and have no symptoms. Even if you "trust" someone, there is no telling, without proper testing, whether he or she has an STI. Therefore, every new sexual encounter places you at risk for contracting an STI. But it is not simply a matter of the number of sexual partners. Casual sexual encounters or sexual encounters that occur under the influence of alcohol are particularly high risk.

Get routinely tested for STIs. Certain STIs can increase the risk of transmission of other STIs. For example, being infected with chlamydia increases the risk of HIV transmission. Be informed about how often you should get screened for STIs and work with your doctor to stay up to date.

Know your partner. Entering into a new sexual relationship should not be a spur-of-the-moment decision, and definitely not one influenced by alcohol, drugs, or social pressures. Before having sexual intercourse, you and your partner should have an open discussion. Ideally, you will agree on the need for condoms and set boundaries and expectations for each other. You should also ask about each other's sexual history, including number of previous sexual partners, experience with condom usage, and history of STIs. If you establish that your partner has risk factors for STIs, insist that he or she get tested before becoming sexually intimate.

How do I use a condom?

Condoms are the only form of protection that can help prevent both STI transmission and pregnancy. Below are a few guidelines for proper condom usage.

Choose the right kind of condom. There are many different types and brands of condoms available—however, only latex or polyurethane condoms provide a highly effective mechanical barrier to STIs. If possible, use a latex condom because they are slightly more reliable. A small number of people have an allergic reaction to latex—these people should use polyurethane condoms instead.

Choose the right kind of lubrication. Applying a lubricant to the outside of a condom can help reduce the chance that the condom will break. Lubricants also prevent irritation and tearing of the skin if there is a lack of natural lubrication during sexual intercourse. Small tears in the vagina or rectum allow STIs to enter the bloodstream. Only water-based lubricants (such as K-Y Jelly) can be used with latex condoms. Oil-based lubricants (such as petroleum jelly, lotions, and body oils) dissolve the latex in condoms and should not be used. With polyurethane condoms, you can use either water-based or oil-based products.

Put the condom on at the right time. The condom should be in place from the beginning to the end of sexual activity and should be used every time you have sex. Use a new condom for each new act of vaginal, anal, and oral intercourse.

Used correctly and consistently, condom usage can dramatically reduce your risk of STIs. However, they are not a foolproof solution. Even with proper usage, condoms can break and expose you to infected bodily fluids. In addition, because condoms do not cover the surrounding skin areas, STIs can still be spread. Thus, condoms should be viewed as one component of a broader STI-prevention strategy.

SECTION II: STI COUNSELING

The USPSTF makes the following recommendations about high-intensity behavioral counseling to prevent STIs:

- routine counseling for all sexually active young people age 19 or younger
- counseling for adults with an STI or a history of infection in the past year and adults with multiple current sexual partners

These recommendations are based on evidence that high-intensity behavioral counseling targeted to sexually active adolescents and adults at increased risk reduces the rate of new infections. Despite this, rates of STI counseling by primary care doctors are low, and by some estimates, only one-third of patients are receiving appropriate counseling. Therefore, if the guidelines above apply to you, talk to your doctor about your sexual practices, and if counseling is available, ask to be referred.

Why do all sexually active adolescents need counseling?

Almost half of STIs occur in adolescents, which places all adolescents at high risk. This is in part due to adolescents being more likely to engage in high-risk behaviors such as having unprotected sex, having multiple sexual partners, and making the decision to engage in sex under the influence of alcohol.

What about adults not at increased risk?

Because of the lower incidence of STIs among adults who are not at increased risk, the potential net benefit of behavioral counseling is likely to be small. Counseling takes up valuable time during the clinic visit and may detract from other preventive health or medical care. To date, the USPSTF has found insufficient evidence for or against STI counseling in adults not at increased risk. If you are interested in STI counseling, talk to your doctor about whether counseling is appropriate for you.

How does STI counseling work?

The USPSTF STI counseling recommendation is relatively new, and it remains to be seen how individual health providers will implement the guideline in their practices. Some providers may offer individual counseling sessions, others group counseling sessions, and still others video or electronic resources—or a combination of these. In the studies that the USPSTF used to formulate their recommendation, successful interventions were delivered through multiple counseling sessions, often in groups, with a total duration from three to nine hours.

The content of counseling will generally include education, risk assessment, skill training, and support for behavioral changes. Educational components may include providing basic information about STIs, dispelling common myths, and introducing preventive strategies. Risk assessment may include identifying risk factors and triggers for unsafe sex and assessing overall riskiness. Skill training may include role playing to increase skills for communication and negotiating about sex, particularly condom use, and learning how to use condoms effectively. Support for behavioral changes may include goal setting, identifying community resources, and establishing social support.

The overall goal is to help you acquire a basic working knowledge of STIs, understand your risk for STIs, learn techniques and strategies for reducing that risk, and develop the confidence and support you need to practice safer sex. Sex is an enjoyable, important part of life. By taking the appropriate preventive measures, you can also make sure it is a safe one.

REFERENCES

American Academy of Family Physicians. "STIs: Common Symptoms and Tips on Prevention." Familydoctor.org. http://familydoctor.org/online/famdocen/home/common/sexinfections/sti/165.html.

Centers for Disease Control and Prevention (CDC). *Sexually Transmitted Disease Surveillance, 2006.* Atlanta, Ga.: U.S. Department of Health and Human Services, November 2007. www.cdc.gov/std/stats06/toc2006.htm.

———. U.S. Department of Health and Human Services. "Sexually Transmitted Diseases." www.cdc.gov/std.

CHAPTER 21

Syphilis Screening

S yphilis is a bacterial infection transmitted through sexual intercourse and from mother to child during pregnancy. While sometimes joked about in popular media, syphilis is a serious illness that if untreated can cause irreversible damage to the brain, nerves, and heart. In pregnancy it can lead to spontaneous abortion, stillbirth, and a disease in the newborn child called *congenital syphilis.*

Syphilis is often called "the great imitator" because many of the signs and symptoms of infection are indistinguishable from those of other diseases. In addition, many of these symptoms resolve on their own despite continued infection, and in some people can be mild and go unnoticed. As a result, without screening, many infected people remain unaware of their illness and stay infected despite the availability of curative antibiotics.

The United States Preventive Services Task Force (USPSTF) recommends screening for syphilis in at-risk individuals and in all women during pregnancy.[1] The following sections provide an introduction to syphilis, explain the importance of screening in certain populations, and detail the screening guidelines. Screening for syphilis in pregnancy is covered in chapter 19.

SECTION I: SYPHILIS 101

Syphilis (SIF-uh-lis) is a sexually transmitted infection (STI) caused by the bacteria *Treponema pallidum.*[2]

How common is syphilis?

Syphilis is currently on the rise. Between 2005 and 2006, the number of cases reported in the United States increased by 12 percent, to 36,000, including 349 cases of congenital syphilis. Most cases occurred in people between 20 and 39 years of age, with the peak ages for women between 20 and 24 years old, and for men between 35 and 39. This increase was especially striking in certain at-risk groups, including men who have sex with men.

How is it spread?

Syphilis is transmitted through direct contact with syphilitic sores, which are usually found on the external genitalia, vagina, anus, and rectum but may also appear on the lips and in the mouth.

The most common way to get syphilis is through sexual contact with an infected person, which includes vaginal, anal, and oral sex. In addition, syphilis can be passed from mother to infant during pregnancy and cause congenital syphilis.

The bacteria that cause syphilis are fragile, so syphilis *cannot* be spread through contact with shared personal items or environmental exposure.

What are the signs and symptoms in adults?

Syphilis progresses through four stages, each of which has distinct signs and symptoms. Furthermore, within a given stage, the signs and symptoms vary significantly. Some people have severe and specific symptoms that promptly lead to diagnosis. Others have mild symptoms that often are overlooked or mistaken for other diseases, which delays diagnosis and treatment. The following overview of the four stages of syphilis presents the characteristic signs and symptoms of each stage. As you read it, keep in mind that regardless of stage, or the presence or resolution of symptoms, people with untreated syphilis remain infected and are at risk for serious health problems and for transmitting the infection to others.

Primary Stage

The first symptom of syphilis is usually a small, firm, round, painless sore called a *chancre* (SHAN-kur). It appears at the place where syphilis entered the body, which is usually the penis, vulva, or vagina but can also include the cervix, tongue, lips, or anus. Sometimes there are multiple chancres, but typically there is one. Its presence may or may not be associated with swelling of nearby lymph nodes. The chancre is highly contagious, and syphilis can be transmitted through contact with it. The time between infection with syphilis and the appearance of the chancre can range from ten to ninety days, although three weeks is most typical. Regardless of whether treatment is received, the chancre disappears in three to six weeks.

Because the chancre is painless, goes away on its own, and can occur in hard-to-see parts of the body, it is common for primary syphilis to go undiagnosed and untreated. If primary syphilis is untreated, it progresses to the secondary stage.

Secondary Stage

The characteristic sign of the secondary stage of syphilis is a nonitchy, rough, reddish brown, spotted rash on the palms and the bottoms of the feet. The rash typically appears two to ten weeks after the chancre appears, as the sore is healing or already healed. However, syphilis is not called the great imitator for nothing. Instead of the typical rash, secondary syphilis may manifest with a different appearance on other parts of the body and can even be so faint as to go unnoticed. Other common symptoms of this stage include fever, swollen lymph glands, sore throat, patchy hair loss, headaches, weight loss, muscle aches, and fatigue.

As with primary syphilis, these signs and symptoms eventually disappear with or without treatment. In addition, because they may also be very mild, they often go unnoticed. Without treatment, however, the infection will progress to the latent and possibly late stages of disease.

Latent Syphilis

The latent, or hidden, stage of syphilis is defined by the absence of clinical signs and symptoms. This stage can last for years. In early latent syphilis, the disease can relapse to secondary syphilis and be transmitted to sexual partners. In late latent syphilis, the infection is quiet, and the risk of infecting sexual partners is low or absent. Without treatment, people with latent syphilis are still infected and remain at risk for developing tertiary syphilis, the most serious stage of the disease.

Tertiary (Late) Stage

Tertiary (or late) syphilis develops in about 15 percent of people who do not receive treatment, sometimes decades after a person is infected. In this stage, the disease causes internal organ damage, affecting the brain, nerves, eyes, heart, blood vessels, liver, bones, and joints. Tertiary syphilis can result in dementia, blindness, deafness, paralysis, numbness, and cardiovascular disease. This damage usually causes profound disability and in some cases death.

How does syphilis affect pregnancy?

Syphilis can be passed from mother to infant during pregnancy. Because the symptoms of syphilis are often mild and fleeting, an estimated 8,000 pregnant women have undiagnosed syphilis each year in the United States.

The effect of syphilis on pregnancy is variable. Untreated early syphilis results in the death of the unborn baby in up to 40 percent of cases. In addition, syphilis can put a woman at risk of giving birth to a baby who dies shortly after birth. Babies who survive develop congenital syphilis, or syphilis acquired at birth. Infants with untreated congenital syphilis can develop a range of health problems, including deformities, seizures, and developmental delays.

How does having syphilis increase the risk of HIV infection?

Another serious complication of syphilis infection is a two- to five-fold increased risk of acquiring HIV if exposed. The sores, ulcers, and breaks in the skin caused by syphilis disrupt natural barriers that provide protection against infections, making it easier to contract HIV.

How is syphilis diagnosed?

There are two primary methods for diagnosing syphilis:

- identifying the syphilis bacteria under a microscope
- performing an antibody blood test for syphilis

The blood test looks for syphilis antibodies—proteins your body produces against invaders. Although this test does not directly detect the bacteria, it will let your doctor know if you have been infected with syphilis. These antibodies can stay around for years, however, even after you have been successfully treated for syphilis. Therefore you should let your doctor know if you have been previously treated.

The decision about which test to use depends on the symptoms and reasons for testing. If you have a skin lesion that has the appearance of a chancre, your doctor may swab the suspected region to examine under a microscope. If instead you have symptoms of syphilis but no identifiable sore, or if you have risk factors for syphilis and are being screened, your doctor will perform a blood test.

Can syphilis be treated?

Yes. A person who has been infected for less than a year requires only a single injection of penicillin to be cured. If you are allergic to penicillin, be sure to tell your doctor. People treated in the early stage often recover without any long-term consequences.

For more advanced syphilis, a longer course of penicillin therapy may be required. If your organs are damaged, treatment won't heal them, but it will prevent further damage.

As important as being treated with antibiotics is preventing yourself from getting reinfected. Because syphilis can be transmitted through sexual contact, there is a high chance that if you are infected with syphilis, so is your partner. Being treated for syphilis does not prevent a new infection. To lower your risk of getting reinfected and to protect your partner, notify him or her that you have tested positive for syphilis. That way, your partner can be tested and, if necessary, treated.

How can I prevent syphilis?

The best way to avoid syphilis infection is to abstain from sexual contact or to be sexually active only with a long-term partner who is also monogamous and found to be free of infection through testing. In addition, keep in mind the following:

- Syphilis is a genital ulcer disease. Men and women can develop genital sores even when they use a condom. Proper use of latex condoms (which also means using them every time you have sex) can reduce the risk of syphilis, but only if the condom completely covers all areas that are or could be infected.

- Usually syphilis is transmitted from people who have no visible sores or rashes and who do not know they are infected. Reducing the number of sexual partners and having new partners tested for STIs before becoming sexually intimate can significantly reduce the risk of syphilis and other STIs.

- Cleaning your genitals (externally or by douching) does not prevent syphilis, or any STI for that matter. Urinating after sex also has no effect on STI transmission.

- If you develop a sore or rash, especially on or near your genitals, or experience unusual discharge, see your doctor. Do not have sexual intercourse until you have been tested.

- Even if you have been treated for syphilis and cured, you can be reinfected by having sex with an infected partner.

- To prevent passing congenital syphilis to their unborn babies, all pregnant women should be tested for syphilis.

SECTION II: SCREENING FOR SYPHILIS IN NONPREGNANT INDIVIDUALS

The USPSTF recommends screening people at increased risk for syphilis infection. This recommendation is based on evidence that screening at-risk groups can accurately detect syphilis infection and lead to antibiotic treatment that ultimately improves health outcomes.

Populations at increased risk for syphilis infection include the following:

- men who have sex with men
- people who exchange sex for drugs or money
- people in adult correctional facilities

People not otherwise specified but who are at increased risk for syphilis (e.g., those who've had unprotected sex with multiple partners or have a history of other STIs) should discuss their risk factors with their doctor and make an individual decision about the benefits and potential harms of screening.

How is screening done?

Usually doctors screen with a nontreponemal test, such as VDRL (venereal disease research laboratory) or RPR (rapid plasma reagin). If either of these tests is positive, doctors perform a confirmatory treponemal serologic test, such as FTA-ABS (fluorescent treponemal antibody absorbed). Samples for all of these screens are obtained through routine blood tests.

All three tests check for antibodies—or proteins the body produces against infection—to syphilis in the blood. The reason they are done sequentially is that the VDRL and RPR tests are generally considered more sensitive for syphilis (fewer false negatives), while the FTA-ABS test is more specific (fewer false positives). The combination provides the best screening tool currently available, although false positives and false negatives still occur.

What are the risks?

The blood tests are safe and have no risks. However, there are potential harms if the screen is positive. False-positive results may lead to anxiety, labeling, and unnecessary testing and treatment. Harms of treatment include a serious allergic reaction to penicillin, side effects of antibiotic use, and the Jarisch-Herxheimer reaction (fever with headache and body aches) that may occur within the first twenty-four hours after treatment.

What happens if the screen is negative?

A negative screen means that you probably do not have syphilis. Because false negatives do occur, you might still have the disease, but the likelihood is probably less than 5 percent.

However, given your risk factors, you are still at risk for contracting syphilis in the future. The USPSTF makes no specific recommendations regarding screening intervals, and therefore when to rescreen is best decided with your doctor. In addition, talk to your doctor about how you can lower your risk of infection. Remember, the same behaviors that put you at risk for syphilis also put you at risk for HIV and other STIs.

What happens if it is positive?

A positive screen is sufficient to diagnose you with syphilis and begin treatment. Because false positives do occur, you might not have syphilis, but the likelihood is probably less than 5 percent.

Treatment will vary with the stage of your infection. For primary and secondary syphilis, the usual treatment is a single injection of penicillin. For those with more advanced disease, longer antibiotic courses are given. While receiving treatment, you must abstain from sexual contact until the syphilis sores are completely healed. In addition, sexual partners should be evaluated and, if necessary, treated.

REFERENCES

Centers for Disease Control and Prevention (CDC). U.S. Department of Health and Human Services. "Sexually Transmitted Diseases." www.cdc.gov/std.

CHAPTER 22

Tobacco Use Counseling

When it comes to health promotion, no topic is more important than tobacco use, because tobacco use, and in particular cigarette smoking, is the number one cause of preventable disease, disability, and death in the United States. It is estimated that each year more than 400,000 adults die prematurely from tobacco-related diseases. And for every person who dies of a tobacco-related disease, twenty more people develop at least one serious illness, including lung disease, cardiovascular disease, and cancer. Countless more are affected daily, because they suffer from chest pain, reduced exercise tolerance, infertility, or simply bad breath. Not to be ignored is the problem of secondhand smoke, which carries health risks to family members, friends, coworkers, and in the case of pregnancy, the unborn child.

At present, nearly everyone who uses tobacco knows it is dangerous, and yet the habit persists because most people find it very difficult to quit smoking. The chemicals in tobacco are addictive, which means that the body becomes accustomed to regular infusions of them and suffers withdrawal symptoms without them, including increased anxiety, decreased concentration, fatigue, headaches, and increased appetite. Most smokers want very much to quit completely but have not been able to break their addiction. Some have tried getting help from their doctors, and others have only tried to quit on their own. For all these people, today there is new hope, because doctors have more ways than ever to help people quit.

Tobacco use is a disease of addiction for most users. Just as no one would try to cure their own cancer, smokers need not manage their addiction themselves. Studies show that through brief behavioral counseling and medications, doctors can help people quit. Compared with smokers who do not receive assistance, smokers who receive treatment are twice as likely to quit. Despite the major health benefits of quitting and the potential impact of health care providers in promoting quitting, less than two-thirds of smokers have ever been asked about their smoking status or been urged to quit by their doctors.

Talking to your doctor about tobacco use is a small and critical first step to quitting. The United States Preventive Services Task Force (USPSTF) recommends that doctors screen all adults for tobacco use and provide tobacco cessation interventions (e.g., counseling and medication) for those who use tobacco products.[1] The following sections provide a brief overview of tobacco use and the dangers of smoking and explain the guidelines for screening and counseling.

SECTION I: TOBACCO USE 101

When people hear the term *tobacco use,* they often assume it means smoking one to two packs of cigarettes a day for thirty years. But tobacco use includes the use of any tobacco-containing products for any period. Tobacco products include cigarettes, cigars, chewing tobacco, hookahs, bidis, and kreteks. Tobacco use can range from three packs a day to one cigarette a month. In this chapter, the terms *tobacco use* and *smoking* are used interchangeably to refer to the use of any tobacco-containing products, whether chewed or smoked.

Another important term to define is *tobacco use cessation,* or *smoking cessation.* Tobacco use cessation means to stop using tobacco or to quit. It also refers to the process of quitting—preparing to quit, quitting, and staying quit.

How common is tobacco use?

One in every five Americans smokes cigarettes; that's 45 million people. Three out of four smokers report that they want to quit completely. Most people who smoke during adulthood began smoking in their teenage years. It is a myth that teenagers smoke for only a few years and then quit.

How dangerous is it?

The facts are clear—smoking is a very dangerous thing to do:

- One in every five Americans dies of conditions caused by tobacco use.
- One half of all lifetime smokers will die early because of their decision to smoke.
- On average, smokers die thirteen to fourteen years earlier than nonsmokers.
- More deaths are caused each year by tobacco use than by HIV/AIDS, illegal drug use, alcohol use, motor vehicle injuries, suicides, and murders *combined.*

What diseases does tobacco cause?

Tobacco harms nearly every organ of the body. The 440,000 tobacco-related deaths each year are the result of different diseases and health problems caused by smoking, as illustrated in figure 22.1 (bottom). The effects of smoking for most people are dose dependent, meaning the more you smoke, the greater the harm done. Quitting has immediate as well as long-term benefits and can even reverse some of the damage caused by smoking. Every few years, when the accumulating research data are reviewed, the list of diseases that we know are caused by or associated with tobacco use grows longer. In recent years, tobacco use has been implicated in acute leukemia, a form of cancer of the blood, and cancers of the cervix, pancreas, kidneys, and stomach; aortic aneurysms; cataracts; pneumonia; and gum disease. The following is only a partial list of diseases caused by tobacco use.[2]

Tobacco and Cancer

Almost everyone knows that cigarettes cause lung cancer. The risk of death from lung cancer is twenty-three times higher among male smokers and thirteen times higher among female smokers than among people who have never smoked. Tobacco use causes many other cancers as well, as illustrated in figure 22.1 (top). Of the over 4,000 chemicals in cigarettes, 43 are known *carcinogens,* or cancer-causing agents. The same carcinogens in tobacco that affect the lungs also affect other organs.

Tobacco and the Cardiovascular System

Tobacco products accelerate atherosclerosis and damage blood vessels. As a result, smoking causes

- coronary heart disease (fourfold higher risk)
- stroke (twofold)
- peripheral vascular disease (tenfold)
- abdominal aortic aneurysm
- congestive heart failure
- sudden cardiac death

Tobacco and the Respiratory System

Smoking causes chronic obstructive pulmonary disease (COPD), which includes chronic bronchitis and emphysema. COPD is the fourth leading cause of death in the United States. An astounding 90 percent of all deaths from

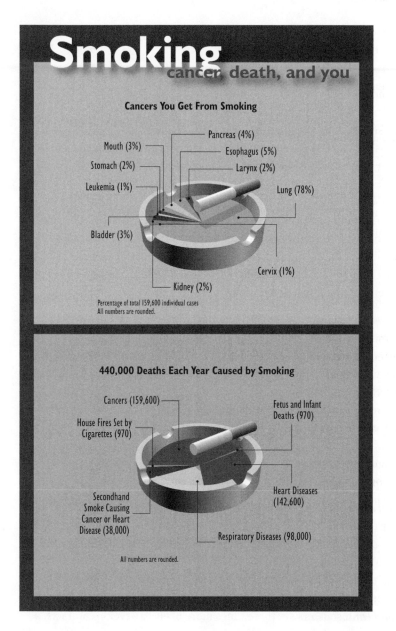

Figure 22.1. Top: Lung cancer is not the only cancer caused by smoking. This panel shows the percentage of tobacco-related cancers by type of cancer. Bottom: Cancer is just one way in which smoking kills people. This panel shows the number of deaths from tobacco use each year by cause of death. Copyright 2004 by the Centers for Disease Control and Prevention. Reprinted with permission. See www.cdc.gov/tobacco/data_statistics/sgr/2004/pdfs/whatitmeanstoyou.pdf.

COPD are caused by cigarette smoking. More generally, smoking harms the lungs and causes

- increased frequency and severity of lung infections, including pneumonia
- permanent stunting of lung development in teenagers who smoke
- increased chronic coughing, wheezing, and asthma
- decreased overall lung function leading to a reduced capacity to exercise and carry out daily activities

Tobacco and Pregnancy

Toxins from tobacco products enter a woman's general circulation and affect her ability to conceive and deliver a baby. In addition, tobacco use has profound effects on the unborn baby. For example, nicotine causes the blood vessels in the umbilical cord to constrict, which decreases the amount of oxygen delivered to the fetus. Some of the more common effects include

- increased difficulty becoming pregnant and increased risk of never becoming pregnant (infertility)
- increased complications during delivery, including placenta previa and placental abruption, and increased risk of a Cesarean section (C-section)
- lower birthweight babies
- increased risk of infant death and disease, including three to four times higher risk of sudden infant death syndrome (SIDS)

Tobacco and Other Diseases

Smoking also increases the risk of the following problems:

- *Fractures:* smokers have lower bone density and increased risk of hip fractures.
- *Dental diseases:* smoking causes half of all cases of periodontitis (gum disease).
- *Sexual problems:* men who smoke are more likely to have erectile dysfunction and poor sexual performance.
- *Eye problems:* smokers are three times more likely to develop cataracts, a leading cause of blindness.
- *Poor wound healing:* after surgery or injury, smokers have more problems with wound healing.
- *Blood clots:* smokers are more likely to develop deep vein thromboses (clots in the leg) and pulmonary emboli (clots in the lung).

Are low-tar or low-nicotine products safer?

No. There is little evidence to suggest that low-tar or low-nicotine cigarettes reduce the harms of smoking.

How about other tobacco products besides cigarettes?

Cigars, pipes, and hookahs are just as harmful as cigarettes. Chewing tobacco and other smokeless tobacco products do not cause the full range of smoking-related diseases, but they are just as harmful as cigarettes in terms of cancer and cardiovascular disease.

After so many years of smoking, is there even any benefit to quitting?

Much of the damage caused by tobacco products is reversible, even after years of use (see figure 22.2). There is a benefit to quitting at any age. Quitting reduces the chance of death from smoking-related diseases by up to 90 percent for those who quit in their thirties. Those who quit at age 50 reduce their risk of premature death by 50 percent. Even those who quit at age 60 or older live substantially longer than those who continue to smoke.

Quitting also has significant health benefits to those around you from decreased exposure to secondhand smoke. It also benefits your pocketbook and gives you money to spend on things other than cigarettes.

Won't quitting make me gain weight?

Gaining weight is a major concern for people considering quitting. Because of the ill health effects of weight gain, it is also a major concern for doctors advising patients to quit. Understand that weight gain is not a direct consequence of quitting. Instead, smokers who quit gain weight largely because of increased cravings that result when the brain "misses" the nicotine it has grown accustomed to getting. There are two lessons from this: one, increased cravings can be satisfied by things other than food; and two, once the brain becomes accustomed to life without nicotine, the increased cravings and associated weight gain go away.

Weight gain is an important concern, but one that can be addressed. Preemptively, doctors often recommend getting into a regular exercise routine at the same time as quitting; this helps prevent weight gain and helps blow off steam from increased anxiety and stress that may be associated with quitting. Doctors also recommend healthier substitutes for junk food snacks, like fruits or chewing gum. If weight gain becomes an issue despite these efforts, your doctor can advise you on plenty of other interventions. The key is to partner

the benefits
of quitting

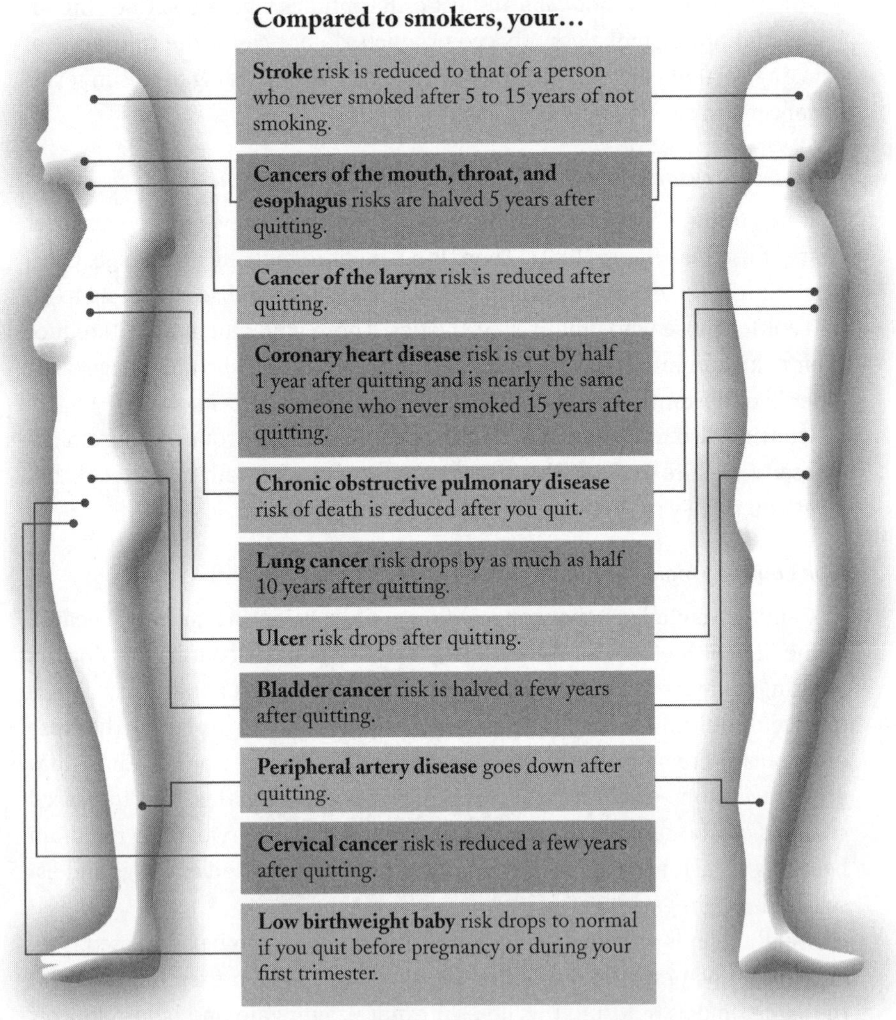

Compared to smokers, your…

Stroke risk is reduced to that of a person who never smoked after 5 to 15 years of not smoking.

Cancers of the mouth, throat, and esophagus risks are halved 5 years after quitting.

Cancer of the larynx risk is reduced after quitting.

Coronary heart disease risk is cut by half 1 year after quitting and is nearly the same as someone who never smoked 15 years after quitting.

Chronic obstructive pulmonary disease risk of death is reduced after you quit.

Lung cancer risk drops by as much as half 10 years after quitting.

Ulcer risk drops after quitting.

Bladder cancer risk is halved a few years after quitting.

Peripheral artery disease goes down after quitting.

Cervical cancer risk is reduced a few years after quitting.

Low birthweight baby risk drops to normal if you quit before pregnancy or during your first trimester.

Figure 22.2. Quitting has a number of health benefits from head to toe. For example, quitting for ten years can decrease the risk of lung cancer by half. Copyright 2004 by the Centers for Disease Control and Prevention. Reprinted with permission. See www.cdc.gov/tobacco/data_statistics/sgr/2004/pdfs/whatitmeanstoyou.pdf.

with your doctor from the start so that as weight gain and other issues arise, you can tackle them with a doctor's support.

The average weight gain after quitting smoking is five pounds. With the above strategies, you can avoid weight gain altogether. However, the bottom line is that the benefits of quitting outweigh any risks from weight gain that may follow quitting.

SECTION II: TOBACCO USE SCREENING AND COUNSELING

The USPSTF recommends screening all adults for tobacco use and providing tobacco cessation interventions (e.g., counseling and medications) for those who use tobacco products. This recommendation is based on evidence that brief smoking cessation interventions are effective in increasing the proportion of smokers who successfully quit smoking and remain tobacco-free after one year.

These recommendations are written for doctors, who are advised to counsel their patients about tobacco cessation. What you can do is talk to your doctor openly about your tobacco use and ask him or her for assistance to quit smoking. Don't wait for your doctor to initiate the conversation. A large population-based study showed that only 15 percent of smokers who saw a physician in the prior year reported being offered tobacco cessation interventions.

How will talking to a doctor help?

Many people see tobacco use as a personal problem. Although many people have successfully quit without any help from their doctor or any medications, studies show that people are much more likely to succeed if they are not alone. Part of the challenge is in our thinking. Most of us think of smoking as a choice. "If I wanted to quit, I would just quit." But as anyone who has tried and failed to quit knows, it is often not about choice. Smoking is a disease of addiction for most people; fortunately, it is also a disease for which we have effective treatments.

Talking to your doctor about smoking can help you quit. Studies show that even brief advice from a doctor can produce cessation rates (or rates of quitting) of 5 to 10 percent. If in addition to advice, a doctor provides counseling and medicines to help people quit, cessation rates increase to as high as 20 to 25 percent, which is twice that of people who do not receive treatment.

Unfortunately, many people try to quit only after receiving a wake-up

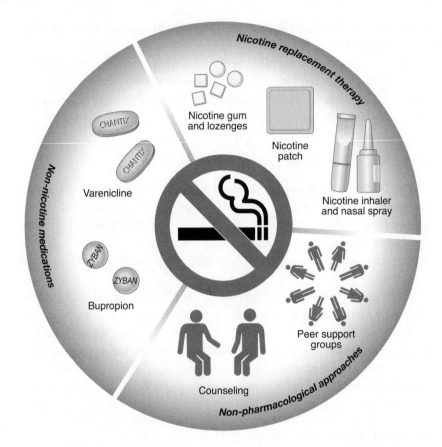

Figure 22.3. There are many effective methods for quitting. No one way works for everyone and often a combination works best. Non-pharmacologic approaches to quitting include counseling and peer-support groups. Nicotine replacement therapies include nicotine gum and lozenges, nicotine patches, and nicotine inhalers and nasal sprays. Non-nicotine medications include bupropion (marketed as Zyban) and varenicline (marketed as Chantix). Which method will work for you?

call—a diagnosis of a dreaded tobacco-related disease. If you are reading this, please know that it is better to quit before that happens to you.

How do doctors help people quit?

There are a variety of interventions to help people quit (see figure 22.3). Doctors are intermediaries to all of these interventions. Through counseling, doctors can motivate people to quit and help them identify and overcome barriers to successful quitting. They also serve as a resource and advocate through the quitting process. In addition, doctors connect people to support groups, smoking cessation programs, and other services; advise people about medications that help with withdrawal symptoms; and provide prescriptions as well as monitoring for those medications that require it.

What if I don't want to quit?

Even if you don't want to quit, talking to your doctor about your tobacco use is important for two reasons:

1. Smoking affects your health in many ways. If you come to your doctor with a cough, you are more likely to have pneumonia if you are a smoker. If you are deciding how to reduce your risk of heart attacks, your doctor is more likely to recommend aspirin if you are a smoker. In short, because smoking affects your health, your doctor needs to know about it.
2. Talking to your doctor may put you on the path to quitting. By providing you clear and strong messages about quitting and by relaying to you the dangers of smoking in a personal way, your doctor may gradually motivate you to quit.

I've tried quitting before. Nothing seems to work. Why should I keep trying?

Trying to quit can be frustrating. Changing any habit can be frustrating. Smoking is even harder than most bad habits because cigarettes are engineered to deliver nicotine, which is strongly addictive. For most people, it takes at least two or three attempts, often more, before they successfully quit. Your chance of eventual success increases every time you try to quit. Try different approaches: one might be exactly the right approach for you, even though other approaches were ineffective. Today doctors have more ways to help you quit smoking than ever before. You can fail a hundred times, but you only need to be successful once.

What medications can help people quit?

There are two categories of medications for smoking cessation: nicotine replacement products and non-nicotine medications. Nicotine is the primary pharmacological agent in tobacco products that makes them addictive. The lack of nicotine drives your cravings for cigarettes and makes quitting difficult. Nicotine replacement products come in several forms: gum, inhaler, lozenge, patch, and nasal spray. By "replacing" the nicotine your body is accustomed to, these products satisfy the nicotine cravings and reduce the symptoms of withdrawal without the harmful effects of tobacco.

Non-nicotine medications are medicines that do not contain nicotine but that have been proven to help people quit. They generally work by changing the chemicals in the brain that make you dependent on tobacco products. The two most common non-nicotine medications are bupropion (marketed as Zyban) and varenicline (Chantix). Bupropion helps reduce nicotine withdrawal symptoms and the urge to smoke. Varenicline reduces nicotine withdrawal symptoms and blocks the effects of nicotine from cigarettes if the user keeps smoking.

These medicines can also be safely used in combination. For example, it is not uncommon for people to use nicotine patches and bupropion at the same time. Medication, along with counseling and other nonpharmacological approaches, in various combinations, provide a tremendous number of ways to quit. Different strategies work for different people, and there is no way of knowing which method will work for you until you try.

Is talking to my doctor really going to help?

Quitting is hard, but one study after another has shown that simply talking to your doctor about smoking—and opening the door to counseling, behavioral interventions, and new medications aimed at helping you quit—is an effective approach to kicking the tobacco habit. Talk to a doctor about your tobacco use and discuss ways he or she can help you quit. Don't wait until the time is right. The time is now. You don't have to do it alone.

REFERENCES

Centers for Disease Control and Prevention (CDC). U.S. Department of Health and Human Services. "Smoking and Tobacco Use." www.cdc.gov/tobacco.

National Center for Chronic Disease Prevention and Health Promotion, Office of Smoking Health. *The Health Consequences of Smoking: A Report of the Surgeon General.* Centers for Disease Control and Prevention, U.S. Department of Health and Human Services. Washington, D.C.: Government Printing Office, 2004. www.surgeongeneral.gov/library/smokingconsequences.

CHAPTER 23

Vaccines for Adults

Infectious diseases are a leading cause of death in the United States. Depending on your age and medical history, you are at risk for different infectious diseases. No age group or risk group is without hazard.

One of the greatest advances in modern medicine has been the development of vaccines. Thanks to vaccines, some diseases such as smallpox have been completely eradicated, while others such as polio, diphtheria, mumps, and rubella have been reduced to diseases so rare that many of us have never heard of them.

Despite these advances, however, thousands of people still die every year from infectious diseases such as influenza, pneumonia, and hepatitis. Countless more become ill, resulting in missed days of work and school, hospitalizations, and disability. With better use of existing vaccines, many of these illnesses would be prevented.

It is surprising to many people that vaccines are not just for children. A handful of vaccines are specifically made and recommended for young adults, middle-aged adults, and adults age 60 or older. Appropriately timed adult immunizations can prevent disability and death related to a host of common infectious illnesses, including pneumococcal disease, meningococcal disease, influenza, and shingles. Unfortunately, because of lack of public awareness and effective systems for vaccine delivery, many adults do not get appropriately vaccinated. Only one in every three adults who should receive the flu shot every year receives it; only one in four adults who should receive the pneumococcal vaccine receives it. For the vaccine against shingles, only one in fifty eligible adults is vaccinated. The result is that many adults suffer needlessly from preventable infectious illnesses.

Unlike childhood vaccines, which are routinely administered to all children of a certain age, the appropriate timing of adult vaccines is based on multiple risk factors. For example, the pneumococcal vaccine (pneumonia vaccine) is recommended for all adults over age 65 and for younger adults with chronic diseases such as diabetes or asthma. Although taking into account multiple risk factors makes vaccination in adults more complicated than in children, by partnering with your doctor you can make sure you are up to date on your immunizations based on the latest recommendations from the Centers for Disease Control and Prevention (CDC).

This chapter will provide you with a starting point for discussing vaccines with your doctor. Section I provides a broad overview on adult vaccines. Section II outlines the latest CDC recommendations. Section III discusses five common adult vaccines in detail. The appendix at the end of the book includes the complete 2009 CDC adult immunization schedule and CDC vaccine information sheets for fourteen commonly recommended vaccines. The HPV vaccine is covered in depth in chapter 6. The hepatitis B vaccine is discussed in chapter 15.

SECTION I: VACCINES 101

Vaccines are any substance administered to produce immunity to, or protection against, a particular disease. Immunization is the process of inducing immunity to a particular disease. Strictly speaking, vaccines are a form of immunization, but in practice, the terms are interchangeable. Here the term vaccine is used.

What exactly is a vaccine?

Let's break down the definition of a vaccine: "any substance administered to produce immunity to a particular disease."

Vaccines are commonly made of one of four *substances*: killed microorganisms (e.g., flu vaccine); live, weakened microorganisms (e.g., measles, mumps, rubella vaccine); toxoids or modified toxins rendered nontoxic (e.g., tetanus vaccine); or subunits of microorganisms (e.g., hepatitis B vaccine). Vaccines must be *administered*. People usually think of getting shots when they think of vaccines, but there are other ways to get vaccinated. For example, the flu vaccine is available in a vaporized form, which is inhaled, as well as in an injectable form, given as a shot. Other vaccines can be administered by mouth.

Vaccines produce *immunity,* or protection. The immune system is adaptable. Most adults are immune to chickenpox. However, when you were born, you didn't have natural protection against it. Usually, we develop immunity to a microorganism after the first time we are exposed to it. That's why people ordinarily get chickenpox only once in their lives. But through vaccination, immunity develops without having to get sick. Thus, today children who get the vaccine against chickenpox are immune from the disease, even though they never had it.

Finally, they provide protection against a *particular* disease. Each vaccine provides protection against one or more microorganisms that cause disease. Getting a vaccine against one microorganism does not usually provide protection against any others. This is true even if the two microorganisms cause the same disease. That is why, for example, the pneumococcal vaccine provides protection against only some causes of pneumonia. Pneumonia is caused by over a dozen different types of bacteria, but the pneumococcal polysaccharide vaccine protects against only the pneumococcus family of bacteria, also called *Streptococcus pneumoniae*, and even then only certain members of that family. Vaccines are so specific that sometimes you need a new shot every time the microorganism mutates, or changes its genetic material. That is why, for example, people who need the flu shot are advised to get it every year. The virus that causes the flu, the influenza virus, mutates every year, so last year's flu shot often does not provide adequate protection against this year's flu.

How do vaccines prevent infection?

Vaccines themselves do not prevent infection. Instead, they rev up the body's immune system, which in turn prevents infection. Vaccines teach the immune system how to recognize a microorganism and how to defend against it. Normally, the immune system learns these skills after the first infection. Thus, the first time the immune system encounters one of these microorganisms, it is slow to respond. But if the same microorganism attacks the body a second time, the immune system is more prepared, often so much so that it prevents the second infection altogether. The trouble is that the first infection can sometimes cause serious harm to the body—even death. Vaccines work by *simulating* the first infection so that when the immune system encounters the microorganism for the first time, it will be as if it were the second time.

Vaccines do this in surprising ways; they basically have the look, smell, and taste of a microorganism without its disease-causing capabilities. Some vaccines, for example, are dead microorganisms; by being vaccinated with these dead microorganisms, the body learns how to recognize them, but because they are dead, they do not harm the body. Other vaccines are living microorganisms that have been weakened, called *attenuated vaccines*. Still others are made of one part of the microorganism, such as its outer coating. The idea behind all of these is the same—to simulate the microorganism without harming the body.

This concept helps explain why the most common side effects of any vaccine are mild flulike symptoms—a low-grade fever, a rash, or just feeling tired and worn out. The purpose of a vaccine is to simulate an actual infection by activating the immune system. When we get sick, the fevers, rashes, and tiredness we experience are not because of the infection; instead they are by-products of the immune system being activated. So the flulike symptoms we sometimes experience after a shot are actually a sign that the immune system is being activated and that the vaccine is working.

I get the flu shot every year and I still get the flu. Do vaccines really work?

No vaccine is 100 percent effective. Most childhood vaccinations prevent 85 percent or more of infections; for the 15 percent or fewer children who still get the infection, the illness is often milder and less dangerous than it would have been without the vaccine. For adult vaccinations, the result is often to prevent life-threatening illness rather than to prevent infection. This is true, for example, with pneumonia. Pneumonia, or infection of the lung, can be caused by many different types of bacteria. But the vaccine against pneumonia, called the *pneumococcal polysaccharide* (PPV23) vaccine, protects against the type of bacteria that causes the most deadly type of pneumonia, pneumococcal pneumonia. So even after receiving the PPV23, you may still get pneumonia, but it is much less likely to be fatal or disabling than it would be otherwise.

The flu shot is a special case. The flu shot protects against a specific microorganism called the influenza virus. But the "flu" as most people know it can be caused by many different viruses. That's why your doctor might say you have "flulike" symptoms without necessarily saying you have the specific "flu" virus. Part of the reason that doctors vaccinate against the influenza virus and not other viruses that cause flulike symptoms is that infection with the influenza virus is the most dangerous. The most important thing to keep in mind is that the flu shot is meant to protect you against life-threatening flu illnesses but unfortunately may not protect you against other, less dangerous but still troublesome flulike illnesses.

Do vaccines have side effects? Can they cause harm?

Vaccines are very safe. Many of the recommended vaccines have been used by doctors for decades. Newer vaccines, although they have not been around as long, are extensively studied for their safety and effectiveness.

That being said, vaccines are not harmless. Every vaccine has potential side effects. The most common side effect is pain and redness at the site of injection. In addition, it is not uncommon for vaccines to cause mild flulike symptoms, such as low-grade fevers and general tiredness. As noted earlier, these symptoms are actually a sign that the vaccine is working. They are generally mild and improve on their own or with over-the-counter remedies. Rarely, vaccines can cause more serious side effects, such as a severe allergic reaction. The specific side effects vary with each vaccine and are listed in the appendix. As with any medication, be sure to tell your doctor if you have any allergies, including a history of a reaction to medications or foods.

The risks of vaccination must be weighed against the risks of not vaccinating. The Centers for Disease Control and Prevention (CDC) recommends a vaccine based on its assessment of the risks and benefits. It is up to you, however, to weigh these risks and benefits and decide what is right for you.

Isn't there a whole controversy around vaccines?

Recently, there has been much controversy around routine immunizations, particularly in children. The issues relate to the continued need for vaccines, their safety, and their effectiveness. Addressing these issues in detail is outside the scope of this book, but a few comments are warranted:

▸ The concern that vaccines cause serious illnesses such as autism is unfounded. As noted above, vaccines rarely can lead to major side effects. However, after extensive review, scientists and doctors as a group have concluded that there is no link between vaccines and autism. While there are those that question this assertion, they are largely outside the walls of medicine and science.

▸ The argument that many vaccines are no longer necessary because they protect against diseases that have now become rare is proving incorrect. Declining rates of vaccination due to parental refusal have led to major outbreaks of measles and pertussis, or whooping cough, over the past few years. At the same time not every disease that vaccines protect against is rare, especially those targeted by adult vaccines. Diseases such as pneumonia, the flu, and shingles are common causes of serious illness in the United States, so vaccination against these diseases is still very important.

In the end, doctors can only counsel patients about medical decisions. Their goal is make sure you have accurate information with which to make informed decisions. But in the end, the choice is up to you.

SECTION II: VACCINE GUIDELINES

The Centers for Disease Control and Prevention (CDC) makes the following recommendations regarding adult vaccinations:

- Adults age 50 or older should receive the influenza vaccine (flu shot) every year during flu season.
- Adults age 60 or older should receive the shingles vaccine once in their lifetime.
- Adults age 65 or older should receive the pneumonia vaccine (PPV23) once in their lifetime, if not received earlier.
- Adults should receive the Td vaccine every ten years. Adults ages 19 through 64 should substitute Tdap for one booster of Td and then resume receiving Td thereafter.
- Women should receive the HPV (human papillomavirus) vaccine series before their 27th birthday.

These are only a subset of the CDC guidelines for adult vaccines. The ones presented above are those that are age based. For each vaccine listed above, people with certain risk factors should receive the vaccine at an earlier age or more frequently. Moreover, there are additional vaccines that only people with certain risk factors should receive. As examples, the meningococcal vaccine is recommended for college students living in dorms; the pneumococcal vaccine is recommended for people with diabetes and other chronic diseases regardless of age; the hepatitis A vaccine is recommended for people with liver disease or who live or travel to countries where hepatitis A is common.

At the same time, some vaccines are unsafe to give to certain people because of a history of an allergic reaction or other medical conditions. As examples, adults who have weakened immune systems should not receive the shingles vaccine and adults with severe allergies to eggs should not receive the flu shot.

The complete 2009 CDC adult immunization schedule is included in the appendix, as are the CDC information sheets for each vaccine. The best way to make sure you are up to date on immunizations is to partner with your doctor.

How often do the recommendations change?

The CDC revises the adult vaccination schedule every year. Most of the recommendations stay the same, but with the pace of medical advancements, at least one or two changes can be expected each year. As a result, it is critical that you and your doctor review the most up-to-date CDC guidelines to determine which vaccinations are recommended for you.

How many people are getting routinely vaccinated?

Rates of immunizations are generally low:[1]

▸ Rates of vaccination against the flu and pneumococcus in people age 65 or older are 69 and 66 percent, respectively.

▸ Only 44 percent of adults over age 65 have received a tetanus shot in the previous decade.

▸ Only 10 percent of females 18 to 26 years old have received at least one dose of the HPV vaccine. Among teenagers, the vaccination rate is 25 percent.

▸ A dismal 2 percent of adults over age 60 have received the shingles vaccine.

As a result, thousands of Americans are being harmed by infections that could have been prevented through routine vaccination.

One of the most important reasons for this is the lack of awareness in the general public about adult vaccines. Hopefully, after reading this chapter, you will take the initiative to talk to your doctor and make sure you are up to date on your vaccinations.

SECTION III: SPECIFIC VACCINES

This section provides a brief introduction to the adult vaccines outlined in section II: pneumococcal polysaccharide, influenza, tetanus-diphtheria, tetanus-diphtheria-pertussis, and shingles vaccines. The HPV vaccine is covered in chapter 6. Much of the information has been heavily adopted from the CDC Vaccine Information Statements—informational sheets on each vaccine that the CDC composes for the general public—which are provided in their original form in the appendix.

What is the pneumococcal polysaccharide vaccine?

The bacteria *S. pneumonia* causes a serious illness called *pneumococcal disease*. It is against this bacteria and this disease that the pneumococcal polysaccharide (PPV23) vaccine provides protection. Pneumococcal disease kills more people in the United States each year than all other vaccine-preventable diseases combined.

Anyone can get pneumococcal disease. However, some people are at greater risk for the disease and for becoming seriously ill or dying from it. This includes adults over 65, young children, and people with chronic health problems such as cardiovascular disease, lung disease, and diabetes.

Pneumococcal disease can lead to serious infections of the lungs (pneumonia), the blood (bacteremia), and the covering of the brain (meningitis). One in twenty people with pneumococcal pneumonia dies from the disease, as do one in five people with pneumococcal bacteremia, and three in ten people with pneumococcal meningitis. People at increased risk for pneumococcal disease are even more likely to become seriously ill or die.

The CDC recommends the vaccine for the following individuals:

- people age 65 or older who have not already received it
- people with chronic medical illness
- people with weakened immune systems
- people who have had their spleen removed

Usually one dose is all that is needed. You may need a second dose if you are over 65 and received your first dose before age 65, or if you have kidney disease, a weakened immune system, a history of an organ or a bone marrow transplant, or had your spleen removed.

What is the influenza vaccine?

Influenza is the virus that causes the flu. Although many other viruses cause flulike symptoms, influenza is the most life threatening. It is against this virus that the influenza vaccine, or flu shot, protects.

Seasonal influenza infects between 5 and 20 percent of the U.S. population each year. Most people who get infected recover in a week or two without complications. But more than 200,000 Americans have complications severe enough to warrant hospitalization each year, and another 36,000 die from influenza-related illness. Anyone can get the influenza virus. Those at greatest risk for having severe complications are people over age 65, young children, and people who live in nursing homes or have chronic medical illness.

The best protection against the flu is annual flu vaccination. The influenza vaccine is 70 to 90 percent effective in healthy adults younger than 65 years. In people older than age 65, the influenza vaccine is 30 to 70 percent effective in preventing hospitalization from influenza. And for those living in nursing homes or long-term care facilities, the vaccine is 80 percent effective in preventing death from influenza.

The CDC recommends the flu vaccine for

- children and adolescents, ages 6 months to 18 years
- women who will be pregnant during the influenza season
- everyone age 50 or older
- anyone who shares a home with a child 5 years old or younger
- residents of nursing homes or long-term care facilities
- people who have a chronic illness, such as diabetes, cardiovascular disease, or asthma
- anyone with a weakened immune system
- people who work in a health care setting

You may receive influenza vaccine anytime before or during the flu season. It is the best to get the vaccine just as it becomes available, typically around September or October, to protect yourself throughout the entire flu season, but getting vaccinated as late as February or March is still beneficial.

There are two vaccines: a live, attenuated influenza vaccine (LAIV) that is sprayed into the nose rather than given as an injection, and an inactivated influenza vaccine that is given by injection. They are equally effective, but the LAIV is restricted to healthy, nonpregnant people ages 2 through 49.

Although the influenza vaccine is generally safe, people with one or more of the following risk factors are at increased risk for harm and should talk to their doctors about whether the vaccine is safe for them:

- allergies to chicken eggs
- history of allergic reaction to a previous dose of flu vaccine
- history of Guillain-Barré syndrome after previous flu vaccination

What is the Td vaccine?

Tetanus and diphtheria are two different diseases that a single vaccine, the Td (tetanus-diphtheria) vaccine, protects against. Both tetanus and diphtheria are life-threatening illnesses caused by bacteria.

Tetanus, or lockjaw, is a disease of the nervous system that is caused by bacteria. Even with the latest medical advances, 10 to 20 percent of those who get tetanus die from the disease, and many more suffer permanent damage. People usually get the disease when the bacteria that cause tetanus get into injured skin via punctures, cuts, burns, or animal bites. The bacteria can get in through even a tiny pinprick or scratch, but deep puncture wounds or cuts like those made by nails or knives are especially prone to infection.

Diphtheria is a bacterial disease that usually affects the skin and pharynx (tonsils, throat, nose). In its early stages, it might be mistaken for a sore throat, but it is a serious, life-threatening illness. Between 5 and 10 percent of the people who develop respiratory diphtheria die from the disease, and many more suffer permanent damage. Diphtheria is passed from person to person through infected droplets, such as when an infected person coughs or sneezes.

The Td vaccine is nearly 100 percent effective in preventing tetanus and 85 percent effective in preventing diphtheria. Because the effectiveness of the tetanus and diphtheria vaccines declines over time, a Td booster shot is periodically required. The CDC recommends the Td vaccine for all adults every ten years. In addition, people who sustain an injury that breaks the skin should consider getting a booster dose if their last shot was more than five years before the injury.

What is the Tdap vaccine?

The Tdap vaccine protects against tetanus, diphtheria, and pertussis. Pertussis, also known as whooping cough, is a serious infection that spreads easily from person to person via respiratory contact. Early symptoms of pertussis are similar to those of the common cold but can progress to coughing spells so severe that it becomes difficult to breathe. Children are particularly vulnerable to serious infection and sometimes suffer cracked ribs and pneumonia, requiring hospitalization. There is no cure for pertussis, and treatment relies on providing supportive care while the infection resolves. Far from uncommon, pertussis is on the rise and affects thousands of children and adults in the United States annually.

The most effective way to prevent pertussis is through vaccination. Although most adults were immunized against pertussis as children, they require a booster shot to keep themselves best protected. The shot is administered through the Tdap (tetanus-diphtheria-acellular pertussis) vaccine.

The CDC recommends that adults 19 to 64 years of age receive a single dose of Tdap in place of a Td (tetanus-diphtheria) booster, and then resume the Td booster thereafter.

What is the shingles vaccine?

Shingles, also called *herpes zoster* or zoster, is a painful skin rash caused by the varicella zoster virus (VZV). This is the same virus that causes chickenpox. The first time someone gets infected with VZV, they develop chickenpox. After a person recovers, the virus stays in the body and never goes away completely. Usually the virus does not cause any problems; however, after years of remaining dormant, VZV can reactivate and cause shingles.

Shingles typically manifests as a painful, burning, sometimes itchy rash. The rash typically follows a bandlike distribution across one side of the face or body. It begins as a red raised area and progresses into blisters that eventually scab over. The rash and associated pain usually clear within two to four weeks. However, one in every five affected people continues to have severe pain at the site of the rash even after the rash clears up and suffer from a condition called *postherpetic neuralgia* (post-her-PET-ik nuh-RAWL-juh). In addition, very rarely, shingles can lead to more serious medical problems, such as pneumonia, encephalitis, or death.

One in three Americans will develop shingles in his or her lifetime, resulting in 1 million cases each year. Anyone who has had chickenpox in the past can develop shingles. However, shingles most commonly occurs in people age 50 or older. People who have medical conditions that keep the immune system from working properly are at greater risk of developing shingles at a younger age and with more severe symptoms.

The shingles vaccine reduces the risk of shingles by half and the risk of postherpetic neuralgia by two-thirds in adults age 60 or older. For people ages 60 to 69, it reduces occurrence by over 60 percent. The CDC recommends a single dose of the shingles vaccine for all adults over age 60, even if they have had shingles.

The shingles vaccine is generally safe, but people with one or more of the following conditions are at increased risk for harm and should talk to their doctors about whether the vaccine is safe for them:

▸ women who are pregnant or might become pregnant
▸ anyone with a weakened immune system
▸ anyone who has ever had a life-threatening allergic reaction to gelatin, the antibiotic neomycin, or any other component of the shingles vaccine

REFERENCES

Centers for Disease Control and Prevention (CDC). U.S. Department of Health and Human Services. "Vaccines and Immunizations." www.cdc.gov/vaccines.
National Commission on Prevention Priorities. Partnership for Prevention. *Preventive Care: A National Profile on Use, Disparities, and Health Benefits.* Press release, August 2007, available at www.prevent.org/content/view/129/72.

Immunization Schedules and Vaccine Information Sheets from the Centers for Disease Control and Prevention

This appendix consists of immunization recommendations and guidelines from the Centers for Disease Control and Prevention (CDC), starting with the 2009 immunization schedules for various age groups:

- ‣ young children (birth, or age 0, through 6 years)
- ‣ older children and adolescents (7 through 18 years)
- ‣ adults (age 19 and older)

Following these schedules are the complete CDC information sheets for the following vaccines:

- ‣ chickenpox (varicella)
- ‣ Td and Tdap
- ‣ hepatitis A
- ‣ hepatitis B
- ‣ *Haemophilus influenzae* type b (Hib)
- ‣ human papillomavirus (HPV)
- ‣ inactivated influenza (injectable)
- ‣ live, intranasal influenza (nasal spray)
- ‣ measles, mumps, and rubella (MMR)
- ‣ pneumococcal conjugate (PCV7)
- ‣ pneumococcal polysaccharide (PPV23)
- ‣ polio (IPV)
- ‣ rotavirus
- ‣ shingles

As the information sheets indicate, some of the vaccines are only for adults, and some are only for children. Use the information included here to inform your discussion with your doctor about which immunizations are right for you and your family.

RECOMMENDED IMMUNIZATION SCHEDULE FOR PERSONS AGED 0 THROUGH 6 YEARS
—United States • 2009 *For those who fall behind or start late, see the catch-up schedule*

VACCINE	Birth	1 month	2 months	4 months	6 months	12 months	15 months	18 months	19–23 months	2–3 years	4–6 years
Hepatitis B[1]	HepB	HepB		see footnote 1	HepB						
Rotavirus[2]			RV	RV	RV[2]						
Diphtheria, Tetanus, Pertussis[3]			DTaP	DTaP	DTaP	see footnote 3	DTaP				DTaP
Haemophilus influenzae type b[4]			Hib	Hib	Hib[4]	Hib					
Pneumococcal[5]			PCV	PCV	PCV	PCV					PPSV
Inactivated Poliovirus			IPV	IPV		IPV					IPV
Influenza[6]						Influenza (Yearly)					
Measles, Mumps, Rubella[7]						MMR		see footnote 7			MMR
Varicella[8]						Varicella		see footnote 8			Varicella
Hepatitis A[9]						HepA (2 doses)				HepA Series	
Meningococcal[10]										MCV	

▨ Range of recommended ages

■ Certain high-risk groups

This schedule indicates the recommended ages for routine administration of currently licensed vaccines, as of December 1, 2008, for children aged 0 through 6 years. Any dose not administered at the recommended age should be administered at a subsequent visit, when indicated and feasible. Licensed combination vaccines may be used whenever any component of the combination is indicated and other components are not contraindicated and if approved by the Food and Drug Administration for that dose of the series. Providers should consult the relevant Advisory Committee on Immunization Practices statement for detailed recommendations, including high-risk conditions: http://www.cdc.gov /vaccines/pubs/acip-list.htm. Clinically significant adverse events that follow immunization should be reported to the Vaccine Adverse Event Reporting System (VAERS). Guidance about how to obtain and complete a VAERS form is available at http://www.vaers.hhs.gov or by telephone, 800-822-7967.

Source: Department of Health and Human Services • Centers for Disease Control and Prevention

FOOTNOTES: Recommended Immunization Schedule for Persons Aged 0 Through 6 Years —UNITED STATES · 2009

For complete statements by the Advisory Committee on Immunization Practices (ACIP), visit www.cdc.gov/vaccines/pubs/ACIP-list.htm.

1. **Hepatitis B vaccine (HepB).** *(Minimum age: birth)*
   At birth:
   - Administer monovalent HepB to all newborns before hospital discharge.
   - If mother is hepatitis B surface antigen (HBsAg)-positive, administer HepB and 0.5 mL of hepatitis B immune globulin (HBIG) within 12 hours of birth.
   - If mother's HBsAg status is unknown, administer HepB within 12 hours of birth. Determine mother's HBsAg status as soon as possible and, if HBsAg-positive, administer HBIG (no later than age 1 week).
   After the birth dose:
   - The HepB series should be completed with either monovalent HepB or a combination vaccine containing HepB. The second dose should be administered at age 1 or 2 months. The final dose should be administered no earlier than age 24 weeks.
   - Infants born to HBsAg-positive mothers should be tested for HBsAg and antibody to HBsAg (anti-HBs) after completion of at least 3 doses of the HepB series, at age 9 through 18 months (generally at the next well-child visit).
   4-month dose:
   - Administration of 4 doses of HepB to infants is permissible when combination vaccines containing HepB are administered after the birth dose.

2. **Rotavirus vaccine (RV).** *(Minimum age: 6 weeks)*
   - Administer the first dose at age 6 through 14 weeks (maximum: 14 weeks 6 days). Vaccination should not be initiated for infants aged 15 weeks or older (i.e., 15 weeks 0 days or older).
   - Administer the final dose in the series by age 8 months 0 days.
   - If Rotarix® is administered at ages 2 and 4 months, a dose at 6 months is not indicated.

3. **Diphtheria and tetanus toxoids and acellular pertussis vaccine (DTaP).** *(Minimum age: 6 weeks)*
   - The fourth dose may be administered as early as age 12 months, provided at least 6 months have elapsed since the third dose.
   - Administer the final dose in the series at age 4 through 6 years.

4. ***Haemophilus influenzae* type b conjugate vaccine (Hib).** *(Minimum age: 6 weeks)*
   - If PRP-OMP (PedvaxHIB® or Comvax® [HepB-Hib]) is administered at ages 2 and 4 months, a dose at age 6 months is not indicated.
   - TriHiBit® (DTaP/Hib) should not be used for doses at ages 2, 4, or 6 months but can be used as the final dose in children aged 12 months or older.

5. **Pneumococcal vaccine.** *(Minimum age: 6 weeks for pneumococcal conjugate vaccine [PCV]; 2 years for pneumococcal polysaccharide vaccine [PPSV])*
   - PCV is recommended for all children aged younger than 5 years. Administer 1 dose of PCV to all healthy children aged 24 through 59 months who are not completely vaccinated for their age.
   - Administer PPSV to children aged 2 years or older with certain underlying medical conditions (see *MMWR* 2000;49[No. RR-9]), including a cochlear implant.

6. **Influenza vaccine.** *(Minimum age: 6 months for trivalent inactivated influenza vaccine [TIV]; 2 years for live, attenuated influenza vaccine [LAIV])*
   - Administer annually to children aged 6 months through 18 years.
   - For healthy nonpregnant persons (i.e., those who do not have underlying medical conditions that predispose them to influenza complications) aged 2 through 49 years, either LAIV or TIV may be used.
   - Children receiving TIV should receive 0.25 mL if aged 6 through 35 months or 0.5 mL if aged 3 years or older.
   - Administer 2 doses (separated by at least 4 weeks) to children aged younger than 9 years who are receiving influenza vaccine for the first time or who were vaccinated for the first time during the previous influenza season but only received 1 dose.

7. **Measles, mumps, and rubella vaccine (MMR).** *(Minimum age: 12 months)*
   - Administer the second dose at age 4 through 6 years. However, the second dose may be administered before age 4, provided at least 28 days have elapsed since the first dose.

8. **Varicella vaccine.** *(Minimum age: 12 months)*
   - Administer the second dose at age 4 through 6 years. However, the second dose may be administered before age 4, provided at least 3 months have elapsed since the first dose.
   - For children aged 12 months through 12 years the minimum interval between doses is 3 months. However, if the second dose was administered at least 28 days after the first dose, it can be accepted as valid.

9. Hepatitis A vaccine (HepA). *(Minimum age: 12 months)*
- Administer to all children aged 1 year (i.e., aged 12 through 23 months). Administer 2 doses at least 6 months apart.
- Children not fully vaccinated by age 2 years can be vaccinated at subsequent visits.
- HepA also is recommended for children older than 1 year who live in areas where vaccination programs target older children or who are at increased risk of infection. See *MMWR* 2006;55(No. RR-7).

10. Meningococcal vaccine. *(Minimum age: 2 years for meningococcal conjugate vaccine [MCV] and for meningococcal polysaccharide vaccine [MPSV])*
- Administer MCV to children aged 2 through 10 years with terminal complement component deficiency, anatomic or functional asplenia, and certain other high-risk groups. See *MMWR* 2005;54(No. RR-7).
- Persons who received MPSV 3 or more years previously and who remain at increased risk for meningococcal disease should be revaccinated with MCV.

RECOMMENDED IMMUNIZATION SCHEDULE FOR PERSONS AGED 7 THROUGH 18 YEARS

—United States • 2009 *For those who fall behind or start late, see the schedule below and the catch-up schedule*

VACCINE	Age		
	7–10 years	11–12 years	13–18 years
Tetanus, Diphtheria, Pertussis[1]	*see footnote 1*	Tdap	Tdap
Human Papillomavirus[2]	*see footnote 2*	HPV (3 doses)	HPV Series
Meningococcal[3]	MCV	MCV	MCV
Influenza[4]	Influenza (Yearly)		
Pneumococcal[5]	PPSV		
Hepatitis A[6]	HepA Series		
Hepatitis B[7]	HepB Series		
Inactivated Poliovirus[8]	IPV Series		
Measles, Mumps, Rubella[9]	MMR Series		
Varicella[10]	Varicella Series		

 Range of recommended ages

 Catch-up immunization

 Certain high-risk groups

This schedule indicates the recommended ages for routine administration of currently licensed vaccines, as of December 1, 2008, for children aged 7 through 18 years. Any dose not administered at the recommended age should be administered at a subsequent visit, when indicated and feasible. Licensed combination vaccines may be used whenever any component of the combination is indicated and other components are not contraindicated and if approved by the Food and Drug Administration for that dose of the series. Providers should consult the relevant Advisory Committee on Immunization Practices statement for detailed recommendations, including high-risk conditions: http://www.cdc.gov/vaccines/pubs/acip-list.htm. Clinically significant adverse events that follow immunization should be reported to the Vaccine Adverse Event Reporting System (VAERS). Guidance about how to obtain and complete a VAERS form is available at http://www.vaers.hhs.gov or by telephone, 800-822-7967.

Source: Department of Health and Human Services • Centers for Disease Control and Prevention

FOOTNOTES: Recommended Immunization Schedule for Persons Aged 7 Through 18 Years —UNITED STATES · 2009

For complete statements by the Advisory Committee on Immunization Practices (ACIP), visit www.cdc.gov/vaccines/pubs/ACIP-list.htm.

1. Tetanus and diphtheria toxoids and acellular pertussis vaccine (Tdap). *(Minimum age: 10 years for BOOSTRIX® and 11 years for ADACEL®)*
- Administer at age 11 or 12 years for those who have completed the recommended childhood DTP/DTaP vaccination series and have not received a tetanus and diphtheria toxoid (Td) booster dose.
- Persons aged 13 through 18 years who have not received Tdap should receive a dose.
- A 5-year interval from the last Td dose is encouraged when Tdap is used as a booster dose; however, a shorter interval may be used if pertussis immunity is needed.

2. Human papillomavirus vaccine (HPV). *(Minimum age: 9 years)*
- Administer the first dose to females at age 11 or 12 years.
- Administer the second dose 2 months after the first dose and the third dose 6 months after the first dose (at least 24 weeks after the first dose).
- Administer the series to females at age 13 through 18 years if not previously vaccinated.

3. Meningococcal conjugate vaccine (MCV).
- Administer at age 11 or 12 years, or at age 13 through 18 years if not previously vaccinated.
- Administer to previously unvaccinated college freshmen living in a dormitory.
- MCV is recommended for children aged 2 through 10 years with terminal complement component deficiency, anatomic or functional asplenia, and certain other groups at high risk. See *MMWR* 2005;54(No. RR-7).
- Persons who received MPSV 5 or more years previously and remain at increased risk for meningococcal disease should be revaccinated with MCV.

4. Influenza vaccine.
- Administer annually to children aged 6 months through 18 years.
- For healthy nonpregnant persons (i.e., those who do not have underlying medical conditions that predispose them to influenza complications) aged 2 through 49 years, either LAIV or TIV may be used.
- Administer 2 doses (separated by at least 4 weeks) to children aged younger than 9 years who are receiving influenza vaccine for the first time or who were vaccinated for the first time during the previous influenza season but only received 1 dose.

5. Pneumococcal polysaccharide vaccine (PPSV).
- Administer to children with certain underlying medical conditions (see *MMWR* 1997;46[No. RR-8]), including a cochlear implant.
- A single revaccination should be administered to children with functional or anatomic asplenia or other immunocompromising condition after 5 years.

6. Hepatitis A vaccine (HepA).
- Administer 2 doses at least 6 months apart.
- HepA is recommended for children older than 1 year who live in areas where vaccination programs target older children or who are at increased risk of infection. See *MMWR* 2006;55 (No. RR-7).

7. Hepatitis B vaccine (HepB).
- Administer the 3-dose series to those not previously vaccinated.
- A 2-dose series (separated by at least 4 months) of adult formulation Recombivax HB® is licensed for children aged 11 through 15 years.

8. Inactivated poliovirus vaccine (IPV).
- For children who received an all-IPV or all-oral poliovirus (OPV) series, a fourth dose is not necessary if the third dose was administered at age 4 years or older.
- If both OPV and IPV were administered as part of a series, a total of 4 doses should be administered, regardless of the child's current age.

9. Measles, mumps, and rubella vaccine (MMR).
- If not previously vaccinated, administer 2 doses or the second dose for those who have received only 1 dose, with at least 28 days between doses.

10. Varicella vaccine.
- For persons aged 7 through 18 years without evidence of immunity (see *MMWR* 2007;56 [No. RR-4]), administer 2 doses if not previously vaccinated or the second dose if they have received only 1 dose.
- For persons aged 7 through 12 years, the minimum interval between doses is 3 months. However, if the second dose was administered at least 28 days after the first dose, it can be accepted as valid.
- For persons aged 13 years and older, the minimum interval between doses is 28 days.

RECOMMENDED ADULT IMMUNIZATION SCHEDULE — United States • 2009 *					
Age Group					
VACCINE	19–26 years	27–49 years	50–59 years	60–64 years	≥65 years
Tetanus, diphtheria, pertussis (Td/Tdap) [1,*]	Substitute 1-time dose of Tdap for Td booster; then boost with Td every 10 yrs				Td booster every 10 yrs
Human papillomavirus (HPV) [2,*]	3 doses (females)				
Varicella [3,*]	2 doses				
Zoster [4]				1 dose	
Measles, mumps, rubella (MMR) [5,*]	1 or 2 doses		1 dose		
Influenza [6,*]	1 dose annually				
Pneumococcal (polysaccharide) [7,8]	1 or 2 doses				1 dose
Hepatitis A [9,*]	2 doses				
Hepatitis B [10,*]	3 doses				
Meningococcal [11,*]	1 or more doses				

*Covered by the Vaccine Injury Compensation Program.

For all persons in this category who meet the age requirements and who lack evidence of immunity (e.g., lack documentation of vaccination or have no evidence of prior infection)

Recommended if some other risk factor is present (e.g., on the basis of medical, occupational, lifestyle, or other indications)

No recommendation

Report all clinically significant postvaccination reactions to the Vaccine Adverse Event Reporting System (VAERS). Reporting forms and instructions on filing a VAERS report are available at www.vaers.hhs.gov or by telephone, 800-822-7967.

Information on how to file a Vaccine Injury Compensation Program claim is available at www.hrsa.gov/vaccinecompensation or by telephone, 800-338-2382. To file a claim for vaccine injury, contact the U.S. Court of Federal Claims, 717 Madison Place, N.W., Washington, D.C. 20005; telephone, 202-357-6400.

Additional information about the vaccines in this schedule, extent of available data, and contraindications for vaccination is also available at www.cdc.gov/vaccines or from the CDC-INFO Contact Center at 800-CDC-INFO (800-232-4636) in English and Spanish, 24 hours a day, 7 days a week.

Use of trade names and commercial sources is for identification only and does not imply endorsement by the U.S. Department of Health and Human Services.

Source: Department of Health and Human Services • Centers for Disease Control and Prevention

VACCINE	Indication								
	Pregnancy	Immuno-compromising conditions (excluding human immuno-deficiency virus [HIV])[13]	HIV Infection[3,12,13] CD4+ T lymphocyte count <200 cells/μl	HIV Infection[3,12,13] CD4+ T lymphocyte count ≥200 cells/μl	Diabetes, heart disease, chronic lung disease, chronic alcoholism	Asplenia[12] (including elective splenectomy and terminal complement component deficiencies)	Chronic liver disease	Kidney failure, end-stage renal disease, receipt of hemodi-alysis	Health-care personnel
Tetanus, diphtheria, pertussis (Td/Tdap)[1,*]	Td	Substitute 1-time dose of Tdap for Td booster; then boost with Td every 10 yrs							
Human papillomavirus (HPV)[2,*]		3 doses for females through 26 yrs							
Varicella[3,*]	Contraindicated			2 doses					
Zoster[4]	Contraindicated			1 dose					
Measles, mumps, rubella (MMR)[5,*]	Contraindicated			1 or 2 doses					
Influenza[6,*]	1 dose TIV annually								1 dose TIV or LAIV annually
Pneumococcal (polysaccharide)[7,8]	1 or 2 doses								
Hepatitis A[9,*]	2 doses								
Hepatitis B[10,*]	3 doses								
Meningococcal[11,*]	1 or more doses								

RECOMMENDED ADULT IMMUNIZATION SCHEDULE — United States · 2009 *

*Covered by the Vaccine Injury Compensation Program.

 For all persons in this category who meet the age requirements and who lack evidence of immunity (e.g., lack documentation of vaccination or have no evidence of prior infection)

 Recommended if some other risk factor is present (e.g., on the basis of medical, occupational, lifestyle, or other indications)

☐ No recommendation

These schedules indicate the recommended age groups and medical indications for which administration of currently licensed vaccines is commonly indicated for adults ages 19 years and older, as of January 1, 2009. Licensed combination vaccines may be used whenever any components of the combination are indicated and when the vaccine's other components are not contraindicated. For detailed recommendations on all vaccines, including those used primarily for travelers or that are issued during the year, consult the manufacturers' package inserts and the complete statements from the Advisory Committee on Immunization Practices (www.cdc.gov/vaccines/pubs/acip-list.htm).

FOOTNOTES: Recommended Adult Immunization Schedule—UNITED STATES · 2009

For complete statements by the Advisory Committee on Immunization Practices (ACIP), visit www.cdc.gov/vaccines/pubs/ACIP-list.htm.

1. Tetanus, diphtheria, and acellular pertussis (Td/Tdap) vaccination

Tdap should replace a single dose of Td for adults aged 19 through 64 years who have not received a dose of Tdap previously.

Adults with uncertain or incomplete history of primary vaccination series with tetanus and diphtheria toxoid-containing vaccines should begin or complete a primary vaccination series. A primary series for adults is 3 doses of tetanus and diphtheria toxoid-containing vaccines; administer the first 2 doses at least 4 weeks apart and the third dose 6–12 months after the second. However, Tdap can substitute for any one of the doses of Td in the 3-dose primary series. The booster dose of tetanus and diphtheria toxoid-containing vaccine should be administered to adults who have completed a primary series and if the last vaccination was received 10 or more years previously. Tdap or Td vaccine may be used, as indicated.

If a woman is pregnant and received the last Td vaccination 10 or more years previously, administer Td during the second or third trimester. If the woman received the last Td vaccination less than 10 years previously, administer Tdap during the immediate postpartum period. A dose of Tdap is recommended for postpartum women, close contacts of infants aged less than 12 months, and all health-care personnel with direct patient contact if they have not previously received Tdap. An interval as short as 2 years from the last Td is suggested; shorter intervals can be used. Td may be deferred during pregnancy and Tdap substituted in the immediate postpartum period, or Tdap may be administered instead of Td to a pregnant woman after an informed discussion with the woman.

Consult the ACIP statement for recommendations for administering Td as prophylaxis in wound management.

2. Human papillomavirus (HPV) vaccination

HPV vaccination is recommended for all females aged 11 through 26 years (and may begin at 9 years) who have not completed the vaccine series. History of genital warts, abnormal Papanicolaou test, or positive HPV DNA test is not evidence of prior infection with all vaccine HPV types. HPV vaccination is recommended for persons with such histories.

Ideally, vaccine should be administered before potential exposure to HPV through sexual activity; however, females who are sexually active should still be vaccinated consistent with age-based recommendations. Sexually active females who have not been infected with any of the four HPV vaccine types receive the full benefit of the vaccination. Vaccination is less beneficial for females who have already been infected with one or more of the HPV vaccine types.

A complete series consists of 3 doses. The second dose should be administered 2 months after the first dose; the third dose should be administered 6 months after the first dose.

HPV vaccination is not specifically recommended for females with the medical indications described in Figure 2, "Vaccines that might be indicated for adults based on medical and other indications." Because HPV vaccine is not a live-virus vaccine, it may be administered to persons with the medical indications described in Figure 2. However, the immune response and vaccine efficacy might be less for persons with the medical indications described in Figure 2 than in persons who do not have the medical indications described or who are immunocompetent. Health-care personnel are not at increased risk because of occupational exposure, and should be vaccinated consistent with age-based recommendations.

3. Varicella vaccination

All adults without evidence of immunity to varicella should receive 2 doses of single-antigen varicella vaccine if not previously vaccinated or the second dose if they have received only one dose unless they have a medical contraindication. Special consideration should be given to those who 1) have close contact with persons at high risk for severe disease (e.g., health-care personnel and family/contacts of persons with immunocompromising conditions) or 2) are at high risk for exposure or transmission (e.g., teachers; child care employees; residents and staff members of institutional settings, including correctional institutions; college students; military personnel; adolescents and adults living in households with children; nonpregnant women of childbearing age; and international travelers).

Evidence of immunity to varicella in adults includes any of the following: 1) documentation of 2 doses of varicella vaccine at least 4 weeks apart; 2) U.S.-born before 1980 (although for health-care personnel and pregnant women, birth before 1980 should not be considered evidence of immunity); 3) history of varicella based on diagnosis or verification of varicella by a health-care provider (for a patient reporting a history of or presenting with an atypical case, a mild case, or both, health-care providers should seek either an epidemiologic link with a typical varicella case or to a laboratory-confirmed case or evidence of laboratory confirmation, if it was performed at the time of acute disease); 4) history of herpes zoster based on health-care provider diagnosis or verification of herpes zoster by a health-care provider; or 5) laboratory evidence of immunity or laboratory confirmation of disease.

Pregnant women should be assessed for evidence of varicella immunity. Women who do not have evidence of immunity should receive the first dose of varicella vaccine upon completion or termination of pregnancy and before discharge from the health-care facility. The second dose should be administered 4–8 weeks after the first dose.

4. Herpes zoster vaccination

A single dose of zoster vaccine is recommended for adults aged 60 years and older regardless of whether they report a prior episode of herpes zoster. Persons with chronic medical conditions may be vaccinated unless their condition constitutes a contraindication.

5. Measles, mumps, rubella (MMR) vaccination

Measles component: Adults born before 1957 generally are considered immune to measles. Adults born during or after 1957 should receive 1 or more doses of MMR unless they have a medical contraindication, documentation of 1 or more doses, history of measles based on health-care provider diagnosis, or laboratory evidence of immunity.

A second dose of MMR is recommended for adults who 1) have been recently exposed to measles or are in an outbreak setting; 2) have been vaccinated previously with killed measles vaccine; 3) have been vaccinated with an unknown type of measles vaccine during 1963–1967; 4) are students in post-secondary educational institutions; 5) work in a health-care facility; or 6) plan to travel internationally.

Mumps component: Adults born before 1957 generally are considered immune to mumps. Adults born during or after 1957 should receive 1 dose of MMR unless they have a medical contraindication, history of mumps based on health-care provider diagnosis, or laboratory evidence of immunity.

A second dose of MMR is recommended for adults who 1) live in a community experiencing a mumps outbreak and are in an affected age group; 2) are students in postsecondary educational institutions; 3) work in a health-care facility; or 4) plan to travel internationally. For unvaccinated health-care personnel born before 1957 who do not have other evidence of mumps immunity, administering 1 dose on a routine basis should be considered and administering a second dose during an outbreak should be strongly considered.

Rubella component: 1 dose of MMR vaccine is recommended for women whose rubella vaccination history is unreliable or who lack laboratory evidence of immunity. For women of childbearing age, regardless of birth year, rubella immunity should be determined and women should be counseled regarding congenital rubella syndrome. Women who do not have evidence of immunity should receive MMR upon completion or termination of pregnancy and before discharge from the health-care facility.

6. Influenza vaccination

Medical indications: Chronic disorders of the cardiovascular or pulmonary systems, including asthma; chronic metabolic diseases, including diabetes mellitus, renal or hepatic dysfunction, hemoglobinopathies, or immunocompromising conditions (including immunocompromising conditions caused by medications or human immunodeficiency virus [HIV]); any condition that compromises respiratory function or the handling of respiratory secretions or that can increase the risk of aspiration (e.g., cognitive dysfunction, spinal cord injury, or seizure disorder or other neuromuscular disorder); and pregnancy during the influenza season. No data exist on the risk for severe or complicated influenza disease among persons with asplenia; however, influenza is a risk factor for secondary bacterial infections that can cause severe disease among persons with asplenia.

Occupational indications: All health-care personnel, including those employed by long-term care and assisted-living facilities, and caregivers of children less than 5 years old.

Other indications: Residents of nursing homes and other long-term care and assisted-living facilities; persons likely to transmit influenza to persons at high risk (e.g., in-home household contacts and caregivers of children aged less than 5 years old, persons 65 years old and older and persons of all ages with high-risk condition[s]); and anyone who would like to decrease their risk of getting influenza. Healthy, nonpregnant adults aged less than 50 years without high-risk medical conditions who are not contacts of severely immunocompromised persons in special care units can receive either intranasally administered live, attenuated influenza vaccine (FluMist®) or inactivated vaccine. Other persons should receive the inactivated vaccine.

7. Pneumococcal polysaccharide (PPSV) vaccination

Medical indications: Chronic lung disease (including asthma); chronic cardiovascular diseases; diabetes mellitus; chronic liver diseases, cirrhosis; chronic alcoholism, chronic renal failure or nephrotic syndrome; functional or anatomic asplenia (e.g., sickle cell disease or splenectomy [if elective splenectomy is planned, vaccinate at least 2 weeks before surgery]); immunocompromising conditions; and cochlear implants and cerebrospinal fluid leaks. Vaccinate as close to HIV diagnosis as possible.

Other indications: Residents of nursing homes or long-term care facilities and persons who smoke cigarettes. Routine use of PPSV is not recommended for Alaska Native or American Indian persons younger than 65 years unless they have underlying medical conditions that are PPSV indications. However public health authorities may consider recommending PPSV for Alaska Natives and American Indians aged 50 through 64 years who are living in areas in which the risk of invasive pneumococcal disease is increased.

8. Revaccination with PPSV

One-time revaccination after 5 years for persons with chronic renal failure or nephrotic syndrome; functional or anatomic asplenia (e.g., sickle cell disease or splenectomy); and for persons with immunocompromising conditions. For persons aged 65 years and older, one-time revaccination if they were vaccinated 5 or more years previously and were aged less than 65 years at the time of primary vaccination.

9. Hepatitis A vaccination

Medical indications: Persons with chronic liver disease and persons who receive clotting factor concentrates.

Behavioral indications: Men who have sex with men and persons who use illegal drugs.

Occupational indications: Persons working with hepatitis A virus (HAV)-infected primates or with HAV in a research laboratory setting.

Other indications: Persons traveling to or working in countries that have high or intermediate endemicity of hepatitis A (a list of countries is available at wwwn.cdc.gov/travel/contentdiseases.aspx) and any person seeking protection from HAV infection.

Single-antigen vaccine formulations should be administered in a 2-dose schedule at either 0 and 6–12 months (Havrix®), or 0 and 6–18 months (Vaqta®). If the combined hepatitis A and hepatitis B vaccine (Twinrix®) is used, administer 3 doses at 0, 1, and 6 months; alternatively, a 4-dose schedule, administered on days 0, 7 and 21 to 30 followed by a booster dose at month 12 may be used.

10. Hepatitis B vaccination

Medical indications: Persons with end-stage renal disease, including patients receiving hemodialysis; persons with HIV infection; and persons with chronic liver disease.

Occupational indications: Health-care personnel and public-safety workers who are exposed to blood or other potentially infectious body fluids.

Behavioral indications: Sexually active persons who are not in a long-term, mutually monogamous relationship (e.g., persons with more than 1 sex partner during the previous 6 months); persons seeking evaluation or treatment for a sexually transmitted disease; current or recent injection-drug users; and men who have sex with men.

Other indications: Household contacts and sex partners of persons with chronic hepatitis B virus (HBV) infection; clients and staff members of institutions for persons with developmental disabilities; international travelers to countries with high or intermediate prevalence of chronic HBV infection (a list of countries is available at www.cdc.gov/travel/contentdiseases.aspx); and any adult seeking protection from HBV infection.

Hepatitis B vaccination is recommended for all adults in the following settings: STD treatment facilities; HIV testing and treatment facilities; facilities providing drug-abuse treatment and prevention services; health-care settings targeting services to injection-drug users or men who have sex with men; correctional facilities; end-stage renal disease programs and facilities for chronic hemodialysis patients; and institutions and nonresidential daycare facilities for persons with developmental disabilities.

If the combined hepatitis A and hepatitis B vaccine (Twinrix®) is used, administer 3 doses at 0, 1, and 6 months; alternatively, a 4-dose schedule, administered on days 0, 7 and 21 to 30 followed by a booster dose at month 12 may be used.

Special formulation indications: For adult patients receiving hemodialysis or with other immunocompromising conditions, 1 dose of 40 μg/mL (Recombivax HB®) administered on a 3-dose schedule or 2 doses of 20 μg/mL (Engerix-B®) administered simultaneously on a 4-dose schedule at 0, 1, 2 and 6 months.

11. Meningococcal vaccination

Medical indications: Adults with anatomic or functional asplenia, or terminal complement component deficiencies.

Other indications: First-year college students living in dormitories; microbiologists who are routinely exposed to isolates of *Neisseria meningitidis*; military recruits; and persons who travel to or live in countries in which meningococcal disease is hyperendemic or epidemic (e.g., the "meningitis belt" of sub-Saharan Africa during the dry season [December–June]), particularly if their contact with local populations will be prolonged. Vaccination is required by the government of Saudi Arabia for all travelers to Mecca during the annual Hajj.

Meningococcal conjugate (MCV) vaccine is preferred for adults with any of the preceding indications who are aged 55 years or younger, although meningococcal polysaccharide vaccine (MPSV) is an acceptable alternative. Revaccination with MCV after 5 years might be indicated for adults previously vaccinated with MPSV who remain at increased risk for infection (e.g., persons residing in areas in which disease is epidemic).

12. Selected conditions for which *Haemophilus influenzae* type b (Hib) vaccine may be used

Hib vaccine generally is not recommended for persons aged 5 years and older. No efficacy data are available on which to base a recommendation concerning use of Hib vaccine for older children and adults. However, studies suggest good immunogenicity in persons who have sickle cell disease, leukemia, or HIV infection or who have had a splenectomy; administering 1 dose of vaccine to these persons is not contraindicated.

13. Immunocompromising conditions

Inactivated vaccines generally are acceptable (e.g., pneumococcal, meningococcal, and influenza [trivalent inactivated influenza vaccine]), and live vaccines generally are avoided in persons with immune deficiencies or immunocompromising conditions. Information on specific conditions is available at www.cdc.gov/vaccines/pubs/acip-list.htm.

CHICKENPOX VACCINE

WHAT YOU NEED TO KNOW

1. Why get vaccinated?

Chickenpox (also called varicella) is a common childhood disease. It is usually mild, but it can be serious, especially in young infants and adults.

- It causes a rash, itching, fever, and tiredness.
- It can lead to severe skin infection, scars, pneumonia, brain damage, or death.
- The chickenpox virus can be spread from person to person through the air, or by contact with fluid from chickenpox blisters.
- A person who has had chickenpox can get a painful rash called shingles years later.
- Before the vaccine, about 11,000 people were hospitalized for chickenpox each year in the United States.
- Before the vaccine, about 100 people died each year as a result of chickenpox in the United States.

Chickenpox vaccine can prevent chickenpox.

Most people who get chickenpox vaccine will not get chickenpox. But if someone who has been vaccinated does get chickenpox, it is usually very mild. They will have fewer blisters, are less likely to have a fever, and will recover faster.

2. Who should get chickenpox vaccine and when?

▶ ROUTINE

Children who have never had chickenpox should get 2 doses of chickenpox vaccine at these ages:

1st Dose: 12–15 months of age

2nd Dose: 4–6 years of age (may be given earlier, if at least 3 months after the 1st dose)

People 13 years of age and older (who have never had chickenpox or received chickenpox vaccine) should get two doses at least 28 days apart.

▶ CATCH-UP

Anyone who is not fully vaccinated, and never had chickenpox, should receive one or two doses of chickenpox vaccine. The timing of these doses depends on the person's age. Ask your provider.

Chickenpox vaccine may be given at the same time as other vaccines.

NOTE: A "combination" vaccine called **MMRV**, which contains both chickenpox and MMR vaccines, may be given instead of the two individual vaccines to people 12 years of age and younger.

3. Some people should not get chickenpox vaccine or should wait

- People should not get chickenpox vaccine if they have ever had a life-threatening allergic reaction to a previous dose of chickenpox vaccine or to gelatin or the antibiotic neomycin.
- People who are moderately or severely ill at the time the shot is scheduled should usually wait until they recover before getting chickenpox vaccine.
- Pregnant women should wait to get chickenpox vaccine until after they have given birth. Women should not get pregnant for 1 month after getting chickenpox vaccine.
- Some people should check with their doctor about whether they should get chickenpox vaccine, including anyone who:
  - Has HIV/AIDS or another disease that affects the immune system
  - Is being treated with drugs that affect the immune system, such as steroids, for 2 weeks or longer
  - Has any kind of cancer
  - Is getting cancer treatment with radiation or drugs
- People who recently had a transfusion or were given other blood products should ask their doctor when they may get chickenpox vaccine.

Ask your provider for more information.

4. What are the risks from chickenpox vaccine?

A vaccine, like any medicine, is capable of causing serious problems, such as severe allergic reactions. The risk of chickenpox vaccine causing serious harm, or death, is extremely small.

Getting chickenpox vaccine is much safer than getting chickenpox disease. Most people who get chickenpox vaccine do not have any problems with it. Reactions are usually more likely after the first dose than after the second.

▶ MILD PROBLEMS

- Soreness or swelling where the shot was given (about 1 out of 5 children and up to 1 out of 3 adolescents and adults)
- Fever (1 person out of 10, or less)
- Mild rash, up to a month after vaccination (1 person out of 25). It is possible for these people to infect other members of their household, but this is extremely rare.

▶ MODERATE PROBLEMS

- Seizure (jerking or staring) caused by fever (very rare)

▶ SEVERE PROBLEMS

▸ Pneumonia (very rare)

Other serious problems, including severe brain reactions and low blood count, have been reported after chickenpox vaccination. These happen so rarely experts cannot tell whether they are caused by the vaccine or not. If they are, it is extremely rare.

NOTE: The first dose of **MMRV** vaccine has been associated with rash and higher rates of fever than MMR and varicella vaccines given separately. Rash has been reported in about 1 person in 20 and fever in about 1 person in 5.

Seizures caused by a fever are also reported more often after MMRV. These usually occur 5–12 days after the first dose.

5. What if there is a moderate or severe reaction?

What should I look for?
▸ Any unusual condition, such as a high fever, weakness, or behavior changes. Signs of a serious allergic reaction can include difficulty breathing, hoarseness or wheezing, hives, paleness, weakness, a fast heart beat or dizziness.

What should I do?
▸ **Call** a doctor, or get the person to a doctor right away.
▸ **Tell** your doctor what happened, the date and time it happened, and when the vaccination was given.
▸ **Ask** your provider to report the reaction by filing a Vaccine Adverse Event Reporting System (VAERS) form.

Or you can file this report through the VAERS website at **www.vaers.hhs.gov**, or by calling **1-800-822-7967**.

VAERS does not provide medical advice.

6. The National Vaccine Injury Compensation Program

A federal program has been created to help people who may have been harmed by a vaccine.

For details about the National Vaccine Injury Compensation Program, call **1-800-338-2382** or visit their website at **www.hrsa.gov/vaccinecompensation**.

7. How can I learn more?

▸ Ask your provider. They can give you the vaccine package insert or suggest other sources of information.
▸ Call your local or state health department.
▸ Contact the Centers for Disease Control and Prevention (CDC):
  - Call **1-800-232-4636 (1-800-CDC-INFO)**
  - Visit CDC website at: **www.cdc.gov/vaccines**

Source: Department of Health and Human Services
Centers for Disease Control and Prevention

Vaccine Information Statement (Interim)
Varicella Vaccine (3/13/08) 42 U.S.C. §300aa-26

TETANUS, DIPHTHERIA (Td) OR TETANUS, DIPHTHERIA, PERTUSSIS (Tdap) VACCINE

WHAT YOU NEED TO KNOW

1. Why get vaccinated?

Children 6 years of age and younger are routinely vaccinated against tetanus, diphtheria and pertussis. But older children, adolescents, and adults need protection from these diseases too. Td (Tetanus, Diphtheria) and Tdap (Tetanus, Diphtheria, Pertussis) vaccines provide that protection.

▶ **TETANUS** (Lockjaw) causes painful muscle spasms, usually all over the body.

- It can lead to tightening of the jaw muscles so the victim cannot open his mouth or swallow. Tetanus kills about 1 out of 5 people who are infected.

▶ **DIPHTHERIA** causes a thick covering in the back of the throat.

- It can lead to breathing problems, paralysis, heart failure, and even death.

▶ **PERTUSSIS** (Whooping Cough) causes severe coughing spells, vomiting, and disturbed sleep.

- It can lead to weight loss, incontinence, rib fractures and passing out from violent coughing. Up to 2 in 100 adolescents and 5 in 100 adults with pertussis are hospitalized or have complications, including pneumonia.

These three diseases are all caused by bacteria. Diphtheria and pertussis are spread from person to person. Tetanus enters the body through cuts, scratches, or wounds.

The United States averaged more than 1,300 cases of tetanus and 175,000 cases of diphtheria each year before vaccines. Since vaccines have been available, tetanus cases have fallen by over 96% and diphtheria cases by over 99.9%.

Before 2005, only children younger than than 7 years of age could get pertussis vaccine. In 2004 there were more than 8,000 cases of pertussis in the U.S. among adolescents and more than 7,000 cases among adults.

2. Td and Tdap vaccines

- Td vaccine has been used for many years. It protects against tetanus and diphtheria.
- Tdap was licensed in 2005. It is the first vaccine for adolescents and adults that protects against all three diseases.

NOTE: At this time, Tdap is licensed for only one lifetime dose per person. Td is given every 10 years, and more often if needed.

These vaccines can be used in three ways: 1) as catch-up for people who did not get all their doses of DTaP or DTP when they were children, 2) as a booster dose every 10 years, and 3) for protection against tetanus infection after a wound.

3. Which vaccine, and when?

▶ ROUTINE: ADOLESCENTS 11 THROUGH 18

- A dose of Tdap is recommended for adolescents who got DTaP or DTP as children and have not yet gotten a booster dose of Td. The preferred age is 11–12.
- Adolescents who have already gotten a booster dose of Td are encouraged to get a dose of Tdap as well, for protection against pertussis. Waiting at least 5 years between Td and Tdap is encouraged, but not required.
- Adolescents who did not get all their scheduled doses of DTaP or DTP as children should complete the series using a combination of Td and Tdap.

▶ ROUTINE: ADULTS 19 AND OLDER

- All adults should get a booster dose of Td every 10 years. Adults under 65 who have never gotten Tdap should substitute it for the next booster dose.
- Adults under 65 who expect to have close contact with an infant younger than 12 months of age (including women who may become pregnant) should get a dose of Tdap. Waiting at least 2 years since the last dose of Td is suggested, but not required.
- Health-care workers under 65 who have direct patient contact in hospitals or clinics should get a dose of Tdap. A 2-year interval since the last Td is suggested, but not required.

New mothers who have never gotten Tdap should get a dose as soon as possible after delivery. If vaccination is needed during pregnancy, Td is usually preferred over Tdap.

▶ PROTECTION AFTER A WOUND

A person who gets a severe cut or burn might need a dose of Td or Tdap to prevent tetanus infection. Tdap may be used for people who have never had a dose. But Td should be used if Tdap is not available, or for:

- anybody who has already had a dose of Tdap,
- children 7 through 9 years of age, or
- adults 65 and older.

Tdap and Td may be given at the same time as other vaccines.

4. Some people should not be vaccinated or should wait

- Anyone who has had a life-threatening allergic reaction after a dose of DTP, DTaP, DT, or Td should not get Td or Tdap.
- Anyone who has a severe allergy to any component of a vaccine should not get that vaccine. Tell your provider if the person getting the vaccine has any severe allergies.
- Anyone who had a coma, or long or multiple seizures within 7 days after a dose of DTP or DTaP should not get Tdap, unless a cause other than the vaccine was found (these people *can* get Td).
- Talk to your provider if the person getting either vaccine:
  - has epilepsy or another nervous system problem,
  - had severe swelling or severe pain after a previous dose of DTP, DTaP, DT, Td, or Tdap vaccine, or
  - has had Guillain-Barré Syndrome (GBS).

Anyone who has a moderate or severe illness on the day the shot is scheduled should usually wait until they recover before getting Tdap or Td vaccine. A person with a mild illness or low fever can usually be vaccinated.

5. What are the risks from Tdap and Td vaccines?

With a vaccine (as with any medicine) there is always a small risk of a life-threatening allergic reaction or other serious problem.

Getting tetanus, diphtheria or pertussis would be much more likely to lead to severe problems than getting either vaccine.

Problems reported after Td and Tdap vaccines are listed below.

▶ **MILD PROBLEMS**
(Noticeable, but did not interfere with activities)

Tdap

- Pain (about 3 in 4 adolescents and 2 in 3 adults)
- Redness or swelling (about 1 in 5)
- Mild fever of at least 100.4°F (up to about 1 in 25 adolescents and 1 in 100 adults)
- Headache (about 4 in 10 adolescents and 3 in 10 adults)
- Tiredness (about 1 in 3 adolescents and 1 in 4 adults)
- Nausea, vomiting, diarrhea, stomach ache (up to 1 in 4 adolescents and 1 in 10 adults)
- Chills, body aches, sore joints, rash, swollen glands (uncommon)

Td

- Pain (up to about 8 in 10)
- Redness or swelling (up to about 1 in 3)
- Mild fever (up to about 1 in 15)
- Headache or tiredness (uncommon)

▶ **MODERATE PROBLEMS**
(Interfered with activities, but did not require medical attention)

Tdap

- Pain at the injection site (about 1 in 20 adolescents and 1 in 100 adults)
- Redness or swelling (up to about 1 in 16 adolescents and 1 in 25 adults)
- Fever over 102°F (about 1 in 100 adolescents and 1 in 250 adults)
- Headache (1 in 300)
- Nausea, vomiting, diarrhea, stomach ache (up to 3 in 100 adolescents and 1 in 100 adults)

Td

- Fever over 102°F (rare)

Tdap or Td

- Extensive swelling of the arm where the shot was given (up to about 3 in 100)

▶ **SEVERE PROBLEMS**
(Unable to perform usual activities; required medical attention)

Tdap

- Two adults had nervous system problems after getting the vaccine during clinical trials. These may or may not have been caused by the vaccine. These problems went away on their own and did not cause any permanent harm.

Tdap or Td

- Swelling, severe pain, and redness in the arm where the shot was given (rare)

A severe allergic reaction could occur after any vaccine. They are estimated to occur less than once in a million doses.

6. What if there is a severe reaction?

What should I look for?

Any unusual condition, such as a high fever or behavior changes. Signs of a severe allergic reaction can include difficulty breathing, hoarseness or wheezing, hives, paleness, weakness, a fast heart beat or dizziness.

What should I do?

- Call a doctor, or get the person to a doctor right away.
- Tell the doctor what happened, the date and time it happened, and when the vaccination was given.
- Ask your provider to report the reaction by filing a Vaccine Adverse Event Reporting System (VAERS) form.

Or you can file this report through the VAERS website at **www.vaers.hhs.gov**, or by calling **1-800-822-7967**.

VAERS does not provide medical advice.

7. The National Vaccine Injury Compensation Program

A federal program exists to help pay for the care of anyone who has a serious reaction to a vaccine.

For details about the National Vaccine Injury Compensation Program, call **1-800-338-2382** or visit their website at **www.hrsa.gov/vaccinecompensation.**

8. How can I learn more?

- Ask your provider. They can give you the vaccine package insert or suggest other sources of information.
- Call your local or state health department.
- Contact the Centers for Disease Control and Prevention (CDC):
  - Call **1-800-232-4636** (**1-800-CDC-INFO**) or
  - Visit CDC's website at **www.cdc.gov/vaccines**

Source: Department of Health and Human Services
Centers for Disease Control and Prevention

Vaccine Information Statement (Interim)
Td & Tdap Vaccines (11/18/08) U.S.C. 42

WHAT YOU NEED TO KNOW

1. What is hepatitis A?

Hepatitis A is a serious liver disease caused by the hepatitis A virus (HAV). HAV is found in the stool of persons with hepatitis A. It is usually spread by close personal contact and sometimes by eating food or drinking water containing HAV.

Hepatitis A can cause:

- mild "flulike" illness
- jaundice (yellow skin or eyes)
- severe stomach pains and diarrhea

People with hepatitis A often have to be hospitalized (up to about 1 person in 5).

Sometimes, people die as a result of hepatitis A (about 3–5 deaths per 1,000 cases).

A person who has hepatitis A can easily pass the disease to others within the same household.

Hepatitis A vaccine can prevent hepatitis A.

2. Who should get hepatitis A vaccine and when?

▶ WHO?

Some people should be routinely vaccinated with hepatitis A vaccine:
- All children 1 year (12 through 23 months) of age.
- Persons 1 year of age and older traveling to or working in countries with high or intermediate prevalence of hepatitis A, such as those located in Central or South America, Mexico, Asia (except Japan), Africa, and eastern Europe. For more information see **www.cdc.gov/travel**.
- Children and adolescents through 18 years of age who live in states or communities where routine vaccination has been implemented because of high disease incidence.
- Men who have sex with men.
- Persons who use street drugs.
- Persons with chronic liver disease.
- Persons who are treated with clotting factor concentrates.
- Persons who work with HAV-infected primates or who work with HAV in research laboratories.

Other people might get hepatitis A vaccine in special situations:
- Hepatitis A vaccine might be recommended for children or adolescents in communities where outbreaks of hepatitis A are occurring.

Hepatitis A vaccine is not licensed for children younger than 1 year of age.

▶ **WHEN?**

For children, the first dose should be given at 12–23 months of age. Children who are not vaccinated by 2 years of age can be vaccinated at later visits.

For travelers, the vaccine series should be started at least one month before traveling to provide the best protection.

Persons who get the vaccine less than one month before traveling can also get a shot called immune globulin (IG). IG gives immediate, temporary protection.

For others, the hepatitis A vaccine series may be started whenever a person is at risk of infection.

Two doses of the vaccine are needed for lasting protection. These doses should be given at least 6 months apart.

Hepatitis A vaccine may be given at the same time as other vaccines.

3. Some people should not get hepatitis A vaccine or should wait

- Anyone who has ever had a severe (life-threatening) **allergic reaction to a previous dose** of hepatitis A vaccine should not get another dose.
- Anyone who has a severe (life-threatening) **allergy to any vaccine component** should not get the vaccine. Tell your doctor if you have any severe allergies. All hepatitis A vaccines contain alum and some hepatitis A vaccines contain 2-phenoxyethanol.
- Anyone who is **moderately or severely ill** at the time the shot is scheduled should probably wait until they recover. Ask your doctor or nurse. People with a **mild illness** can usually get the vaccine.
- Tell your doctor if you are **pregnant**. The safety of hepatitis A vaccine for pregnant women has not been determined. But there is no evidence that it is harmful to either pregnant women or their unborn babies. The risk, if any, is thought to be very low.

4. What are the risks from hepatitis A vaccine?

A vaccine, like any medicine, could possibly cause serious problems, such as severe allergic reactions. The risk of hepatitis A vaccine causing serious harm, or death, is extremely small.

Getting hepatitis A vaccine is much safer than getting the disease.

▶ **MILD PROBLEMS**

- Soreness where the shot was given (about 1 out of 2 adults, and up to 1 out of 6 children)
- Headache (about 1 out of 6 adults and 1 out of 25 children)
- Loss of appetite (about 1 out of 12 children)
- Tiredness (about 1 out of 14 adults)

If these problems occur, they usually last 1 or 2 days.

▶ **SEVERE PROBLEMS**

- Serious allergic reaction, within a few minutes to a few hours of the shot (very rare)

5. What if there is a moderate or severe reaction?

What should I look for?

- Any unusual condition, such as a high fever or behavior changes. Signs of a serious allergic reaction can include difficulty breathing, hoarseness or wheezing, hives, paleness, weakness, a fast heart beat or dizziness.

What should I do?

- **Call** a doctor, or get the person to a doctor right away.
- **Tell** your doctor what happened, the date and time it happened, and when the vaccination was given.
- **Ask** your doctor, nurse, or health department to report the reaction by filing a Vaccine Adverse Event Reporting System (VAERS) form.

Or you can file this report through the VAERS website at **www.vaers.hhs.gov**, or by calling **1-800-822-7967.**

VAERS does not provide medical advice.

6. The National Vaccine Injury Compensation Program

In the event that you or your child has a serious reaction to a vaccine, a federal program has been created to help pay for the care of those who have been harmed.

For details about the National Vaccine Injury Compensation Program, call **1-800-338-2382** or visit their website at **www.hrsa.gov/vaccinecompensation.**

7. How can I learn more?

- Ask your doctor or nurse. They can give you the vaccine package insert or suggest other sources of information.
- Call your local or state health department.
- Contact the Centers for Disease Control and Prevention (CDC):
  - Call **1-800-232-4636 (1-800-CDC-INFO)**
  - Visit CDC websites at: **www.cdc.gov/hepatitis** or **www.cdc.gov/nip**

Source: Department of Health and Human Services
Centers for Disease Control and Prevention

Vaccine Information Statement (Interim)
Hepatitis (3/21/06) 42 U.S.C. § 300aa-26

HEPATITIS B VACCINE

WHAT YOU NEED TO KNOW

1. What is hepatitis B?

Hepatitis B is a serious disease that affects the liver. It is caused by the hepatitis B virus (HBV). HBV can cause:

Acute (short-term) illness. This can lead to:
- loss of appetite
- tiredness
- pain in muscles, joints, and stomach
- diarrhea and vomiting
- jaundice (yellow skin or eyes)

Acute illness is more common among adults. Children who become infected usually do not have acute illness.

Chronic (long-term) infection. Some people go on to develop chronic HBV infection. This can be very serious, and often leads to:

- liver damage (cirrhosis)   - liver cancer   - death

Chronic infection is more common among infants and children than among adults. People who are infected can spread HBV to others, even if they don't appear sick.

- In 2005, about 51,000 people became infected with hepatitis B.
- About 1.25 million people in the United States have chronic HBV infection.
- Each year about 3,000 to 5,000 people die from cirrhosis or liver cancer caused by HBV.

Hepatitis B virus is spread through contact with the blood or other body fluids of an infected person. A person can become infected by:
- contact with a mother's blood and body fluids at the time of birth;
- contact with blood and body fluids through breaks in the skin such as bites, cuts, or sores;
- contact with objects that could have blood or body fluids on them such as toothbrushes or razors;
- having unprotected sex with an infected person;
- sharing needles when injecting drugs;
- being stuck with a used needle on the job.

2. Hepatitis B vaccine: Why get vaccinated?

Hepatitis B vaccine can prevent hepatitis B, and the serious consequences of HBV infection, including liver cancer and cirrhosis.

Routine hepatitis B vaccination of U.S. children began in 1991. Since then, the reported incidence of acute hepatitis B among children and adolescents has dropped by more than 95%—and by 75% in all age groups.

Hepatitis B vaccine is made from a part of the hepatitis B virus. It cannot cause HBV infection.

Hepatitis B vaccine is usually given as **a series of 3 or 4 shots.** This vaccine series gives long-term protection from HBV infection, possibly lifelong.

3. Who should get hepatitis B vaccine and when?

▶ CHILDREN AND ADOLESCENTS

- All children should get their first dose of hepatitis B vaccine **at birth** and should have completed the vaccine series by 6–18 months of age.
- Children and adolescents through 18 years of age who did not get the vaccine when they were younger should also be vaccinated.

▶ ADULTS

- All unvaccinated adults **at risk for HBV infection** should be vaccinated. This includes:
  - sex partners of people infected with HBV,
  - men who have sex with men,
  - people who inject street drugs,
  - people with more than one sex partner,
  - people with chronic liver or kidney disease,
  - people with jobs that expose them to human blood,
  - household contacts of people infected with HBV,
  - residents and staff in institutions for the developmentally disabled,
  - kidney dialysis patients,
  - people who travel to countries where hepatitis B is common,
  - people with HIV infection.
- Anyone else who wants to be protected from HBV infection may be vaccinated.

4. Who should NOT get hepatitis B vaccine?

- Anyone with a life-threatening allergy to **baker's yeast**, or to any other **component of the vaccine**, should not get hepatitis B vaccine. Tell your provider if you have any severe allergies.
- Anyone who has had a life-threatening allergic reaction to a **previous dose of hepatitis B vaccine** should not get another dose.
- Anyone who is **moderately or severely ill** when a dose of vaccine is scheduled should probably wait until they recover before getting the vaccine.

Your provider can give you more information about these precautions. Pregnant women who need protection from HBV infection may be vaccinated.

5. Hepatitis B vaccine risks

Hepatitis B is a very safe vaccine. Most people do not have any problems with it.

The following **mild problems** have been reported:

- Soreness where the shot was given (up to about 1 person in 4)
- Temperature of 99.9°F or higher (up to about 1 person in 15)

Severe problems are extremely rare. Severe allergic reactions are believed to occur about once in 1.1 million doses.

A vaccine, like any medicine, *could* cause a serious reaction. But the risk of a vaccine causing serious harm, or death, is extremely small. More than 100 million people have gotten hepatitis B vaccine in the United States.

6. What if there is a moderate or severe reaction?

What should I look for?

- Any unusual condition, such as a high fever or behavior changes. Signs of a serious allergic reaction can include difficulty breathing, hoarseness or wheezing, hives, paleness, weakness, a fast heart beat or dizziness.

What should I do?

- **Call** a doctor, or get the person to a doctor right away.
- **Tell** your doctor what happened, the date and time it happened, and when the vaccination was given.
- **Ask** your doctor, nurse, or health department to report the reaction by filing a Vaccine Adverse Event Reporting System (VAERS) form.

Or you can file this report through the VAERS website at **www.vaers.hhs.gov,** or by calling **1-800-822-7967.**

VAERS does not provide medical advice.

7. The National Vaccine Injury Compensation Program

In the event that you or your child has a serious reaction to a vaccine, a federal program has been created to help pay for the care of those who have been harmed.

For details about the National Vaccine Injury Compensation Program, call 1-800-338-2382 or visit their website at **www.hrsa.gov/vaccinecompensation.**

8. How can I learn more?

- Ask your doctor or nurse. They can give you the vaccine package insert or suggest other sources of information.
- Call your local or state health department.
- Contact the Centers for Disease Control and Prevention (CDC):
  - Call **1-800-232-4636 (1-800-CDC-INFO)**
  - Visit CDC websites at: **www.cdc.gov/ncidod/diseases/hepatitis**
    www.cdc.gov/vaccines
    www.cdc.gov/travel

Source: Department of Health and Human Services
Centers for Disease Control and Prevention

Vaccine Information Statement (Interim)
Hepatitis B (7/18/07) 42 U.S.C. § 300aa-26

HAEMOPHILUS INFLUENZAE
Type b (Hib) VACCINE

WHAT YOU NEED TO KNOW

1. What is Hib disease?

Haemophilus influenzae **type b (Hib) disease is a serious disease caused by a bacteria.** It usually strikes children under 5 years old.

Your child can get Hib disease by being around other children or adults who may have the bacteria and not know it. The germs spread from person to person. If the germs stay in the child's nose and throat, the child probably will not get sick. But sometimes the germs spread into the lungs or the bloodstream, and then Hib can cause serious problems.

Before Hib vaccine, Hib disease was the leading cause of bacterial meningitis among children under 5 years old in the United States. Meningitis is an infection of the brain and spinal cord coverings, which can lead to lasting brain damage and deafness. Hib disease can also cause:

- pneumonia
- severe swelling in the throat, making it hard to breathe
- infections of the blood, joints, bones, and covering of the heart
- death

Before Hib vaccine, about 20,000 children in the United States under 5 years old got severe Hib disease each year and nearly 1,000 people died.

Hib vaccine can prevent Hib disease.

Many more children would get Hib disease if we stopped vaccinating.

2. Who should get Hib vaccine and when?

▶ **CHILDREN SHOULD GET HIB VACCINE AT:**

- 2 months of age
- 4 months of age
- 6 months of age*
- 12–15 months of age

* Depending on what brand of Hib vaccine is used, your child might not need the dose at 6 months of age. Your doctor or nurse will tell you if this dose is needed.

If you miss a dose or get behind schedule, get the next dose as soon as you can. There is no need to start over.

Hib vaccine may be given at the same time as other vaccines.

▶ **OLDER CHILDREN AND ADULTS**

Children over 5 years old usually do not need Hib vaccine. But some older children or adults with special health conditions should get it. These conditions include sickle cell disease, HIV/AIDS, removal of the spleen, bone marrow transplant, or cancer treatment with drugs. Ask your doctor or nurse for details.

3. Some people should not get Hib vaccine or should wait

- People who have ever had a life-threatening allergic reaction to a previous dose of Hib vaccine should not get another dose.
- Children less than 6 weeks of age should not get Hib vaccine.
- People who are moderately or severely ill at the time the shot is scheduled should usually wait until they recover before getting Hib vaccine.

Ask your doctor or nurse for more information.

4. What are the risks from Hib vaccine?

A vaccine, like any medicine, is capable of causing serious problems, such as severe allergic reactions. The risk of Hib vaccine causing serious harm or death is extremely small.

Most people who get Hib vaccine do not have any problems with it.

▶ MILD PROBLEMS

- Redness, warmth, or swelling where the shot was given (up to 1/4 of children)
- Fever over 101° (up to 1 out of 20 children)

If these problems happen, they usually start within a day of vaccination. They may last 2–3 days.

5. What if there is a moderate or severe reaction?

What should I look for?
- Any unusual condition, such as a serious allergic reaction, high fever or behavior changes. Signs of a serious allergic reaction can include difficulty breathing, hoarseness or wheezing, hives, paleness, weakness, a fast heart beat, or dizziness within a few minutes to a few hours after the shot.

What should I do?
- **Call** a doctor, or get the person to a doctor right away.
- **Tell** your doctor what happened, the date and time it happened, and when the vaccination was given.
- **Ask** your doctor, nurse, or health department to report the reaction by filing a Vaccine Adverse Event Reporting System (VAERS) form.

Or you can file this report through the VAERS website at **www.vaers.org,** or by calling **1-800-822-7967.**

VAERS does not provide medical advice

6. The National Vaccine Injury Compensation Program

In the rare event that you or your child has a serious reaction to a vaccine, a federal program has been created to help you pay for the care of those who have been harmed.

For details about the National Vaccine Injury Compensation Program, call **1-800-338-2382** or visit the program's website at **www.hrsa.gov/osp/vicp**.

7. How can I learn more?

- ‣ Ask your doctor or nurse. They can give you the vaccine package insert or suggest other sources of information.
- ‣ Call your local or state health department's immunization program.
- ‣ Contact the Centers for Disease Control and Prevention (CDC):
   - Call **1-800-232-4636 (1-800-CDC-INFO)**
   - Visit the National Immunization Program's website at **www.cdc.gov/nip**

Source: Department of Health and Human Services
Centers for Disease Control and Prevention

Vaccine Information Statement
Hib (12/16/98) 42 U.S.C. § 300aa-26

HPV (HUMAN PAPILLOMA-VIRUS) VACCINE

WHAT YOU NEED TO KNOW

1. What is HPV?

Genital human papillomavirus (HPV) is the most common sexually transmitted virus in the United States.

There are about 40 types of HPV. About 20 million people in the U.S. are infected, and about 6.2 million more get infected each year. HPV is spread through sexual contact.

Most HPV infections don't cause any symptoms, and go away on their own. But HPV is important mainly because it can cause **cervical cancer** in women. Every year in the U.S. about 10,000 women get cervical cancer and 3,700 die from it. It is the 2nd leading cause of cancer deaths among women around the world.

HPV is also associated with several less common types of cancer in both men and women. It can also cause genital warts and warts in the upper respiratory tract.

More than 50% of sexually active men and women are infected with HPV at sometime in their lives.

There is no treatment for HPV infection, but the conditions it causes can be treated.

2. HPV Vaccine—Why get vaccinated?

HPV vaccine is an inactivated (not live) vaccine which protects against 4 major types of HPV.

These include 2 types that cause about 70% of cervical cancer and 2 types that cause about 90% of genital warts. *HPV vaccine can prevent most genital warts and most cases of cervical cancer.*

Protection from HPV vaccine is expected to be long-lasting. But vaccinated women still need cervical cancer screening because the vaccine does not protect against all HPV types that cause cervical cancer.

3. Who should get HPV vaccine and when?

▶ ROUTINE VACCINATION

- ▸ HPV vaccine is routinely recommended for girls **11–12 years of age.** Doctors may give it to girls as young as 9 years.

Why is HPV vaccine given to girls at this age? It is important for girls to get HPV vaccine **before** their first sexual contact—because they have not been exposed to HPV. For these girls, the vaccine can prevent almost 100% of disease caused by the 4 types of HPV targeted by the vaccine.

However, if a girl or woman is already infected with a type of HPV, the vaccine will not prevent disease from that type.

▶ **CATCH-UP VACCINATION**

▸ The vaccine is also recommended for girls and women **13–26 years of age** who did not receive it when they were younger.

HPV vaccine is given as a 3-dose series:

1st Dose:	Now
2nd Dose:	2 months after Dose 1
3rd Dose:	6 months after Dose 1

Additional (booster) doses are not recommended.
HPV vaccine may be given at the same time as other vaccines.

4. Some girls or women should not get HPV vaccine or should wait

▸ Anyone who has ever had a life-threatening **allergic reaction** to **yeast**, to **any other component of HPV vaccine**, or to a **previous dose of HPV vaccine** should not get the vaccine. Tell your doctor if the person getting the vaccine has any severe allergies.
▸ **Pregnant women** should not get the vaccine. The vaccine appears to be safe for both the mother and the unborn baby, but it is still being studied. Receiving HPV vaccine when pregnant is **not** a reason to consider terminating the pregnancy. Women who are breastfeeding may safely get the vaccine.

Any woman who learns that she was pregnant when she got HPV vaccine is encouraged to call the **HPV vaccine in pregnancy registry** at 800-986-8999. Information from this registry will help us learn how pregnant women respond to the vaccine.

▸ People who are mildly ill when the shot is scheduled can still get HPV vaccine. People with **moderate or severe illnesses** should wait until they recover.

5. What are the risks from HPV vaccine?

HPV vaccine does not appear to cause any serious side effects.
However, a vaccine, like any medicine, could possibly cause serious problems, such as severe allergic reactions. The risk of **any** vaccine causing serious harm, or death, is extremely small.
Several **mild problems** may occur with HPV vaccine:

▸ Pain at the injection site (about 8 people in 10)
▸ Redness or swelling at the injection site (about 1 person in 4)
▸ Mild fever (100°F) (about 1 person in 10)
▸ Itching at the injection site (about 1 person in 30)
▸ Moderate fever (102°F) (about 1 person in 65)

These symptoms do not last long and go away on their own.

Life-threatening allergic reactions from vaccines are very rare. If they do occur, it would be within a few minutes to a few hours after the vaccination.

Like all vaccines, HPV vaccine will continue to be monitored for unusual or severe problems.

6. What if there is a severe reaction?

What should I look for?
- Any unusual condition, such as a high fever or behavior changes. Signs of a serious allergic reaction can include difficulty breathing, hoarseness or wheezing, hives, paleness, weakness, a fast heart beat or dizziness.

What should I do?
- **Call** a doctor, or get the person to a doctor right away.
- **Tell** your doctor what happened, the date and time it happened, and when the vaccination was given.
- **Ask** your doctor, nurse, or health department to report the reaction by filing a Vaccine Adverse Event Reporting System (VAERS) form.

Or you can file this report through the VAERS website at **www.vaers.hhs.gov,** or by calling **1-800-822-7967.**

VAERS does not provide medical advice.

7. How can I learn more?

- Ask your doctor or nurse. They can show you the vaccine package insert or suggest other sources of information.
- Call your local or state health department.
- Contact the Centers for Disease Control and Prevention (CDC):
  - Call **1-800-232-4636 (1-800-CDC-INFO)**
  - Visit CDC's website at **www.cdc.gov/vaccines**

Source: Department of Health and Human Services
Centers for Disease Control and Prevention

Vaccine Information Statement (Interim)
Human Papillomavirus (HPV) Vaccine (2/2/07)

INACTIVATED INFLUENZA VACCINE

WHAT YOU NEED TO KNOW

1. Why get vaccinated?

Influenza ("flu") is a contagious disease.
It is caused by the influenza virus, which can be spread by coughing, sneezing, or nasal secretions.

Other illnesses can have the same symptoms and are often mistaken for influenza. But only an illness caused by the influenza virus is really influenza.

Anyone can get influenza, but rates of infection are highest among children. For most people, it lasts only a few days.

It can cause:

- ▸ fever
- ▸ cough
- ▸ sore throat
- ▸ headache
- ▸ chills
- ▸ muscle aches
- ▸ fatigue

Some people get much sicker. Influenza can lead to pneumonia and can be dangerous for people with heart or breathing conditions. It can cause high fever, diarrhea and seizures in children. On average, 226,000 people are hospitalized every year because of influenza and 36,000 die—mostly elderly.

Influenza vaccine can prevent influenza.

2. Inactivated influenza vaccine

There are two types of influenza vaccine:

1. Inactivated (killed) vaccine, or the "flu shot" is given by injection into the muscle. **2. Live, attenuated** (weakened) influenza vaccine is sprayed into the nostrils. *This vaccine is described in a separate Vaccine Information Statement.*

Influenza viruses are always changing. Because of this, influenza vaccines are updated every year, and an annual vaccination is recommended.

Each year scientists try to match the viruses in the vaccine to those most likely to cause flu that year. When there is a close match the vaccine protects most people from serious influenza-related illness. But even when there is not a close match, the vaccine provides some protection. Influenza vaccine will not prevent "influenza-like" illnesses caused by other viruses.

It takes up to 2 weeks for protection to develop after the shot. Protection lasts up to a year.

Some inactivated influenza vaccine contains a preservative called thimerosal. Some people have suggested that thimerosal may be related to developmental problems in children. In 2004 the Institute of Medicine reviewed many studies looking into this theory and concluded that there is no evidence of such a relationship. Thimerosal-free influenza vaccine is available.

3. Who should get inactivated influenza vaccine?

All children 6 months and older and all older adults:

- **All children** from 6 months through 18 years of age.
- Anyone **50 years of age or older.**

Anyone who is at risk of complications from influenza, or more likely to require medical care:

- Women who will be **pregnant** during influenza season.

- Anyone with **long-term health problems** with:
  - heart disease
  - kidney disease
  - liver disease
  - lung disease
  - metabolic disease, such as diabetes
  - asthma
  - anemia, and other blood disorders

- Anyone with a **weakened immune system** due to:
  - HIV/AIDS or other diseases affecting the immune system
  - long-term treatment with drugs such as steroids
  - cancer treatment with x-rays or drugs

- Anyone with certain **muscle or nerve disorders** (such as seizure disorders or cerebral palsy) that can lead to breathing or swallowing problems.

- Anyone 6 months through 18 years of age on **long-term aspirin treatment** (they could develop Reye Syndrome if they got influenza).

- **Residents of nursing homes** and **other chronic-care facilities.**

Anyone who lives with or cares for people at high risk for influenza-related complications:

- **Health care providers.**
- **Household contacts and caregivers of children** from birth up to 5 years of age.
- **Household contacts and caregivers** of
  - people 50 years and older, or
  - anyone with medical conditions that put them at higher risk for severe complications from influenza.

Health care providers may also recommend a yearly influenza vaccination for:

- People who provide **essential community services.**
- People living in **dormitories, correctional facilities**, or under other **crowded conditions**, to prevent outbreaks.
- People at high risk of influenza complications who **travel** to the Southern hemisphere between April and September, or to the tropics or in organized tourist groups at any time.

Influenza vaccine is also recommended for anyone who wants to **reduce the likelihood of becoming ill** with influenza or **spreading influenza to others.**

4. When should I get influenza vaccine?

Plan to get influenza vaccine in October or November if you can. But getting vaccinated in December, or even later, will still be beneficial in most years. You can get the vaccine as soon as it is available, and for as long as illness is occurring in your community. Influenza can occur any time from November through May, but it most often peaks in January or February.

Most people need one dose of influenza vaccine each year. **Children younger than 9 years of age getting influenza vaccine for the first time**—or who got influenza vaccine for the first time last season but got only one dose—should get 2 doses, at least 4 weeks apart, to be protected.

Influenza vaccine may be given at the same time as other vaccines, including pneumococcal vaccine.

5. Some people should talk with a doctor before getting influenza vaccine

Some people should not get inactivated influenza vaccine or should wait before getting it.

- Tell your doctor if you have any **severe** (life-threatening) allergies. Allergic reactions to influenza vaccine are rare.
  - Influenza vaccine virus is grown in eggs. People with a severe egg allergy should not get the vaccine.
  - A severe allergy to any vaccine component is also a reason to not get the vaccine.
  - If you have had a severe reaction after a previous dose of influenza vaccine, tell your doctor.

- Tell your doctor if you ever had Guillain-Barré Syndrome (a severe paralytic illness, also called GBS). You may be able to get the vaccine, but your doctor should help you make the decision.

- People who are moderately or severely ill should usually wait until they recover before getting flu vaccine. If you are ill, talk to your doctor or nurse about whether to reschedule the vaccination. People with a **mild illness** can usually get the vaccine.

6. What are the risks from inactivated influenza vaccine?

A vaccine, like any medicine, could possibly cause serious problems, such as severe allergic reactions. The risk of a vaccine causing serious harm, or death, is extremely small.

Serious problems from influenza vaccine are very rare. The viruses in inactivated influenza vaccine have been killed, so you cannot get influenza from the vaccine.

▶ **MILD PROBLEMS:**

- soreness, redness, or swelling where the shot was given
- fever   • aches

If these problems occur, they usually begin soon after the shot and last 1–2 days.

▶ **SEVERE PROBLEMS:**

- Life-threatening allergic reactions from vaccines are very rare. If they do occur, it is usually within a few minutes to a few hours after the shot.
- In 1976, a type of influenza (swine flu) vaccine was associated with Guillain-Barré Syndrome (GBS). Since then, flu vaccines have not been clearly linked to GBS. However, if there is a risk of GBS from current flu vaccines, it would be no more than 1 or 2 cases per million people vaccinated. This is much lower than the risk of severe influenza, which can be prevented by vaccination.

7. What if there is a severe reaction?

What should I look for?

- Any unusual condition, such as a high fever or behavior changes. Signs of a serious allergic reaction can include difficulty breathing, hoarseness or wheezing, hives, paleness, weakness, a fast heart beat or dizziness.

What should I do?

- **Call** a doctor, or get the person to a doctor right away.
- **Tell** your doctor what happened, the date and time it happened, and when the vaccination was given.
- **Ask** your doctor, nurse, or health department to report the reaction by filing a Vaccine Adverse Event Reporting System (VAERS) form.

Or you can file this report through the VAERS website at **www.vaers.hhs.gov**, or by calling **1-800-822-7967.**

VAERS does not provide medical advice.

8. The National Vaccine Injury Compensation Program

A federal program exists to help pay for the care of anyone who has a serious reaction to a vaccine.

For more information about the National Vaccine Injury Compensation Program, call **1-800-338-2382** or visit their website at **www.hrsa.gov/ vaccinecompensation**.

How can I learn more?

- Ask your immunization provider. They can give you the vaccine package insert or suggest other sources of information.
- Call your local or state health department.
- Contact the Centers for Disease Control and Prevention (CDC):
  - Call **1-800-232-4636 (1-800-CDC-INFO)**
  - Visit CDC's website at **www.cdc.gov/flu**

Source: Department of Health and Human Services Centers for Disease Control and Prevention

Vaccine Information Statement Inactivated Influenza Vaccine (7/24/08) 42 U.S.C. § 300aa-26

LIVE, INTRANASAL INFLUENZA VACCINE

WHAT YOU NEED TO KNOW

1. Why get vaccinated?

Influenza ("flu") is a contagious disease.

It is caused by the influenza virus, which can be spread by coughing, sneezing, or nasal secretions.

Other illnesses can have the same symptoms and are often mistaken for influenza. But only an illness caused by the influenza virus is really influenza.

Anyone can get influenza, but rates of infection are highest among children. For most people, it lasts only a few days. It can cause:

- fever
- cough
- sore throat
- headache
- chills
- muscle aches
- fatigue

Some people get much sicker. Influenza can lead to pneumonia and can be dangerous for people with heart or breathing conditions. It can cause high fever, diarrhea, and seizures in children. On average, 226,000 people are hospitalized every year because of influenza and 36,000 die—mostly elderly.

Influenza vaccine can prevent influenza.

2. Live, attenuated influenza vaccine—LAIV (nasal spray)

There are two types of influenza vaccine:

1. **Live, attenuated** influenza vaccine (LAIV) contains live but attenuated (weakened) influenza virus. It is sprayed into the nostrils. 2. **Inactivated** influenza vaccine, sometimes called the "flu shot," is given by injection. *Inactivated influenza vaccine is described in a separate Vaccine Information Statement.*

Influenza viruses are always changing. Because of this, influenza vaccines are updated every year, and an annual vaccination is recommended.

Each year scientists try to match the viruses in the vaccine to those most likely to cause flu that year. When there is a close match the vaccine protects most people from serious influenza-related illness. But even when there is not a close match, the vaccine provides some protection. Influenza vaccine will *not* prevent "influenza-like" illnesses caused by other viruses.

It takes up to 2 weeks for protection to develop after the vaccination. Protection lasts up to a year.

LAIV does not contain thimerosal or other preservatives.

3. Who can get LAIV?

LAIV is approved for **people from 2 through 49 years of age**, who are not pregnant and do not have certain health conditions (see #4, below). Influenza vaccination is recommended for people who can spread influenza to others at high risk, such as:

- **Household contacts and out-of-home caregivers** of children up to 5 years of age, and people 50 and older.
- Physicians and nurses, and family members or anyone else in **close contact with people at risk** of serious influenza.

Health care providers may also recommend a yearly influenza vaccination for:
- People who provide **essential community services**.
- People living in **dormitories, correctional facilities**, or under other crowded conditions, to prevent outbreaks.

Influenza vaccine is also recommended for anyone who wants to **reduce the likelihood of becoming ill** with influenza or **spreading influenza to others**.

4. Some people should *not* get LAIV

LAIV is not licensed for everyone. The following people should get the **inactivated** vaccine (flu shot) instead:

- **Adults 50 years of age and older or children between 6 months and 2 years of age.** (Children younger than 6 months should not get *either* influenza vaccine.)

- Children younger than 5 with asthma or one or more episodes of **wheezing** within the past year.

- People who have **long-term health problems** with:
  - heart disease
  - lung disease
  - asthma
  - kidney or liver disease
  - metabolic disease, such as diabetes
  - anemia, and other blood disorders

- Anyone with certain **muscle or nerve disorders** (such as seizure disorders or cerebral palsy) that can lead to breathing or swallowing problems.

- Anyone with a **weakened immune system.**

- Children or adolescents on **long-term aspirin treatment**.

- **Pregnant women.**

Tell your doctor if you ever had **Guillain-Barré syndrome** (a severe paralytic illness also called GBS). You may be able to get the vaccine, but your doctor should help you make the decision.

The flu shot is preferred for people (including health-care workers, and family members) in **close contact with anyone who has a severely weakened immune system** (requiring care in a protected environment, such as a bone marrow transplant unit). People in close contact with those whose immune systems are less severely weakened (including those with HIV) may get LAIV.

Anyone with a **nasal condition** serious enough to make breathing difficult, such as a very stuffy nose, should get the flu shot instead.

Some people should talk with a doctor before getting *either* influenza vaccine:

- Anyone who has ever had a <u>serious</u> allergic reaction to **eggs** or another vaccine component, or to a **previous dose** of influenza vaccine. LAIV also contains **MSG, arginine, gentamicin,** and **gelatin.**

▸ People who are moderately or severely ill should usually wait until they recover before getting flu vaccine. If you are ill, talk to your doctor or nurse about whether to reschedule the vaccination. People with a **mild illness** can usually get the vaccine.

5. When should I get influenza vaccine?

Plan to get influenza vaccine in October or November if you can. But getting it in December, or even later, will still be beneficial most years. You can get the vaccine as soon as it is available, and for as long as illness is occurring in your community. Influenza can occur from November through May, but it most often peaks in January or February.

Most people need one dose of influenza vaccine each year. **Children younger than 9 years of age getting influenza vaccine for the first time**—or who got influenza vaccine for the first time last season but got only one dose—should get 2 doses, at least 4 weeks apart, to be protected.

LAIV may be given at the same time as other vaccines.

6. What are the risks from LAIV?

A vaccine, like any medicine, could possibly cause serious problems, such as severe allergic reactions. The risk of a vaccine causing serious harm, or death, is extremely small.

Live influenza vaccine viruses rarely spread from person to person. Even if they do, they are not likely to cause illness.

LAIV is made from weakened virus and does not cause influenza. The vaccine *can* cause mild symptoms in people who get it (see below).

▸ **MILD PROBLEMS:**

Some children and adolescents 2–17 years of age have reported mild reactions, including:

▸ runny nose, nasal congestion or cough   ▸ fever
▸ headache and muscle aches   ▸ wheezing
▸ abdominal pain or occasional vomiting or diarrhea

Some adults 18–49 years of age have reported:

▸ runny nose or nasal congestion   ▸ sore throat
▸ cough, chills, tiredness/weakness   ▸ headache

These symptoms did not last long and went away on their own. Although they can occur after vaccination, they may not have been caused by the vaccine.

▸ **SEVERE PROBLEMS:**

▸ Life-threatening allergic reactions from vaccines are very rare. If they do occur, it is usually within a few minutes to a few hours after the vaccination.

▸ If rare reactions occur with any product, they may not be identified until thousands, or millions, of people have used it. Millions of doses of LAIV have been distributed since it was licensed, and no serious problems have been identified. Like all vaccines, LAIV will continue to be monitored for unusual or severe problems.

7. What if there is a severe reaction?

What should I look for?

‣ Any unusual condition, such as a high fever or behavior changes. Signs of a serious allergic reaction can include difficulty breathing, hoarseness or wheezing, hives, paleness, weakness, a fast heart beat or dizziness.

What should I do?

‣ **Call** a doctor, or get the person to a doctor right away.
‣ **Tell** your doctor what happened, the date and time it happened, and when the vaccination was given.
‣ **Ask** your doctor, nurse, or health department to report the reaction by filing a Vaccine Adverse Event Reporting System (VAERS) form.

Or you can file this report through the VAERS website at **www.vaers.hhs.gov**, or by calling **1-800-822-7967.**

VAERS does not provide medical advice.

8. The National Vaccine Injury Compensation Program

A federal program exists to help pay for the care of anyone who has a serious reaction to a vaccine.

For more information about the National Vaccine Injury Compensation Program, call **1-800-338-2382** or visit their website at **www.hrsa.gov/vaccinecompensation.**

9. How can I learn more?

‣ Ask your immunization provider. They can give you the vaccine package insert or suggest other sources of information.
‣ Call your local or state health department.
‣ Contact the Centers for Disease Control and Prevention (CDC):
  - Call **1-800-232-4636 (1-800-CDC-INFO)**
  - Visit CDC's website at **www.cdc.gov/flu**

Source: Department of Health and Human Services Centers for Disease Control and Prevention

Vaccine Information Statement Live, Attenuated Influenza Vaccine (7/24/08) 42 U.S.C. § 300aa-26

MEASLES, MUMPS & RUBELLA VACCINES

WHAT YOU NEED TO KNOW

1. Why get vaccinated?

Measles, mumps, and rubella are serious diseases.

▶ **MEASLES**

- Measles virus causes rash, cough, runny nose, eye irritation, and fever.
- It can lead to ear infection, pneumonia, seizures (jerking and staring), brain damage, and death.

▶ **MUMPS**

- Mumps virus causes fever, headache, and swollen glands.
- It can lead to deafness, meningitis (infection of the brain and spinal cord covering), painful swelling of the testicles or ovaries, and, rarely, death.

▶ **RUBELLA** (German Measles)

- Rubella virus causes rash, mild fever, and arthritis (mostly in women).
- If a woman gets rubella while she is pregnant, she could have a miscarriage or her baby could be born with serious birth defects.

You or your child could catch these diseases by being around someone who has them. They spread from person to person through the air.

Measles, mumps, and rubella (MMR) vaccine can prevent these diseases.

Most children who get their MMR shots will not get these diseases. Many more children would get them if we stopped vaccinating.

2. Who should get MMR vaccine and when?

Children should get 2 doses of MMR vaccine:
– The first at **12–15 months of age**
– and the second at **4–6 years of age.**

These are the recommended ages. But children can get the second dose at any age, as long as it is at least 28 days after the first dose.

Some **adults** should also get MMR vaccine:

Generally, anyone 18 years of age or older who was born after 1956 should get at least one dose of MMR vaccine, unless they can show that they have had either the vaccines or the diseases.

Ask your provider for more information.

MMR vaccine may be given at the same time as other vaccines.

Note: A "combination" vaccine called **MMRV**, which contains both MMR and varicella (chickenpox) vaccines, may be given instead of the two individual vaccines to people 12 years of age and younger.

3. Some people should not get MMR vaccine or should wait

▸ People should not get MMR vaccine who have ever had a life-threatening allergic reaction to gelatin, the antibiotic neomycin, or to a previous dose of MMR vaccine.

▸ People who are moderately or severely ill at the time the shot is scheduled should usually wait until they recover before getting MMR vaccine.

▸ Pregnant women should wait to get MMR vaccine until after they have given birth. Women should avoid getting pregnant for 4 weeks after getting MMR vaccine.

▸ Some people should check with their doctor about whether they should get MMR vaccine, including anyone who:
- Has HIV/AIDS, or another disease that affects the immune system
- Is being treated with drugs that affect the immune system, such as steroids, for 2 weeks or longer.
- Has any kind of cancer
- Is taking cancer treatment with x-rays or drugs
- Has ever had a low platelet count (a blood disorder)

▸ People who recently had a transfusion or were given other blood products should ask their doctor when they may get MMR vaccine.

Ask your provider for more information.

4. What are the risks from MMR vaccine?

A vaccine, like any medicine, is capable of causing serious problems, such as severe allergic reactions. The risk of MMR vaccine causing serious harm, or death, is extremely small.

Getting MMR vaccine is much safer than getting any of these three diseases. Most people who get MMR vaccine do not have any problems with it.

▸ MILD PROBLEMS

▸ Fever (up to 1 person out of 6)
▸ Mild rash (about 1 person out of 20)
▸ Swelling of glands in the cheeks or neck (rare)

If these problems occur, it is usually within 7–12 days after the shot. They occur less often after the second dose.

▸ MODERATE PROBLEMS

▸ Seizure (jerking or staring) caused by fever (about 1 out of 3,000 doses)
▸ Temporary pain and stiffness in the joints, mostly in teenage or adult women (up to 1 out of 4)

- Temporary low platelet count, which can cause a bleeding disorder (about 1 out of 30,000 doses)

▶ **SEVERE PROBLEMS** (Very Rare)

- Serious allergic reaction (less than 1 out of a million doses)
- Several other severe problems have been known to occur after a child gets MMR vaccine. But this happens so rarely, experts cannot be sure whether they are caused by the vaccine or not. These include:
  - Deafness
  - Long-term seizures, coma, or lowered consciousness
  - Permanent brain damage

Note: The first dose of **MMRV** vaccine has been associated with rash and higher rates of fever than MMR and varicella vaccines given separately. Rash has been reported in about 1 person in 20 and fever in about 1 person in 5.

Seizures caused by a fever are also reported more often after MMRV. These usually occur 5–12 days after the first dose.

5. What if there is a moderate or severe reaction?

What should I look for?

- Any unusual condition, such as a high fever, weakness, or behavior changes. Signs of a serious allergic reaction can include difficulty breathing, hoarseness or wheezing, hives, paleness, weakness, a fast heart beat or dizziness.

What should I do?

- **Call** a doctor, or get the person to a doctor right away.
- **Tell** your doctor what happened, the date and time it happened, and when the vaccination was given.
- **Ask** your provider to report the reaction by filing a Vaccine Adverse Event Reporting System (VAERS) form.

Or you can file this report through the VAERS website at **www.vaers.hhs. gov**, or by calling **1-800-822-7967**.

VAERS does not provide medical advice.

6. The National Vaccine Injury Compensation Program

A federal program has been created to help people who may have been harmed by a vaccine.

For details about the National Vaccine Injury Compensation Program, call **1-800-338-2382** or visit their website at **www.hrsa.gov/vaccine compensation**.

7. How can I learn more?

- Ask your provider. They can give you the vaccine package insert or suggest other sources of information.

- Call your local or state health department.
- Contact the Centers for Disease Control and Prevention (CDC):
  - Call **1-800-232-4636 (1-800-CDC-INFO)**
  - Visit CDC website at: **www.cdc.gov/vaccines**

Source: Department of Health and Human Services Centers for Disease Control and Prevention

Vaccine Information Statement (Interim), MMR Vaccine (3/13/08) 42 U.S.C. § 300aa-26

PNEUMOCOCCAL CONJUGATE VACCINE

WHAT YOU NEED TO KNOW

1. Pneumococcal disease

Infection with *Streptococcus pneumoniae* bacteria can make children very sick. It causes blood infections, pneumonia, and bacterial meningitis, mostly in young children. (Meningitis is an infection of the covering of the brain.) Pneumococcal meningitis kills about 3 people in 10 who get it.

Pneumococcal meningitis can also lead to other health problems, including deafness and brain damage.

Before there was a vaccine, pneumococcal infection caused:

- over 700 cases of meningitis,
- 13,000 blood infections,
- about 5 million ear infections, and
- about 200 deaths

every year in the United States in children under 5.

Children younger than 2 years of age are at highest risk for serious disease.

Pneumococcal bacteria are spread from person to person through close contact.

Pneumococcal infections can be hard to treat because some strains of the bacteria have become resistant to the drugs that have been used to treat them. This makes **prevention** of pneumococcal infections, through vaccination, even more important.

2. Pneumococcal conjugate vaccine (PCV)

There are 91 strains of pneumococcal bacteria. Pneumococcal conjugate vaccine (PCV) protects against 7 of them. These 7 strains are responsible for most severe pneumococcal infections among children. Since PCV came into use, severe pneumococcal disease has dropped by nearly 80% among children under 5.

PCV can also prevent some cases of pneumonia and some ear infections. But pneumonia and ear infections have many causes, and PCV only works against those caused by pneumococcal bacteria.

PCV is given to infants and toddlers . . . to protect them when they are at greatest risk for serious diseases caused by pneumococcal bacteria.

Older children and adults with certain chronic illnesses may get a different vaccine called pneumococcal *polysaccharide* vaccine. There is a separate Vaccine Information Statement for that vaccine.

3. Who should get PCV and when?

▶ **INFANTS AND CHILDREN UNDER 2 YEARS OF AGE**

PCV is routinely given as a series of 4 doses, one dose at each of these ages:

- 2 months   - 6 months
- 4 months   - 12–15 months

Children who miss their shots at these ages should still get the vaccine. The number of doses and the intervals between doses will depend on the child's age. Ask your health care provider for details.

▶ **CHILDREN 2 THROUGH 4 YEARS OF AGE**

- Healthy children between their 2nd and 5th birthdays who have not completed the PCV series should get 1 dose.

- Children with medical conditions such as:
  - sickle cell disease,
  - a damaged spleen or no spleen,
  - cochlear implants,
  - HIV/AIDS or other diseases that affect the immune system (such as diabetes, cancer, or liver disease), or
  - chronic heart or lung disease . . .

  or children who take medications that affect the immune system, such as chemotherapy or steroids . . . should get 1 or 2 doses of PCV, if they have not already completed the 4-dose series. Ask your health care provider for details.

PCV may be given at the same time as other vaccines.

4. Some children should not get PCV or should wait

Children should not get pneumococcal conjugate vaccine if they had a serious (life-threatening) allergic reaction to a previous dose of this vaccine, or if they have a severe allergy to any vaccine component. Tell your health-care provider if your child has ever had a severe reaction to any vaccine, or has any severe allergies.

Children with minor illnesses, such as a cold, may be vaccinated. But children who are moderately or severely ill should usually wait until they recover before getting the vaccine.

5. What are the risks from PCV?

Any medicine, including a vaccine, could possibly cause a serious problem, such as a severe allergic reaction. However, the risk of any vaccine causing serious harm, or death, is extremely small.

In studies (nearly 60,000 doses), pneumococcal conjugate vaccine was associated with only mild reactions:

- Up to about 1 infant out of 4 had redness, tenderness, or swelling where the shot was given.
- Up to about 1 out of 3 had a fever greater than 100.4°F, and up to about 1 in 50 had a higher fever (over 102.2°F).
- Some children also became fussy or drowsy, or had a loss of appetite.

No serious reactions have been associated with this vaccine.

Life-threatening allergic reactions from vaccines are very rare. If they do occur, it would be within a few minutes to a few hours after the vaccination.

6. What if there is a severe reaction?

What should I look for?

- Any unusual condition, such as a high fever or behavior changes. Signs of a severe allergic reaction can include difficulty breathing, hoarseness or wheezing, hives, paleness, weakness, a fast heart beat or dizziness.

What should I do?

- **Call** a doctor, or get the person to a doctor right away.
- **Tell** the doctor what happened, the date and time it happened, and when the vaccination was given.
- **Ask** your provider to report the reaction by filing a Vaccine Adverse Event Reporting System (VAERS) form.

Or you can file this report through the VAERS website at **www.vaers.hhs. gov**, or by calling **1-800-822-7967**.

VAERS does not provide medical advice.

7. The National Vaccine Injury Compensation Program

A federal program exists to help pay for the care of anyone who has a serious reaction to a vaccine.

For more information about the National Vaccine Injury Compensation Program, call **1-800-338-2382** or visit their website at **www.hrsa.gov/ vaccinecompensation**.

8. How can I learn more?

- Ask your provider. They can give you the vaccine package insert or suggest other sources of information.
- Call your local or state health department.
- Contact the Centers for Disease Control and Prevention (CDC):
  - Call **1-800-232-4636** (**1-800-CDC-INFO**) or
  - Visit CDC's website at **www.cdc.gov/vaccines**

Source: Department of Health and Human Services Centers for Disease Control and Prevention

Vaccine Information Statement (Interim), Pneumococcal Conjugate Vaccine (12/9/08) 42 U.S.C. § 300aa-26

PNEUMOCOCCAL POLYSACCHARIDE VACCINE

WHAT YOU NEED TO KNOW

1. Why get vaccinated?

Pneumococcal disease is a serious disease that causes much sickness and death. In fact, pneumococcal disease kills more people in the United States each year than all other vaccine preventable diseases combined. Anyone can get pneumococcal disease. However, some people are at greater risk from the disease. These include people 65 and older, the very young, and people with special health problems such as alcoholism, heart or lung disease, kidney failure, diabetes, HIV infection, or certain types of cancer.

Pneumococcal disease can lead to serious infections of the lungs (pneumonia), the blood (bacteremia), and the covering of the brain (meningitis). About 1 out of every 20 people who get pneumococcal pneumonia dies from it, as do about 2 people out of 10 who get bacteremia and 3 people out of 10 who get meningitis. People with the special health problems mentioned above are even more likely to die from the diease.

Drugs such as penicillin were once effective in treating these infections; but the disease has become more resistant to these drugs, making treatment of pneumococcal infections more difficult. This makes prevention of the disease through vaccination even more important.

2. Pneumococcal polysaccharide vaccine (PPV)

The pneumococcal polysaccharide vaccine (PPV) protects against 23 types of pneumococcal bacteria. Most healthy adults who get the vaccine develop protection to most or all of these types within 2 to 3 weeks of getting the shot. Very old people, children under 2 years of age, and people with some long-term illnesses might not respond as well or at all.

3. Who should get PPV?

- All adults 65 years of age or older.

- Anyone over 2 years of age who has a long-term health problem such as:
  - heart disease
  - lung disease
  - sickle cell disease
  - diabetes
  - alcoholism
  - cirrhosis
  - leaks of cerebrospinal fluid

- Anyone over 2 years of age who has a disease or condition that lowers the body's resistance to infection, such as:
  - Hodgkin's disease
  - lymphoma, leukemia
  - kidney failure
  - multiple myeloma
  - nephrotic syndrome
  - HIV infection or AIDS
  - damaged spleen, or no spleen
  - organ transplant

- Anyone over 2 years of age who is taking any drug or treatment that lowers the body's resistance to infection, such as:
  - long-term steroids
  - certain cancer drugs
  - radiation therapy

- Alaskan Natives and certain Native American populations.

4. How many doses of PPV are needed?

Usually one dose of PPV is all that is needed.
However, under some circumstances a second dose may be given.

- A second dose is recommended for those people aged 65 and older who got their first dose when they were under 65, if 5 or more years have passed since that dose.

- A second dose is also recommended for people who:
  - have a damaged spleen or no spleen
  - have sickle-cell disease
  - have HIV infection or AIDS
  - have cancer, leukemia, lymphoma, multiple myeloma
  - have kidney failure
  - have nephrotic syndrome
  - have had an organ or bone marrow transplant
  - are taking medication that lowers immunity (such as chemotherapy or long-term steroids)

Children 10 years old and younger may get this second dose 3 years after the first dose. Those older than 10 should get it 5 years after the first dose.

5. Other facts about getting the vaccine

- Otherwise healthy children who often get ear infections, sinus infections, or other upper respiratory diseases do not need to get PPV because of these conditions.
- PPV may be less effective in some people, especially those with lower resistance to infection. But these people should still be vaccinated, because they are more likely to get seriously ill from pneumococcal disease.

- **Pregnancy**: The safety of PPV for pregnant women has not yet been studied. There is no evidence that the vaccine is harmful to either the mother or the fetus, but pregnant women should consult with their doctor before being vaccinated.Women who are at high risk of pneumococcal disease should be vaccinated before becoming pregnant, if possible.

6. What are the risks from PPV?

PPV is a very safe vaccine.

About half of those who get the vaccine have very mild side effects, such as redness or pain where the shot is given.

Less than 1% develop a fever, muscle aches, or more severe local reactions. Severe allergic reactions have been reported very rarely.

As with any medicine, there is a very small risk that serious problems, even death, could occur after getting a vaccine.

Getting the disease is much more likely to cause serious problems than getting the vaccine.

7. What if there is a serious reaction?

What should I look for?

- Severe allergic reaction (hives, difficulty breathing, shock)

What should I do?

- **Call** a doctor, or get the person to a doctor right away.
- **Tell** your doctor what happened, the date and time it happened, and when the vaccination was given.
- **Ask** your doctor, nurse, or health department to report the reaction by filing a Vaccine Adverse Event Reporting System (VAERS) form.

Or you can file this report through the VAERS website at **www.vaers.org**, or by calling **1-800-822-7967.**

VAERS does not provide medical advice.

8. How can I learn more?

- Ask your doctor or nurse. They can give you the vaccine package insert or suggest other sources of information.
- Call your local or state health department.
- Contact the Centers for Disease Control and Prevention (CDC):
  - Call **1-800-232-4636 (1-800-CDC-INFO)** or
  - Visit the National Immunization Program website at **www.cdc.gov/nip**

Source: Department of Health and Human Services
Centers for Disease Control and Prevention

Vaccine Information Statement,
Pneumococcal Vaccine (7/29/97)

WHAT YOU NEED TO KNOW

1. What is polio?

Polio is a disease caused by a virus. It enters a child's (or adult's) body through the mouth. Sometimes it does not cause serious illness. But sometimes it causes *paralysis* (can't move arm or leg). It can kill people who get it, usually by paralyzing the muscles that help them breathe.

Polio used to be very common in the United States. It paralyzed and killed thousands of people a year before we had a vaccine for it.

2. Why get vaccinated?

Inactivated Polio Vaccine (IPV) can prevent polio.

History: A 1916 polio epidemic in the United States killed 6,000 people and paralyzed 27,000 more. In the early 1950's there were more than 20,000 cases of polio each year. **Polio vaccination was begun in 1955.** By 1960 the number of cases had dropped to about 3,000, and by 1979 there were only about 10. The success of polio vaccination in the U.S. and other countries sparked a world-wide effort to eliminate polio.

Today: No wild polio has been reported in the United States for over 20 years. But the disease is still common in some parts of the world. It would only take one case of polio from another country to bring the disease back if we were not protected by vaccine. If the effort to eliminate the disease from the world is successful, some day we won't need polio vaccine. Until then, we need to keep getting our children vaccinated.

ORAL POLIO VACCINE: NO LONGER RECOMMENDED

There are two kinds of polio vaccine: **IPV**, which is the shot recommended in the United States today, and a live, oral polio vaccine (**OPV**), which is drops that are swallowed.

Until recently OPV was recommended for most children in the United States. OPV helped us rid the country of polio, and it is still used in many parts of the world.

Both vaccines give immunity to polio, but OPV is better at keeping the disease from spreading to other people. However, for a few people (about one in 2.4 million), OPV actually causes polio. Since the risk of getting polio in the United States is now extremely low, experts believe that using oral polio vaccine is no longer worth the slight risk, except in limited circumstances which your doctor can describe. The polio shot (IPV) does not cause polio. **If you or your child will be getting OPV, ask for a copy of the OPV Supplemental Vaccine Information Statement.**

3. Who should get polio vaccine and when?

IPV is a shot, given in the leg or arm, depending on age.
Polio vaccine may be given at the same time as other vaccines.

▶ **CHILDREN**

Most people should get polio vaccine when they are children. Children get 4 doses of IPV, at these ages:

- A dose at 2 months
- A dose at 4 months
- A dose at 6–18 months
- A booster dose at 4–6 years

▶ **ADULTS**

Most adults do not need polio vaccine because they were already vaccinated as children. But three groups of adults are at higher risk and *should* consider polio vaccination:

(1) people traveling to areas of the world where polio is common,
(2) laboratory workers who might handle polio virus, and
(3) health care workers treating patients who could have polio.

Adults in these three groups who **have never been vaccinated against polio** should get 3 doses of IPV:

- The first dose at any time,
- The second dose 1 to 2 months later,
- The third dose 6 to 12 months after the second.

Adults in these three groups who have **had 1 or 2 doses** of polio vaccine in the past should get the remaining 1 or 2 doses. It doesn't matter how long it has been since the earlier dose(s).

Adults in these three groups who **have had 3 or more doses** of polio vaccine (either IPV or OPV) in the past may get a booster dose of IPV.

Ask your health care provider for more information.

4. Some people should not get IPV or should wait.

These people should not get IPV:

- Anyone who has ever had a life-threatening allergic reaction to the antibiotics **neomycin, streptomycin** or **polymyxin B** should not get the polio shot.
- Anyone who has a severe allergic reaction to a polio shot should not get another one.

These people should wait:

- Anyone who is moderately or severely ill at the time the shot is scheduled should usually wait until they recover before getting polio vaccine. People with minor illnesses, such as a cold, *may* be vaccinated.

Ask your health care provider for more information.

5. What are the risks from IPV?

Some people who get IPV get a sore spot where the shot was given. The vaccine used today has never been known to cause any serious problems, and most people don't have any problems at all with it.

However, a vaccine, like any medicine, could cause serious problems, such as a severe allergic reaction. *The risk of a polio shot causing serious harm, or death, is extremely small.*

6. What if there is a serious reaction?

What should I look for?

Look for any unusual condition, such as a serious allergic reaction, high fever, or unusual behavior.

If a serious allergic reaction occurred, it would happen within a few minutes to a few hours after the shot. Signs of a serious allergic reaction can include difficulty breathing, weakness, hoarseness or wheezing, a fast heart beat, hives, dizziness, paleness, or swelling of the throat.

What should I do?

- **Call** a doctor, or get the person to a doctor right away.
- **Tell** your doctor what happened, the date and time it happened, and when the vaccination was given.
- **Ask** your doctor, nurse, or health department to report the reaction by filing a Vaccine Adverse Event Reporting System (VAERS) form.

Or you can file this report through the VAERS website at **www.vaers.org**, or by calling **1-800-822-7967.**

VAERS does not provide medical advice.

Reporting reactions helps experts learn about possible problems with vaccines.

7. The National Vaccine Injury Compensation Program

In the rare event that you or your child has a serious reaction to a vaccine, there is a federal program that can help pay for the care of those who have been harmed.

For details about the National Vaccine Injury Compensation Program, call **1-800-338-2382** or visit the program's website at **http: //www.hrsa.gov/osp/vicp.**

8. How can I learn more?

- Ask your doctor or nurse. They can give you the vaccine package insert or suggest other sources of information.
- Call your local or state health department's immunization program.
- Contact the Centers for Disease Control and Prevention (CDC):
  - Call **1-800-232-4636 (1-800-CDC-INFO)**
  - Visit the National Immunization Program's website at **http: //www.cdc.gov/nip**

Source: Department of Health and Human Services
Centers for Disease Control and Prevention

Vaccine Information Statement, Polio
(1/1/2000) 42 U.S.C. § 300aa-26

WHAT YOU NEED TO KNOW

1. What is rotavirus?

Rotavirus is a virus that causes severe diarrhea, mostly in babies and young children. It is often accompanied by vomiting and fever.

Rotavirus is not the only cause of severe diarrhea, but it is one of the most serious. Before rotavirus vaccine was used, rotavirus was responsible for:

- more than 400,000 doctor visits,
- more than 200,000 emergency room visits,
- 55,000 to 70,000 hospitalizations, and
- 20–60 deaths in the United States each year.

Almost all children in the U.S. are infected with rotavirus before their 5th birthday.

Children are most likely to get rotavirus diarrhea between November and May, depending on the part of the country.

Your baby can become infected by being around other children who have rotavirus diarrhea.

2. Rotavirus vaccine

Better hygiene and sanitation have not reduced rotavirus diarrhea very much in the United States. The best way to protect your baby is with rotavirus vaccine.

Rotavirus vaccine is an oral (swallowed) vaccine, not a shot.

Rotavirus vaccine will not prevent diarrhea or vomiting caused by other germs, but it is very good at preventing diarrhea and vomiting caused by rotavirus. Most babies who get the vaccine will not get rotavirus diarrhea at all, and almost all of them will be protected from *severe* rotavirus diarrhea.

Babies who get the vaccine are also much less likely to be hospitalized or to see a doctor because of rotavirus diarrhea.

3. Who should get rotavirus vaccine and when?

There are two brands of rotavirus vaccine. A baby should get either 2 or 3 doses, depending on which brand is used.

The doses are recommended at these ages:

First Dose:	2 months of age
Second Dose:	4 months of age
Third Dose:	6 months of age (if needed)

The first dose may be given as early as 6 weeks of age, and should be given by age 14 weeks 6 days. The last dose should be given by 8 months of age.

Rotavirus vaccine may be given at the same time as other childhood vaccines. Babies who get the vaccine may be fed normally afterward.

4. Some babies should not get rotavirus vaccine or should wait

- A baby who has had a severe (life-threatening) allergic reaction to a dose of rotavirus vaccine should not get another dose. A baby who has a severe (life-threatening) allergy to any component of rotavirus vaccine should not get the vaccine. Tell your doctor if your baby has any severe allergies that you know of, including a severe allergy to latex.

- Babies who are moderately or severely ill at the time the vaccination is scheduled should probably wait until they recover. This includes babies who have moderate or severe diarrhea or vomiting. Ask your doctor or nurse. Babies with mild illnesses should usually get the vaccine.

- Check with your doctor if your baby's immune system is weakened because of:
  - HIV/AIDS, or any other disease that affects the immune system
  - treatment with drugs such as long-term steroids
  - cancer, or cancer treatment with x-rays or drugs

In the late 1990s a different type of rotavirus vaccine was used. This vaccine was found to be associated with an uncommon type of bowel obstruction called "intussusception," and it was taken off the market.

The new rotavirus vaccines have not been associated with intussusception.

However, babies who have had intussusception, from any cause, are at higher risk for getting it again. If your baby has ever had intussusception, discuss this with your doctor.

5. What are the risks from rotavirus vaccine?

A vaccine, like any medicine, could possibly cause serious problems, such as severe allergic reactions. The risk of any vaccine causing serious harm, or death, is extremely small.

Most babies who get rotavirus vaccine do not have any problems with it.

▶ MILD PROBLEMS

Babies may be slightly more likely to be irritable, or to have mild, temporary diarrhea or vomiting after getting a dose of rotavirus vaccine than babies who did not get the vaccine.

Rotavirus vaccine does not appear to cause any serious side effects.

If rare reactions occur with any new product, they may not be identified until thousands, or millions, of people have used it. Like all vaccines, rotavirus vaccine will continue to be monitored for unusual or severe problems.

6. What if there is a moderate or severe reaction?

What should I look for?
- Any unusual condition, such as a high fever or behavior changes. Signs of a serious allergic reaction can include difficulty breathing, hoarseness or wheezing, hives, paleness, weakness, a fast heart beat or dizziness.

What should I do?
- **Call** a doctor, or get the person to a doctor right away.
- **Tell** your doctor what happened, the date and time it happened, and when the vaccination was given.
- **Ask** your doctor, nurse, or health department to report the reaction by filing a Vaccine Adverse Event Reporting System (VAERS) form.

Or you can file this report through the VAERS website at **www.vaers.hhs.gov**, or by calling **1-800-822-7967**.

VAERS does not provide medical advice.

7. The National Vaccine Injury Compensation Program

A federal program has been created to help people who may have been harmed by a vaccine.

For details about the National Vaccine Injury Compensation Program, call **1-800-338-2382** or visit their website at **www.hrsa.gov/vaccinecompensation**.

8. How can I learn more?

- Ask your doctor or nurse. They can give you the vaccine package insert or suggest other sources of information.
- Call your local or state health department.
- Contact the Centers for Disease Control and Prevention (CDC):
  - Call **1-800-232-4636 (1-800-CDC-INFO)**
  - Visit CDC's National Immunization Program website at: **www.cdc.gov/vaccines**

Source: Department of Health and Human Services Centers for Disease Control and Prevention

Vaccine Information Statement (Interim)
Rotavirus (8/28/08)

SHINGLES VACCINE

WHAT YOU NEED TO KNOW

1. What is shingles?

Shingles is a painful skin rash, often with blisters. It is also called Herpes Zoster.

A shingles rash usually appears on one side of the face or body and lasts from 2 to 4 weeks. Its main symptom is pain, which can be quite severe. Other symptoms of shingles can include fever, headache, chills and upset stomach. Very rarely, a shingles infection can lead to pneumonia, hearing problems, blindness, brain inflammation (encephalitis) or death.

For about 1 person in 5, severe pain can continue even after the rash clears up. This is called **post-herpetic neuralgia**.

Shingles is caused by the Varicella Zoster virus, the same virus that causes chickenpox. Only someone who has had a case of chickenpox—or gotten chickenpox vaccine—can get shingles. The virus stays in your body. It can reappear many years later to cause a case of shingles.

You can't catch shingles from another person with shingles. However, a person who has never had chickenpox (or chickenpox vaccine) could get **chickenpox** from someone with shingles. This is not very common.

Shingles is far more common in people 50 and older than in younger people. It is also more common in people whose immune systems are weakened because of a disease such as cancer, or drugs such as steroids or chemotherapy. At least 1 million people a year in the United States get shingles.

2. Shingles vaccine

A vaccine for shingles was licensed in 2006. In clinical trials, the vaccine prevented shingles in about half of people 60 years of age and older. It can also reduce the pain associated with shingles.

A **single dose** of shingles vaccine is indicated for adults **60 years of age and older**.

3. Some people should not get shingles vaccine or should wait

A person should not get shingles vaccine who:

- has ever had a life-threatening **allergic reaction** to **gelatin**, the antibiotic **neomycin**, or **any other component of shingles vaccine**. Tell your doctor if you have any severe allergies.

- has a **weakened immune system** because of
  - HIV/AIDS or another disease that affects the immune system,
  - treatment with drugs that affect the immune system, such as steroids,
  - cancer treatment such as radiation or chemotherapy,
  - a history of cancer affecting the bone marrow or lymphatic system, such as leukemia or lymphoma.

- has active, untreated **tuberculosis.**

- is **pregnant**, or might be pregnant. Women should not become pregnant until at least three months after getting shingles vaccine.

Someone with a minor illness, such as a cold, may be vaccinated. But anyone who is moderately or severely ill should usually wait until they recover before getting the vaccine. This includes anyone with a temperature of 101.3°F or higher.

4. What are the risks from shingles vaccine?

A vaccine, like any medicine, could possibly cause serious problems, such as severe allergic reactions. However, the risk of a vaccine causing serious harm, or death, is extremely small.

No serious problems have been identified with shingles vaccine.

▶ MILD PROBLEMS

- Redness, soreness, swelling, or itching at the site of the injection (about 1 person in 3)
- Headache (about 1 person in 70)

Like all vaccines, shingles vaccine is being closely monitored for unusual or severe problems.

5. What if there is a moderate or severe reaction?

What should I look for?

- Any unusual condition, such as a high fever or behavior changes. Signs of a serious allergic reaction can include difficulty breathing, hoarseness or wheezing, hives, paleness, weakness, a fast heart beat or dizziness. These usually occur within the first few hours after vaccination.

What should I do?

- **Call** a doctor, or get the person to a doctor right away.
- **Tell** your doctor what happened, the date and time it happened, and when the vaccination was given.
- **Ask** your doctor, nurse, or health department to report the reaction by filing a Vaccine Adverse Event Reporting System (VAERS) form.

Or you can file this report through the VAERS website at **www.vaers.hhs.gov**, or by calling **1-800-822-7967.**

VAERS does not provide medical advice.

6. How can I learn more?

▸ Your provider can give you the vaccine package insert or suggest other sources of information.
▸ Call your local or state health department.
▸ Contact the Centers for Disease Control and Prevention (CDC):
  - Call **1-800-232-4636 (1-800-CDC-INFO)**
  - Visit CDC's website at **www.cdc.gov/nip**

Source: Department of Health and Human Services
Centers for Disease Control and Prevention

Vaccine Information Statement (Interim)
Shingles Vaccine (9/11/06)

INTRODUCTION: **About This Book**

1. Partnership for Prevention, "New Study: Boosting 5 Preventive Services Would Save 100,000 Lives Each Year," August 7, 2007, www.prevent.org/content/view/131/72.

CHAPTER 1. **Abdominal Aortic Aneurysm Screening**

1. USPSTF, release date February 2005.

CHAPTER 2. **Alcohol Misuse Counseling**

1. USPSTF, release date April 2004.

2. This section is based on the National Institute of Alcohol Abuse and Alcoholism's *Rethinking Drinking,* 2009.

3. The following statistics are adapted from "Quick Stats: General Information on Alcohol Use and Health," a CDC web page, www.cdc.gov/alcohol/quickstats/general_info.htm.

CHAPTER 3. **Aspirin to Prevent Cardiovascular Disease**

1. USPSTF, release date March 2009.

CHAPTER 4. **Blood Pressure Screening**

1. USPSTF, release date December 2007.

CHAPTER 5. **Breast Cancer Preventive Services**

1. USPSTF, release dates November 2009, September 2005, and July 2002, respectively for each bulleted recommendation.

2. From the Surveillance Epidemiology and End Results (SEER) website, http://seer.cancer.gov, accessed October 1, 2008. SEER is a service of the National Cancer Institute, which is a branch of the National Institutes of Health.

3. Adapted from the National Cancer Institute's *What You Need to Know About Breast Cancer,* 2005, www.cancer.gov/cancertopics/types/breast.

4. "American Cancer Society Guidelines for Breast Screening with MRI as an Adjunct to Mammography," 2007.

5. Vogel VG, et al. "Effects of Tamoxifen vs. Raloxifene on the Risk of Developing Invasive Breast Cancer and Other Disease Outcomes: The NSABP Study of Tamoxifen and Raloxifene (STAR) P-2 trial," *JAMA* 295, no. 3 (June 2006): 2727-41. Epub 2006, Jun 5.

CHAPTER 6. Cervical Cancer Screening and HPV

1. From the Surveillance Epidemiology and End Results (SEER) website, http://seer.cancer.gov, accessed February 20, 2008. SEER is a service of the National Cancer Institute (NCI), which is a branch of the National Institutes of Health (NIH).

2. USPSTF, release date January 2003.

3. CDC, "Quadrivalent Human Papillomavirus Vaccine," 2007.

4. Because the HPV vaccine is relatively new, and most of the guidance is coming directly from the CDC, this section is largely based on patient-oriented materials from the CDC website, www.cdc.gov/std/hpv/STDFact-HPV-vaccine-young-women.htm.

CHAPTER 7. Chlamydia Screening

1. USPSTF, release date June 2007.

2. Much of the information in this section has been adapted from the CDC fact sheet "Chlamydia," updated December 2007, www.cdc.gov/std/Chlamydia/STDFact-Chlamydia.htm.

CHAPTER 8. Cholesterol Screening

1. USPSTF, release date June 2008.

CHAPTER 9. Colon Cancer Screening

1. Screening with high-sensitivity fecal occult blood testing (FOBT) using Hemoccult II has been shown in randomized controlled trials to reduce mortality of colorectal cancer by 15 to 33 percent. Other screening methods, including colonoscopies, sigmoidoscopies, and newer FOBT tests, have not been subjected to similar trials that might provide mortality reduction estimates. Thus this figure largely reflects FOBT data, and to date the exact mortality benefit of other screening methods is unknown.

2. USPSTF, release date October 2008.

3. This section is based on "What You Need to Know about Cancer of the Colon and Rectum," an NCI publication revised May 2006.

4. Levin et al., "Screening and Surveillance for the Early Detection of Colorectal Cancer and Adenomatous Polyps, 2008: A Joint Guideline," 2008.

CHAPTER 10. Depression Screening

1. "Suffering" is difficult to quantify. Health economists commonly measure suffering using disability-adjusted life-years, or DALYs, as was the case for this WHO statistic. DALYs for a disease are the sum of the years of life lost due to premature death and the years of life lost due to disability. In other words, they take into account the fact that diseases shorten lifespan but also reduce quality of life.

2. USPSTF, release dates May 2002 (adults), March 2009 (adolescents).

CHAPTER 11. Diabetes Screening

1. USPSTF, release date June 2008.

2. The following statistics were adapted from the "National Diabetes Fact Sheet," a CDC webpage, www.cdc.gov/diabetes/pubs/factsheet07.htm.

CHAPTER 12. **Early Childhood Preventive Health**

1. USPSTF, release dates May 2005 (eye drops), March 2008 (PKU and CH), September 2007 (sickle cell disease), July 2008 (hearing loss), May 2006 (iron supplementation), April 2004 (fluoride supplementation), and May 2004 (visual acuity).

2. This section is largely based on patient-oriented materials put together by the National Institute on Deafness and Other Communication Disorders, www.nidcd.nih.gov/health/hearing/screened.asp.

3. As of July 16, 2009, specific water quality reports are at www.epa.gov/safewater/dwinfo/index.html.

4. Material in this section is adapted from Cooper and Cooper, "All About Amblyopia (lazy eye)," available at www.strabismus.org/amblyopia_lazy_eye.html.

5. Centers for Disease Control and Prevention, *Epidemiology and Prevention of Vaccine-Preventable Diseases,* Atkinson W, Wolfe S, Hamborsky J, McIntyre L, eds. 11th ed. Washington DC: Public Health Foundation, 2009.

6. Information obtained from the Washington State Department of Health website, www.doh.wa.gov/.

7. Atkinson et al., "Poliomyelitis," in *Epidemiology,* 2009, available at www.cdc.gov/vaccines/pubs/pinkbook/downloads/polio.pdf.

CHAPTER 13. **Gonorrhea Screening**

1. USPSTF, release date May 2005.

2. Much of the information in this section has been adapted from the CDC fact sheet, "Gonorrhea," updated December 2007, www.cdc.gov/std/gonorrhea/stdfact-gonorrhea.htm.

CHAPTER 14. **Healthy Eating Counseling**

1. U.S. Department of Health and Human Services, *Healthy People 2010: Understanding and Improving Health,* 2nd ed. Washington, DC: U.S. Government Printing Office, November 2000.

2. USPSTF, release date January 2003.

3. U.S. Department of Health and Human Services and U.S. Department of Agriculture. *Dietary Guidelines for Americans,* 2005. 6th Edition. Washington, DC: U.S. Government Printing Office, January 2005.

CHAPTER 15. **Hepatitis B Vaccination and Screening**

1. USPSTF, release date June 2009.

2. CDC, "Hepatitis B Vaccination Recommendations for Adults," 2006, www.cdc.gov/hepatitis/HBV/VaccAdults.htm, and CDC, "Hepatitis B Vaccination Recommendations for Infants, Children, and Adolescents," 2005, www.cdc.gov/hepatitis/HBV/VaccChildren.htm.

3. CDC, "Recommendations for Identification and Public Health Management of Persons with Chronic Hepatitis B Virus Infection," 2008, www.cdc.gov/hepatitis/HBV/TestingChronic.htm.

CHAPTER 16. **HIV Screening**

1. USPSTF, release date June 2005. An April 2007 amendment confirms that the USPSTF makes no recommendation for or against screening nonpregnant adolescents and adults who are not at increased risk for HIV infection.

CHAPTER 17. **Obesity Screening and Counseling**

1. USPSTF, release date December 2003.

2. The following text is from U.S. Department of Health and Human Services, *The Surgeon General's Call to Action to Prevent and Decrease Overweight and Obesity*, 2001, www.surgeongeneral.gov/topics/obesity.

3. NHLBI, *Clinical Guidelines on the Identification, Evaluation, and Treatment of Overweight and Obesity in Adults*, September 1998.

CHAPTER 18. **Osteoporosis Screening**

1. USPSTF, release date September 2002.

2. The "bone bank account" analogy is from the National Institute of Arthritis and Musculoskeletal Disease patient-oriented materials: www.niams.nih.gov/Health_Info/Bone/Bone_Health/default.asp.

3. Parts of this section were adapted from "Osteoporosis Overview," a document prepared by the NIH Osteoporosis and Related Diseases National Resource Center, available at www.niams.nih.gov/Health_Info/Bone/Osteoporosis/overview.pdf.

CHAPTER 19. **Pregnancy Preventive Health**

1. USPSTF, release dates May 2009 (folate supplementation), July 2008 (asymptomatic bacteriuria), July 2007 (chlamydia), May 2005 (gonorrhea), July 2005 (HIV), June 2009 (hepatitis B), February 2004 (Rh[D] typing), May 2009 (syphilis), May 2006 (iron deficiency anemia), November 2003 (tobacco use), April 2004 (alcohol misuse), and October 2008 (breastfeeding).

2. The following information was adapted from the 2005 AAP policy statement "Breastfeeding and the Use of Human Milk" and Moreland J, Coombs J. Promoting and supporting breast-feeding, *Am Fam Physician* 2000 Apr 1;61(7):2093–100, 2103–4.

3. This section has been adapted from the CDC fact sheet, "STDs and Pregnancy," updated December 2007.

CHAPTER 20. **Sexually Transmitted Infection Counseling**

1. USPSTF, release date October 2008.

2. Centers for Disease Control and Prevention. *Sexually Transmitted Disease Surveillance, 2006*. Atlanta, GA: U.S. Department of Health and Human Services, November 2007, www.cdc.gov/std/stats06/toc2006.htm. For HIV and hepatitis B, there are additional modes of transmission other than sexual contact (e.g., needle sharing). The estimates provided are the total number of new cases, not only those acquired through sexual contact.

CHAPTER 21. **Syphilis Screening**

1. USPSTF, release date July 2004.

2. Much of this section is based on the CDC fact sheet "Syphilis," updated December 2007, available at www.cdc.gov/std/Syphilis/STDFact-Syphilis.htm.

CHAPTER 22. **Tobacco Use Counseling**

1. USPSTF, release date April 2009.

2. Most of the statistics in this section are from the 2004 surgeon general's report

The Health Consequences of Smoking, available at www.surgeongeneral.gov/library/smokingconsequences.

CHAPTER 23. Vaccines for Adults

1. The following statistics are from the 2008 Adult Immunization News Conference, www.nfid.org/pressconfs/adultimm08.shtml.